Geriatric Nursing Research Digest

Joyce J. Fitzpatrick, PhD, RN, FAAN, is Professor of Nursing, Frances Payne Bolton School of Nursing at Case Western Reserve University in Cleveland, Ohio, where she was Dean from 1982 to 1997. Dr. Fitzpatrick is widely published in nursing literature, having received the American Journal of Nursing Book of the Year Award ten times. She is the Editor of the *Annual Review of Nursing Research* series, now in its eighteenth volume, and in 1997 she was appointed Editor of the National League for Nursing's journal *Nursing and Health Care Perspectives.* She also is Consulting Editor of the Springer journal *Nursing Leadership Forum.* Dr. Fitzpatrick was president of the American Academy of Nursing from 1997–99.

Terry T. Fulmer, PhD, RN, FAAN, is Professor of Nursing, New York University Division of Nursing where she is also the director of the Muriel and Virginia Pless Center for Nursing Research and the Co-Director of the John A. Hartford Institute for Geriatric Nursing. She is certified in Gerontological Nursing by the American Nurses Association, was elected a Fellow in the American Academy of Nursing in 1989. Dr. Fulmer is a fellow of the New York Academy of Medicine, and The Gerontological Society of America. She is President of the Eastern Nursing Research Society and has received over 12 million dollars in fellowship and research funding. Dr. Fulmer is widely published in the nursing and health care literature having over 150 publications.

Meredith Wallace, PhDc, RN, CS-ANP, is Assistant Professor in the Department of Nursing at Southern Connecticut State University in New Haven, Connecticut. She is a Ph.D. candidate at New York University, Division of Nursing.

Ellen Flaherty, PhDc, RN, CS-GNP, is the Project Director of the John A. Hartford Institute for Geriatric Nursing at New York University. She is a Ph.D. candidate at New York University, Division of Nursing.

Geriatric Nursing Research Digest

Joyce J. Fitzpatrick, PhD, RN, FAAN
Terry Fulmer, PhD, RN, FAAN
Editors

Meredith Wallace, PhDc, RN, CS-ANP
Associate Editor

Ellen Flaherty, PhDc, RN, CS-GNP
Assistant Editor

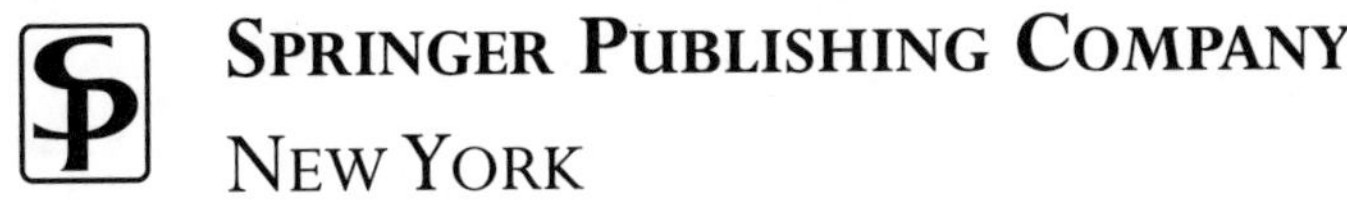

Springer Publishing Company
New York

No part of this publication may be reproduced, stored in a retrieval system, or transmitted in any form or by any means, electronic, mechanical, photocopying, recording, or otherwise, without the prior permission of Springer Publishing Company, Inc.

Springer Publishing Company, Inc.
536 Broadway
New York, NY 10012-3955

Acquisitions Editor: Sheri W. Sussman
Production Editor: Jeanne W. Libby
Cover design by James Scotto-Lavino

00 01 02 03 04/5 4 3 2 1

Library of Congress Cataloging-in-Publication Data

Geriatric nursing research digest / Joyce J. Fitzpatrick and Terry Fulmer, editors.
    p. cm.
    Includes bibliographical references and index.
    ISBN 0-8261-1332-X (hardcover)
    1. Geriatric nursing. I. Fitzpatrick, Joyce J., 1944– II. Fulmer, Terry T.
    [DNLM: 1. Geriatric Nursing—United States. 2.Research—United States. WY 152
G3699 2000]
RC954.G468 2000
610.73'65—dc21
                                           00-020175
                                            CIP

Printed in the United States of America

CONTENTS

VI   Cognitive and Neurobehavioral Issues in Aging — 313

CONTRIBUTORS

Lauren S. Aaronson, PhD, RN, FAAN
Associate Dean for Research and Professor
University of Kansas
School of Nursing
Kansas City, KS

Barbara W. Abraham, BS, RN, MPH
Gerontology Consultant
Trumbull, CT

Jerilyn K. Allen ScD, RN
Associate Professor
The Johns Hopkins University
School of Nursing
Baltimore, MD

Elaine J. Amella, PhD, RN, CS, GNP
Assistant Professor
Medical University of South Carolina
College of Nursing
Charleston, SC

Patricia G. Archbold, PhD, RN, FAAN
Professor
Oregon Health Sciences University
School of Nursing
Portland, OR

Cornelia K. Beck, PhD, RN, FAAN
Professor
Department of Geriatrics
University of Arkansas School for Medical Sciences
Little Rock, AR

Nancy Bergstrom, PhD, RN, FAAN
Professor
University of Nebraska Medical Center
College of Nursing
Omaha, NE

Carol E. Blixen, PhD, RN
Senior Nurse Researcher
Cleveland Clinic Foundation
Department of Nursing Education and Research
Cleveland, OH

Eleanor J. Bond, PhD, RN
Associate Professor
University of Washington
Department of Biobehavioral Nursing and Health Systems
Seattle, WA

Barbara L. Brush, PhD, RN
Assistant Professor
Boston College
School of Nursing
Chestnut Hill, MA

Kathleen C. Buckwalter, PhD, RN, FAAN
Professor
University of Iowa
College of Nursing
Iowa City, IA

Vern L. Bullough, PhD, RN, FAAN
Visiting Professor
University of Southern California
Department of Nursing
Northridge, CA

Victoria Champion, DNS, RN, FAAN
Associate Dean of Research
Indiana University
School of Nursing
Indianapolis, IN

Deborah Chyun, PhD, RN
Assistant Professor & Director of
    Adult Advanced Practice Nurs-
    ing Specialty
Yale University School of Nursing
New Haven, CT

Kathleen Byrne Colling, PhD, RN
University of Michigan
School of Nursing
Ann Arbor, MI

Inge B. Corless, PhD, RN, FAAN
Associate Professor and Director
Massachusetts General Hospital
Institute of Health Professions
Boston, MA

Marie J. Cowan, PhD, RN, FAAN
Professor and Dean
University of California, Los
    Angeles
School of Nursing
Los Angeles, CA

Diane Cronin-Stubbs, PhD, RN, FAAN
Professor
Rush University College of Nursing
Riverside, IL

Sabina De Geest, PhD, RN, NFESC
Assistant Professor
Catholic University of Leuven
Center for Health Services and
    Nursing Research
School of Public Health
Kapucijnenvoer 35/4
B-3000 Leuven, Belgium

Alice S. Demi, DNS, RN, FAAN
Professor
Georgia State University
School of Nursing
Atlanta, GA

Karen E. Dennis, PhD, RN, FAAN
Associate Professor
University of Maryland
School of Nursing
Baltimore, MD

Deborah Dillon McDonald, PhD, RN
Associate Professor
University of Connecticut
School of Nursing
Storrs, CT

Karen Hassey Dow, PhD, RN
Associate Professor
University of Central Florida
School of Nursing
Orlando, FL

Annemarie Dowling-Castronovo, MA, RN, CS-GNP
Instructor
New York University
Division of Nursing
New York, NY

Jacqueline Dunbar-Jacob, PhD, RN, FAAN
Professor
University of Pittsburgh
School of Nursing
Pittsburgh, PA

Carol Edelman, APRN, RN, CS
Director of Out-patient Services
Waverny Care Center
New Canaan, CT

Ophelia Empleo-Frazier, MSN, RN, CS-GNP
Lecturer
Yale University
School of Nursing
New Haven, CT

Lois K. Evans, DNSc, RN, FAAN
Associate Professor
University of Pennsylvania
School of Nursing
Philadelphia, PA

Karen Feldt, PhD, RN, GNP
Assistant Professor
University of Minnesota
School of Nursing
Minneapolis, MN

Donna Fick, PhD, RN, CS
Assistant Professor
Medical College of Georgia
School of Medicine &
Research Scientist, Department of
Veterans Affairs
Augusta, GA

Ellen Flaherty, PhDc, RN, CS-GNP
Project Director, Hartford Institute
for Geriatric Nursing
New York University
Division of Nursing
New York, NY

Marilyn Frank-Stromborg, EdD, JD, RN, FAAN
Professor
Northern Illinois University
Dekalb, IL

Terry Fulmer, PhD, RN, FAAN
Professor & Co-Director Hartford
Institute for Geriatric Nursing
New York University
Division of Nursing
New York, NY

Susan Gardner, MSN, RN
University of Iowa
College of Nursing
Iowa City, IA

Carol Gaskamp, MA, RN
Associate Professor
Kansas Newman College
Division of Nursing
Wichita, KS

Linda A. Gerdner, PhD, RN
Post Doctoral Fellow
VA Health Services Research and
Development
University of Arkansas for Medical
Sciences
Little Rock, AR

Marion Good, PhD, RN
Associate Professor
Case Western Reserve University
Frances Payne Bolton School of
Nursing
Cleveland, OH

Margaret Grey, DrPH, RN, FAAN
Associate Dean for Research and
Doctoral Studies
Yale University
School of Nursing
New Haven, CT

Margaret Heitkemper, PhD, RN, FAAN
Professor
University of Washington
Department of Biobehavioral Nursing and Health
Seattle, WA

Marion M. Hemstrom, DNSc, RN
Assistant Professor
Case Western Reserve University
Frances Payne Bolton School of Nursing
Cleveland, OH

Eileen Hermann, RN, MSN
Director of Education
The Connecticut VNA
Wallingford, CT

Martha N. Hill, PhD, RN, FAAN
Professor
Johns Hopkins University
School of Nursing
Baltimore, MD

Mary Hujer, MSN, RN, CS
Clinical Nurse Specialist
Cleveland Clinic Foundation
Division of Nursing
Cleveland, OH

Ann Hurley, DNSc, RN, FAAN
Associate Director for Education and Evaluation
Geriatric Research Education and Clinical Center
Edith Nourse Rogers Memorial Veterans Hospital
Bedford, MA

Ada Jacox, PhD, RN, FAAN
Professor and Associate Dean for Research
Wayne State University
College of Nursing
Detroit, MI

Monica E. Jarrett, PhD, RN
Research Associate Professor
University of Washington
Department of Biobehavioral Nursing and Health
Seattle, WA

Julie E. Johnson
Director and Associate Professor
Orvis School of Nursing
University of Nevada
Reno, NV

Susan J. Kelly, PhD, RN
Professor and Dean
Georgia State University
College of Health and Human Services
Atlanta, GA

Christine T. Kovner, PhD, RN, FAAN
Associate Professor
New York University
Division of Nursing
New York, NY

Kathleen Krichbaum, PhD, RN
Associate Professor
University of Minnesota
School of Nursing
Minneapolis, MN

Helen Lach, MSN, RN, CS
Gerontological Nurse Specialist
Division of Geriatrics & Gerontology
Washington University
School of Medicine
St. Louis, MO

Hae-OK Lee, DNSc, RN
Assistant Professor
Case Western Reserve University
School of Nursing
Cleveland, OH

Adrianne Linton, PhD, RN
Associate Professor
The University of Texas Health Science Center at San Antonio
School of Nursing
San Antonio, TX

Brenda L. Lyon, DNS, RN, FAAN
Associate Professor
Indiana University School of Nursing
Adult Health Nursing
Indianapolis, IN

Meridean Maas, PhD, RN, FAAN
Professor
University of Iowa
College of Nursing
Iowa City, IA

Ellen K. Mahoney, DNS, RN, CS
Associate Professor
Boston College
School of Nursing
Chestnut Hill, MA

Arlene Mann, MSN, RN, CS
Clinical Nurse Specialist
Cleveland Clinic Foundation
Cleveland, OH

Mary Ann Matteson, PhD, RN, FAAN
Thelma and Joe Crow Endowed Professor
Department of Family Nursing Care
The University of Texas Health Science Center at San Antonio
School of Nursing
San Antonio, TX

Kathleen A. McCormick, PhD, RN, FAAN
Agency of Health Care Policy and Research
Rockville, MD

Graham McDougall, PhD, RN
Associate Professor
Case Western Reserve University
School of Nursing
Cleveland, OH

Elizabeth McGann, DNSc (candidate), RN, CS
Assistant Professor and Chairperson
Department of Nursing
Quinnipiac College
Hamden, CT

Sue E. Meiner, EdD, RN, CS, GNP
Research Patient Coordinator
Washington University
School of Medicine - Division of Geriatrics
St. Louis, MO

Mathy Mezey, EdD, RN, FAAN
Professor and Director
Hartford Institute for Geriatric Nursing
New York University
Division of Nursing
New York, NY

Nancy Houston Miller, RN, BSN
Associate Director
Stanford University School of Medicine
Division of Cardiovascular Medicine
Palo Alto, CA

Lorraine Mion, PhD, RN
Director, Outcomes Research
Department of Geriatrics & Adult Development
Mount Sinai–
New York University Medical Center
New York, NY

Pamela H. Mitchell, PhD, RN, FAAN
Professor
School of Nursing
University of Washington
Seattle, WA

Ethel Mitty, EdD, RN
Rudin Professor of Geriatric
    Nursing
New York University
Division of Nursing
New York, NY

Patricia Moritz, PhD, RN, FAAN
Associate Professor
University of Colorado Health Sci-
    ences Center
School of Nursing
Denver, CO

Kathleen Ondus, MSN, RN, CS
Clinical Nurse Specialist
Cleveland Clinic Foundation
Division of Nursing
Cleveland, OH

Louiselle Ouellet, MSN, RN
Professor
University of New Brunswick
Faculty of Nursing
Fredericton, New Brunswick,
    Canada

Mary H. Palmer, PhD, RNC, FAAN
Associate Professor and Director of
    the Office of Research
Rutgers University
College of Nursing
Newark, NJ

Sally Phillips, PhD, RN
Director, Nursing Doctorate
    Program
University of Colorado
Health Sciences Center
Denver, CO

Eileen Porter, PhD, RN
Assistant Professor
Sinclair School of Nursing
University of Missouri - Columbia
Columbia, MO

Lorrie L. Powel, MS, RN
PhD Student
University of Maryland
School of Nursing
Baltimore, MD

Gloria C. Ramsey, RN, BSN, JD
Project Director
New York University
Division of Nursing
New York, NY

Barbara Resnick, PhD, CRNP
Assistant Professor
University of Maryland
School of Nursing
Baltimore, MD

Barbara A. Ritgert, MA, CCC-SLP
Senior Speech-Language
    Pathologist
University of Maryland Medical
    Systems
The James Lawrence Kernan Reha-
    bilitation Hospital
Department of Rehabilitation
    Services
Baltimore, MD

Beverly L. Roberts, PhD, RN, FAAN
Associate Professor
Case Western Reserve University
Frances Payne Bolton School of
    Nursing
Cleveland, OH

Marlene M. Rosenkoetter, RN, PhD, FAAN
Professor
Gerontology Program
College of Arts and Sciences
University of North Carolina at Wilmington
Wilmington, NC

Meredeth A. Rowe, PhD, RN
Associate Professor
Binghamton University
Decker School of Nursing
Binghamton, NY

Kathy Rush, PhDc, MSc BN
Professor
University of New Brunswick
Faculty of Nursing
Fredericton, New Brunswick, Canada

Dina Shah, BSN, RN
Senior Staff Nurse
Department of Surgery
New York University Medical Center
New York, NY

Marianne Shaughnessy, PhD, CRNP
Assistant Professor
University of Maryland at Baltimore
School of Nursing
Baltimore, MD

Mary Shelkey, PhDc, RN
Assistant Professor
Seattle University
School of Nursing
Seattle, WA

Valorie M. Shue, BA
Research Assistant
Department of Psychiatry
University of Arkansas for Medical Sciences
Little Rock, AR

Carol E. Smith, RN, PhD
Professor
University of Kansas
School of Nursing
Kansas City, KS

Gwi-Ryung Son, RN, MN
Case Western Reserve University
School of Nursing
Cleveland, OH

Janet Specht, PhD, RN
Research Scientist
University of Iowa
College of Nursing
Iowa City, IA

Joanne Sabol Stevenson, PhD, RN, FAAN
Professor and Associate Dean
Rugters University
College of Nursing
Newark, NJ

Barbara J. Stewart, PhD, RN
Professor
Oregon Health Sciences University
School of Nursing
Portland, OR

Neville E. Strumpf, PhD, RN, FAAN
Associate Professor
University of Pennsylvania
School of Nursing
Philadelphia, PA

Eleanor J. Sullivan, PhD, RN, FAAN
Professor
University of Kansas
School of Nursing
St. Louis, MO

Patricia A. Tabloski, PhD, RNCS, GNP
CMC Associate Professor
Boston College
School of Nursing
Chestnut Hill, MA

Susan Dale Tannenbaum, RN, BSN
Staff Nurse- Cardiac Unit
Johns Hopkins University
School of Nursing
Baltimore, MD

Ann Gill Taylor, RN, EdD, FAAN
Professor of Nursing
University of Virginia
Center for the Study of Complementary and Alternative Therapies
Charlottesville, VA

Carol Lynn Thompson, PhD, RN
Associate Professor and Chair
University of Tennessee
College of Nursing
Memphis, TN

Antonia M. Villarruel, PhD, RN, FAAN
University of Pennsylvania
College of Nursing
Philadelphia, PA

Ladislov Volicer, PhD, MD
Boston University
School of Medicine
Boston, MA
Geriatric Research Education and Clinical Center

Edith Nourse Rogers Memorial Veterans Hospital
Bedford, MA

Meredith Wallace, PhDc, RN, CS-ANP
Assistant Professor
Southern Connecticut State University
Department of Nursing
New Haven, CT

Ann L. Whall, PhD, RN, FAAN
Professor
University of Michigan
School of Nursing
Ann Arbor, MI

Sarah A. Wilson, PhD, RN
Associate Professor
Marquette University
College of Nursing
Milwaukee, WI

May L. Wykle, PhD, RN, FAAN
Professor and Associate Dean for Community
Case Western Reserve University
Frances Payne Bolton School of Nursing
Cleveland, OH

Jaclene A. Zauszniewski, PhD, RN
Associate Professor
Case Western Reserve University
Frances Payne Bolton School of Nursing
Cleveland, OH

Cora Zembrzuski, PhDc, RN
Director of Program Development
The Connecticut VNA
Wallingford, CT

PREFACE

This Geriatric Nursing Research Digest represents an important resource for the future care of the elderly: a synopsis of geriatric nursing research. As nurses strive for evidence-based practice and look for proven ways to enhance the care of elderly persons, we also must aim to achieve the highest level of science possible. The geriatric nurse researchers who have authored the individual entries are in the forefront of the geriatric nursing field and experts on the topic area. In the introductory sections to each group of entries, we have asked experts to describe the relevance of this set of research entries to clinical practice. Thus, it is our expectation that this Digest will be useful to both clinicians and researchers.

It is readily apparent how much our knowledge base has grown over the past several years. As recently as ten years ago, if an older person was incontinent, we would insert a catheter. If a patient was confused, we would apply a restraint; and if a patient was agitated, we would use sedating medications. Through new research, we now know that far better care is possible and should be expected. We believe that this Digest provides information that forms the foundation for better care of the older adult. In the future, as new knowledge is generated through geriatric nursing and health care research, we can expect even more significant breakthroughs. As our science base continues to evolve in both sophistication and breadth, avenues such as the Geriatric Nursing Research Digest will keep both clinicians and researchers apprised of our scientific and clinical progress and will take an important step forward in translating nursing's contributions to the public.

This Digest includes six sections; each entry has been placed in a section based on conceptual consistency of the content. The sections include: health promotion and risk reduction, normalcy throughout the life span, issues in environments of care, geriatric emotional health, pathological conditions, and cognitive and neurobehavioral issues in aging. Each author was asked to identify and describe the most significant research in the selected area. All entries were kept to the succinct style originally used in the *Encyclopedia of Nursing Research,* and references were limited to those that were deemed classic in the research on aging or representative of the most recent research in the topic area.

It is our goal to guide both future research in geriatric nursing and professional nursing care of the elderly. Also, the Digest is designed for beginning students in geriatric nursing, to help them improve their understanding of the field, and advanced students in geriatric nursing, to lead them to research questions and further examples of evidence-based practice.

This Digest would not have been possible without the expert assistance of two PhD students in nursing at New York University. We were fortunate to have Meredith Wallace join us as Associate Editor and Ellen Flaherty as Assistant Editor of this Digest. Thank you Meredith and Ellen for your attention to detail in pursuing this project with us.

JOYCE J. FITZPATRICK
TERRY FULMER

Part I

HEALTH PROMOTION AND RISK REDUCTION

INTRODUCTION

The World Health Organization stated over 40 years ago that "Health in the elderly is best measured in terms of function" and that "the degree of fitness" rather than the extent of pathology may be used as a measure of the amount of services the aged will require from the community (WHO, 1959). Since that time, the U.S. Department of Health and Human Services published *Healthy People 2000 Mid-Course Review* and 1995 revisions in which it challenged healthcare providers to work toward goals that promote health and prevent disease among all age groups (Edelman & Mandle, 1998). The overall goals for older adults in the Healthy People 2000 document are to increase the life span and to reduce morbidity and mortality (Edelman & Mandle, 1998). A specific goal for health promotion within this document is to facilitate well-being for the older person on a daily basis (Ruffing-Rahal, 1991).

The National Research Council recommended a major refocus in health systems with development of specific health promotion models so that older persons might enjoy extended years of vigor and autonomy (Gilford, 1998). Maintaining quality of life and health is a major category designated by the U.S. Surgeon General for nationwide implementation in the year 2000; designated programs are addressing physical fitness, nutrition, chronic diseases, infectious diseases, mental health, and social support (Office of Disease Prevention and Health Promotion, 1987; Walker, S. N., 1989). Clinical data shows that among adults aged 65 to 74, 95% require no assistance in basic Activities of Daily Living (ADL); and 65% of adults older than 85 still care for their own needs without outside help (Rubel, Reinsch, Tobis, & Hurrell, 1994). Other studies have shown that health-promoting measures can prevent or postpone 80% of all health problems, that physical exercise by the elderly can increase functional status by 67% and decrease the need for mental health care by 10%, and that promotion of self-care activities can reduce primary care visits by 30% to 40% (Kimble & Longe, 1989).

The relevance of health promotion for older adults is underscored by their tendency toward health consciousness and the pursuit of fully independent lifestyles (Platakis, 1987). In addition, there is a growing body of evidence indicating that preventive measures are useful to young and old alike. Health Watch, an ongoing longitudinal study of health and aging (Schmidt, 1993) has provided evidence that diet, activity, extended family, and spirituality are the four most significant healthy behavior determinants of the elderly. Today the focus on improvement of function remains the primary focus of health promotion activities with the elderly.

As always, critical questions arise about financial support to health promotion initiatives. It is well known that our current reimbursement system provides incentives for the delivery of procedure-oriented care rather than preventive care. Since the enactment of Medicare in 1965, the major insurer for older adults, health services and their costs have escalated. The majority of expenditures are illness related and of an acute, institutional nature (Ruffing-Rahal, 1991). Older adults spend almost 20% of their annual income on healthcare (Select Committee on Aging, 1989). Few programs address the needs of older adults from the perspective of well-being and wholeness. However, the Medicare program does incorporate a few selected preventive care services such as a pneumococcal vaccine, a hepatitis B vaccine for persons at intermediate or high risk of contracting Hepatitis B, screening mammograms, and screening pap smears. Cost estimate for preventive, health-promoting services costs the Medicare program $3.99 to $5.10 per enrollee per month.

In addition to the Medicare program, the Federal government sponsors a program in health promotion and disease prevention through the issuing of Block grants which provides about $135 million to the States to support a variety of health-promoting and prevention initiatives. Beyond the year 2000, expenditures for health-promotion spending will slow sharply as heightened scrutiny of providers results in tighter controls for Medicare. Further, the Balanced Budget Act will further limit growth in other health services for older adults even though health promotion has been identified as an intervention with important payoffs in terms of cost savings and quality of life (Ruffing-Rahal, 1991).

Nurses have long been committed to the inclusion of health-promotion activities within their practices. The American Nurses Association has stated that an essential feature of nursing practice is attention to the full range of human experiences and responses to health and illness (ANA, 1995). While the concepts of health promotion and disease prevention are not new to most nurses, there has recently been a dramatic resurgence of interest in this area. Health promotion is defined in the Cumulative Index of Nursing and Allied Health Literature (CINAHL) as "the process of fostering awareness, influencing attitudes and identifying alternatives so that individuals can make informed choices and change their behavior to achieve an optimum level of physical and mental health and improve their physical and social environment" (Travis & Ryan, 1988). The U.S. Preventive Services Task Force has recently released a guide with the stated purpose of provision of a premier reference source on the effectiveness of preventive services to improve health at all ages (U.S. Preventive Services Task Force, 1996).

The PEW Health Professions Commission Report states that competencies needed by all practitioners by the year 2005 will be:

- Ability to care for community populations;
- Focus on accountability;
- Ability to provide preventive services;
- Focus on healthy lifestyles;
- Ability to manage information. (Murray & Zentner, 1997)

Gerontological nurses practice in many settings including ambulatory care, home care, hospitals, nursing homes, and a variety of community settings. There is an abundance of evidence indicating that despite the setting, gerontological nurses provide a comprehensive approach to the care of the older person including health promotion, functional assessment, expert care in acute and chronic illness, and goal-directed rehabilitation. Although aging is a normal developmental process, it is often depicted as a pathological phenomenon, closely associated with disease, decrement and loss of function, and death. Gerontologists have long noted that chronological age and illness are not synonymous. However, until recently there were few studies to guide nurses and other health professionals in our health-promotion efforts. The majority of early studies of health promotion excluded older persons entirely or included convenience samples of frail older persons recruited from hospital or clinic populations. These limited studies and biased samples often produced less than dramatic results which may have contributed to "ageism" in the research and practice of nursing, further emphasizing the inability of older persons to grow, change, and undertake new healthcare practices in later life. Recent research supported by the MacArthur Foundation emphasizes three major points regarding the maintenance of mental and physical function in old age: (a) many of the fears about functional loss are exaggerated; (b) much functional loss can be prevented; (c) many functional losses can be regained (Rowe & Kahn, 1998). Thus, the dual goals of health promotion activities with older persons are not only to add years of life, but also to add increased vitality, health and function in those years.

As we enter the twenty-first century, previously unimagined numbers of people are aging in America. In 1900, approximately 4% of the U.S. population were over 65 years of age. Today that percentage has climbed to 13%. The older person reaching retirement age of 65 now can expect to live on average another 17 years; an increase of a full 5 years from the turn of the century (Rowe & Kahn, 1998). Our population of older persons today is better educated, more affluent, and possesses higher expectations regarding their quality of life than their elders. Many older persons today hope for and expect high quality, disease-free years for their entire lives. No one envisions spending years of their life in a nursing home as a frail dependent person. Most older persons dread loss of function and independence, and becoming a burden on their children. There is mounting evidence that nursing interventions to prevent illness and promote health are more effective than recognized by healthcare professionals. In general, elderly adults perceive health-promotion activities as beneficial, engage in health-promoting behaviors more frequently than younger adults, and participate in community-based and other health-promotion programs (Heidrich, 1998). All of these factors underscore the need for continued research and dialogue concerning health promotion for older adults.

Within the medical model, ample evidence exists that risk factors for coronary heart disease (smoking, obesity, hypertension, and cholesterol) may be substantially reduced by health-promotion activities in middle-aged and elderly men (Haapanen-Neimi, Vuori, & Pasanen, 1999). Influenza immunization rates can be improved for high-risk elderly patients by computerized reminders to physicians before flu season (Hak, van Essen, Stalman, & de Melker, 1998). Within the nursing model, there is growing evidence documenting the effectiveness of nursing interventions to promote health. Elderly women who were long-term sleep medication users were successfully tapered and withdrawn from their medication using a supportive protocol (Tabloski, Cooke, & Thoman, 1998). Hope in nursing home residents can be improved by implementing a caring, health-promotion philosophy of practice rather than an institutional philosophy of cure and treatment (Zorn, 1997). Disability in older persons with osteoarthritis was reduced by health-promotion interventions designed to increase the self-care capabilities of older persons with arthritic pain in the knee and hip (Hopman-Rock et al., 1997). A collaborative health-promotion project between a nursing education program and a community hospital demonstrated that student nurses can function productively to increase safety, reduce sensory deprivation, improve exercise, and address a variety of crucial psychosocial issues (Slaninka & Galbraith, 1998).

Peer-led senior health education programs were found to increase perceived social support and subjective health in a group of older adults (Kocken & Voorham, 1998). Parish nurses are addressing the significance of social support and spirituality for sustained health-promoting behaviors in the elderly (Boland, 1998). The process and standards for achieving a "good death" or a positive process of dying for elderly persons is being studied and developed by nurses in recognition that dying is the natural end to a long life and may be viewed as a means to promoting health in the family circle (*Journal of Gerontological Nursing*, 1998). Many more examples exist including the studies contained in this chapter.

One of the most significant activities undertaken by gerontological nurses at all levels involves health promotion. Both nurses and older adults share collaborative roles in this vital undertaking (Benfield & Williams,

1999). The nurse should assess risk factors, identify positive health behaviors, provide education, act as a role model, and inform patients of resources. The older patient should provide information about personal needs and preferences, evaluate his/her own health practices, seek professional advice as necessary, and try honestly to engage in positive health behaviors. Together, the nurse and patient can agree on goals, select appropriate interventions, and monitor progress and outcomes.

In spite of the growing recognition of the importance of disease prevention with the older adult, there is little in the way of a unified, systematic policy for individual, community, and national interventions for health promotion. The accumulated results of studies on healthy aging have shown that it is possible to identify important modifiable risk factors that cause a great amount of illness and disability. Much of the underlying disease pathology begins in childhood and young adult life, but we are learning that it is never too late to benefit from intervention, as evidenced by trials of blood pressure reduction and smoking cessation with older adults. It therefore seems quite plausible to make intervention involving these known risk factors the first step of a systematic policy for promotion of healthy aging. The National Research Panel on Statistics for an Aging Population recommended a major refocus in health systems to enlarge the potential span of vigorous health in older persons (Gilford, 1998). Such a model would focus on personal autonomy, functional self care, social integration, and sense of self. The incorporation of such wellness values offer the older person a healthier transition to old age including dying with dignity. All of the concepts discussed above bring a challenging vision for the future of gerontological nursing (Burggraf & Barry, 1998). Nursing education, practice, and research, that build upon our unique expertise in caring, can address issues of health promotion and, nurses can contribute to quality healthcare for older persons.

Patricia A. Tabloski
Carole A. Edelman

ADHERENCE/COMPLIANCE

Adherence refers to the degree to which behavior corresponds to a recommended therapeutic regimen (Haynes, Taylor, & Sackett, 1979). Numerous terms have been used to describe this behavior, including compliance, therapeutic alliance, and patient cooperation. Although the literature is filled with discussions of the acceptability of these terms and the differences between them, most investigators view the terms as synonymous and independent of the decision to engage in a particular therapeutic regimen. The most complete literature can be obtained from structured databases with the term *compliance.*

Adherence to health care regimens has been discussed in the literature since the days of Plato. However, little systematic attention was given to this phenomenon until the 1970s, when there was a proliferation of research. One of the first reviews of the literature was published in *Nursing Research* (Marston, 1970). Since that time there has been a profusion of research from a variety of disciplines. The majority of the research has focused on patient adherence, although there is a smaller body of literature on the adherence of research staff to clinical protocols and a growing body of literature on provider adherence to treatment guidelines.

One of the issues that continues to arise in discussions of patient adherence is patient autonomy. Is nonadherence a patient right or responsibility? This argument presumes that the patient is aware of his or her own behavior and has consciously decided not to follow a treatment regimen. The literature suggests that fewer than 20% of patients with medication regimens consciously decide not to engage in a treatment program. Those patients who have decided to follow the regimen but do not carry it out are unaware of episodic lapses in behavior or have difficulty integrating the health care regimen into their lives. The most common reasons given by patients for lapses in adherence are forgetting and being too busy. This group comprises on average 40% to 60% or more of patients in a treatment regimen.

The problem of nonadherence is costly in terms of dollars and lives. The National Pharmacy Council estimates that nonadherence to pharmacological therapies costs approximately $100 billion annually (Grahl, 1994). Although the cost of nonadherence to nonpharmacological therapies has not been estimated, the contribution to morbidity and mortality is high. Failures to quit smoking, to lose and maintain weight, to exercise regularly, to engage in safe sex practices, to avoid excess alcohol, and to use seat belts contribute significantly to declines in functional ability as well as to early mortality. Further data suggest that nonadherence to pharmacological as well as nonpharmacological therapies contributes to excess hospitalizations and complication rates (Dunbar-Jacob & Schlenk, 1996).

Poor adherence, then, is a significant problem of direct relevance to nursing. Nurse practitioners may prescribe or recommend therapies. Home health and community nurses provide education and assistance in carrying out health care advice. Hospital, clinic, and office nurses provide education regarding treatment plans. There is a need for intervention studies that will guide practice as nurses prepare and support patients in the conduct of treatment regimens.

Research on adherence is primarily focused on descriptive studies. In a review of the research conducted within nursing over the past 24 years

(1972–1996), only 21 distinct adherence intervention studies were identified. The majority of the studies addressed adult patients (16 of 21). The studies focused on medication (5) or visit adherence (5), with less attention given to general regimen adherence (4), cancer screening (3), exercise (2), and immunization (1). The majority of the studies used either an educational intervention or "nurse follow-up or visit." Two studies addressed modification of behaviors contributing to adherence, and four studies were theoretically driven. Three studies used the health belief model and one Orem's self-care theory. Only one study examined intervention effectiveness over time. Thus, the state of the research on adherence in nursing is rudimentary. The research on adherence is limited by the lack of attention to intervention studies, the narrow focus of the interventions, and the limited amount of theoretically driven research. This latter point may be related to the small number of theoretical frameworks addressed in the intervention research on adherence.

Future research on adherence should address strategies by which nurses can improve adherence to treatment regimens with attention directed toward various age groups, clinical populations, and regimen behaviors. The research would benefit from theoretical approaches to the problems of patient adherence and to the design of intervention strategies. Effective strategies delivered by nurses have considerable promise of a favorable impact on health outcomes and costs (Dunbar-Jacob & Schlenk, 1996).

This paper was supported in part by the National Institute of Nursing Research grant (5 P30 NR03924) and the National Heart, Lung, and Blood Institute grant (1 UO1HL48992).

JACQUELINE DUNBAR-JACOB

See also:
MEDICATIONS IN ELDERLY
EXERCISE

BREAST CANCER SCREENING

Breast cancer is a disease for which there is no foreseeable cure, and indications are that incidence will remain high. The American Cancer Society estimates that more than 180,000 women will be diagnosed with breast cancer in 1997, and almost 44,000 will die (Parker, Tong, Bolden, & Wingo, 1997). Although breast cancer remains a significant form of cancer mortality for women, in 1996 an overall decrease in mortality was reported. Because treatment is extremely effective with Stage I tumors, increases in mammography screening have influenced breast cancer mortality. When discovered early, breast cancer victims may anticipate a 95% chance for complete cure. Prospective mortality-based studies have demonstrated the effectiveness of mammography screening, particularly in women 50–70 years of age, and therefore most organizations recommend periodic screening beginning at age 50.

Recently, mammography recommendations have been expanded to include women 40 to 49. Two Swedish trials (Anderson, 1997; Bjurstam, Bjorneld, & Duffy, 1997) and a meta-analysis (Smart, Hendrick, Rutledge, & Smith, 1995) have shown a mortality-based advantage for women in their 40s. Consequently, both the American Cancer Society and the National Cancer Institute now recommend screening beginning at age 40. Obviously, breast cancer screening by mammography does not magically become effective at age 40 or 50 or 60, and one mistake that fueled controversy was comparing one decade to another. Comparing women aged 40 to 49 with women 50 and over creates artificial boundaries that cause much confusion. Now that the American Cancer Society and National Cancer Institute are in agreement, energy may be focused on other issues.

The effectiveness of clinical breast examination is not as clear as that of mammography, although it is currently recommended. Some studies demonstrating a mortality decrease for mammography have included clinical breast examination, but the independent effect of the latter has been studied. In addition, the efficacy of breast self-examination (BSE) has been documented although not in randomized, prospective mortality-based trials. To date, retrospective studies have found that BSE may detect an earlier stage of disease or smaller tumor size. Gastrin and colleagues (Gastrin et al., 1994) reported a significantly lower mortality for a sample population of 28,785 women enrolled in a BSE program, compared to what was expected with the general Finnish population. Preliminary results of a randomized study for BSE have indicated no benefit, although definitive conclusions cannot be made (Thomas, Gao, Self, et al., 1997).

Despite its apparent effectiveness, breast cancer screening is not used to its fullest advantage. According to the National Cancer Institute's *Cancer Facts* for 1996, one-time screening rates may approach 70% to 74%, but rates were lower for minorities and women over 65. The rates for consistent mammography screening at recommended intervals are not good. Rates for mammography in 1996 ranged from 40% to 51% for women aged 50–64 and from 30% to 42% for women 65 and over. Rates for clinical breast examination were somewhat higher, ranging between 60% and 75%. Recent data indicate that women may report BSE practice as frequently as seven to eight times a year but have low proficiency scores. In one study, mean proficiency scores were a little over half of what an optimal examination score would be (Champion, 1995).

Relevance to Nursing

It is obvious that breast cancer screening has the potential to reduce mortality and morbidity from this dreaded disease. Breast cancer screening rates, although increasing, are not optimal. Most problematic is the fact that women do not follow current recommendations for screening. Minority rates for follow-up are dismal, and access to care is a real issue. This health-promoting detection activity is of primary importance to nurses in all areas of practice. Nurses are in an optimal position to increase all three screening methods (mammography, clinical breast examination, and BSE). Interventions to promote mammography and teach BSE can be carried out during general health promotion or while women are being seen for other reasons. Clinical breast examination is a skill that should be learned by all nurse practitioners and conducted yearly on all women aged 20 and over.

Theoretical Variables Related to Breast Cancer Screening

Several important theoretical variables have been tested for relationships to breast cancer screening—in particular, mammography and BSE. The theory that has generated the most research is the *health belief model.* The *health belief model* was initially conceptualized in the early 1950s to predict preventive behaviors such as influenza inoculations (Rosenstock, 1966). As originally formulated, the *health belief model* included the variable of perceived threat to health, which included the concepts of risk of contracting the disease (perceived susceptibility) and personal cost should the disease be contracted (perceived seriousness). In addition, benefits and barriers to taking a preventive action were predicted to influence the health behavior. In 1988, the concept of self-efficacy, or perceived confidence in carrying out a preventive behavior, was added to the health belief model.

Other theories that have been used to predict breast cancer screening have included Fishbein and Ajzen's (1975) theory of reasoned action, which postulates that two major concepts are related to breast cancer screening: (a) beliefs and evaluations of these beliefs and (b) social influence. Social influence is also composed of two components: beliefs of significant others and the influence of significant others on the individual. Most recently, the transtheoretical model has been tested with mammography use and found to predict behavior (Prochaska et al., 1994). This model defines the outcome in terms of stages of preparedness to engage in a health-promoting activity. In addition to the factors involved in these models, descriptive research suggests that breast cancer screening is influenced by knowledge, previous health habits, particular demographic characteristics, and health care systems. For example, physician recommendation has proved to be highly predictive of mammography use in many studies.

Studies of Breast Cancer Screening

A number of studies spanning over a decade have used various models to predict mammography screening. In general, attitudinal variables such as perceived susceptibility, perceived benefits to screening, and perceived barriers to screening have been predictive of mammography. Rakowski and co-workers (Rakowski et al., 1992) found that perceived pros (benefits) and cons (barriers) varied across stages of mammography. The most consistent predictors of mammography use have been physician recommendation and barriers. The latter have included perceived lack of need, fear of results, fear of radiation, cost, pain, time, and inconvenience. Recently, the transtheoretical model has been used for predicting mammography by postulating that women move through a series of stages from precontemplation, or not thinking about mammography, to maintenance of mammography over time.

Descriptive studies to predict BSE have spanned the past two decades. Again, the variables of perceived susceptibility, benefits, and barriers have been significantly related to BSE. A less significant prediction of BSE compliance has been physician recommendation. Instead, women who were taught personally and returned a demonstration have been found to comply at higher rates. A major problem with BSE research has been the measurement of outcomes. In many earlier studies women were asked how many times they examined their breasts, and this was used as the operational measure of compliance. Later, self-report proficiency scales were widely used. Research has shown that there is often little correlation between reported frequency and proficiency, indicating that even if women practice BSE, they may not be doing it proficiently enough to detect lumps.

Actual measurement of BSE proficiency also has been problematic. The best studies have used trained observers to watch women either complete BSE or identify silicon lumps embedded in models. Subjective norms, as identified in the theory of reasoned action, have been predictive in some studies. In summary, most research has identified low to moderate correlations between attitudinal variables and BSE. Perceived confidence for completing self-examination has been one of the strongest predictors.

Interventions for Breast Cancer Screening

Intervention research for both mammography and BSE has systematically built on the descriptive studies of earlier decades. Interventions have ranged from multistrategy community interventions to individual patient-oriented interventions. Many of the individually focused interventions targeted perceptions of risk, benefits, and barriers. Multistrategy interventions often targeted physician recommendation, which had been found to be an important predictor of mammography screening. Various ways of delivering messages have been tried, including the media, telephone delivery, tailored letters or postcards, and in-person counseling. Access has been identified as a problem, as shown by the fact that persons in health maintenance organizations (HMOs) consistently have higher rates of mammography screening than do patients in private medical practice. Access-enhancing interventions have included the use of mobile vans, which provide easier access for women with transportation problems. Costs of mammography for indigent women continue to be a problem, although agencies such as the American Cancer Society and Little Red Door have helped to defray these costs. Social network interventions have been effective with minority groups. Peer leaders can sometimes be important links for low-income, African American, or Hispanic women. In summary, most interventions, but especially those based on sound theory, have been successful in increasing mammography.

Interventions addressing BSE often focus on teaching women the correct skills for practice. Many of the interventions use educational strategies, with or without counseling, related to the theoretical constructs of perceived susceptibility, benefits, and barriers. Many studies have used reminder systems or self-prompts to increase practice. Interventions have ranged from handing out pamphlets to one-to-one teaching sessions with return demonstrations. Studies using models to identify lumps have been the most vigorous. Studies that include personal demonstrations, guided feedback, and both cognitive and personal instruction evidence the greatest increase in proficiency.

Implications for Practice

Descriptive and intervention studies based on similar theories of breast cancer screening have extended over the past two decades. The major difference in relation to promoting mammography is the addition of physician recommendation. Physician recommendation is important both because medical advice is related to mammography and because an order may be necessary to obtain a mammogram. For BSE, personal teaching has been found to be a most important predictor. We now know enough about breast cancer screening to make certain recommendations for nursing practice. For both BSE and mammography, clinicians must take into account the individual's perceptions about her susceptibility to breast cancer. If this perceived susceptibility is unrealistically low, efforts must be made to paint a more accurate picture. Perceived benefits and barriers to both mammography and BSE also should be addressed and individualized strategies developed. For BSE teaching, the set of skills needed to complete this exam and observation of proficiency will be important. A major future direction related to mammography will be to increase interval compliance.

Breast cancer screening research has broad implications for increasing other health behaviors, such as colorectal or prostate screening. Preventive behaviors such as the use of skin protection and adherence to low-fat diets can also be targeted for intervention trials. Finally, nurses must actively encourage public policy decisions that increase screening access for all people

VICTORIA CHAMPION

See also:
BREAST CANCER
CANCER CARE: CHEMOTHERAPY
CANCER SURVIVORSHIP

ELDER ABUSE

Elder mistreatment is a complex syndrome that can lead to morbid or even fatal outcomes for those afflicted. *Mistreatment* is the term used to describe outcomes from such actions as abuse, neglect, exploitation, and abandonment of the elderly, and it affects all socioeconomic, cultural, ethnic, and religious groups. It is estimated that between 700,000 and 1.2 million cases of elder mistreatment occur annually in this country (Pillemer & Finkelhor, 1988). The National Center on Elder Abuse 1991 survey, conducted by adult protective service agencies and state units on aging, documented an estimate of over 250,000 reports of elder mistreatment in that year (Tatara, 1993).

The term *elder mistreatment* has been defined by Hudson (1989) as "destructive behavior that is directed toward an older adult, occurs within the context of a relationship connoting trust and is of sufficient intensity and/ or frequency to produce harmful physical, psychological, social and/or financial effects of unnecessary suffering, injury, pain, loss and/or violation of human rights and poorer quality of life for the older adult" (p. 16). In her seminal study, Hudson (1991) conducted a three-round Delphi survey with a national panel of 63 elder mistreatment experts to develop a taxonomy that now serves as the basis for research in the field and her ongoing program of nursing research (Hudson, 1991, 1994; Hudson & Carlson, 1994). Abuse is aggressive or invasive behavior, actions, or threats inflicted on an older adult and resulting in harmful effects for the older adult. Neglect is the failure of a responsible party to act so as to provide what is prudently deemed adequate and reasonable assistance that is warranted to ensure that the older adult's basic physical, psychological, social, and financial needs are met; the neglect results in harmful effects for the older adult (Hudson, 1989).

Physical abuse may include hitting, kicking, punching, and other physical contact. *Neglect* is the term used for inadequate care, which may be intentional or unintentional. Intentional neglect is the omission of appropriate care, which can readily lead to serious functional decline or death, for example, the intentional withholding of food or medicine. Unintentional neglect is a different situation. It occurs when an individual providing care to an elder person does not have the requisite knowledge and skills to provide such care appropriately. Finally, self-neglect, which is reportable in some states, occurs when an elder, either knowingly or unknowingly, lives in such a manner that his or her health is likely to deteriorate or already has done so.

Exploitation is fraudulent activity in connection with an older person's property or assets, and abandonment is defined as the deliberate and abrupt withdrawal of services in caring for an elderly person. Restriction as a form of elder mistreatment has recently been examined in an investigation of caregiver behaviors that have fewer social sanctions but may be equally deleterious to the older person (Fulmer & Gurland, 1996).

Nationally, the leading reason for mistreatment referral is neglect of elders, which accounts for over half of all cases that reach adult protective services hotlines or offices. Evidence suggests that only 1 in 14 elder mistreatment cases is reported to some public agency. Underreporting of elder mistreatment is a concern because elders may have disease symptoms or age-related changes that mask or mimic mistreatment symptoms, making assessment of mistreatment complex. Moreover, few clinicians have been trained in elder mistreatment assessment and intervention, which has also led to underreporting. Elder mistreatment is not new, but the term and the related literature have developed only in the past two decades. With an unprecedented number of individuals living beyond the age of 65 and even beyond the age of 85, clinicians and nurses must be sensitive to the possibility of elder mistreatment.

Theories for elder mistreatment causality have been posited. The dependency theory refers to the amount of care an elder person requires and is related to stressed caregiver research, which describes overwhelmed caregivers who lose their control or stop providing reasonable care. Conversely, there are data that reflect the caregiver's dependency on the elder (for shelter, money, etc.), which puts the elder at risk. Transgenerational violence theory refers to children who learn violent behavior as normal and then become violent and abusive as they grow older. This might be viewed from a learning theory perspective, although some have looked at it as a retribution act: an adult child may strike back at a parent or caregiver who was once abusive. The psychopathology of the abuser theory refers to any nonnormal caregiver, such as substance abusers (alcohol, drugs), psychiatrically impaired individuals, or mentally retarded caregivers. The number of mentally retarded elders over 65 years of age has grown substantially over the past decade, creating situations where mentally retarded or disabled offspring become caregivers for very elderly parents.

Elder mistreatment is a relatively new construct within the domain of family violence research. Early studies looked at the prevalence of elder mistreatment from a variety of perspectives: acute care, community nursing care, and the nursing home setting. Differences in operational definitions, methodological concerns, and the lack of national random samples have made it difficult to understand the conditions under which elder mistreatment is likely to occur. The National Committee for the Prevention of Elder Abuse has pointed out "that such basic questions as to the prevalence and incidence of abuse, risk factors and barriers to seeking and accepting help have not been answered" (Tatara, 1993, p. 37). Although reporting of elder abuse and neglect has been improved and there has been an increase in education and training, there is still a great need for empowerment of elders, preventive measures, and improved systems coordination.

Recent work by Hudson and Carlson (1994) provided a lexicon for elder mistreatment, operationalizing terms that can be used more effectively in practice. The outcome variables in elder mistreatment are challenging to name. Bruises have multiple causality in elders, who may be taking coumadin or have a history of frequent falling. Elders with cognitive impairment may report abuse appropriately, but no credence is given because of their deteriorated mental status. There is no Denver developmental screen for aging that enables the clinician to understand what an 80-year-old looks like and what conditions are likely to represent elder mistreatment. More researchers must be attracted to this field in order to conduct the studies that can begin to clarify the multiplicity of variables.

Signs and symptoms of elder mistreatment might include unexplained bruises, fractures, burns, poor hydration, reports of hitting or any other violent behavior against the elder, sexually transmitted disease in institutionalized elders, unexplained loss of money or goods, evidence of fearfulness around a caregiver, or the subjective report of abuse. It is especially difficult to evaluate the demented elder for mistreatment; a careful and thorough interdisciplinary team approach is required.

The American Medical Association's *Diagnostic and Treatment Guidelines on Elder Abuse and Neglect* (Aravanis et al., 1992) provides guidelines for the assessment of abuse and neglect of elders as well as flowcharts for assessing and intervening in elder mistreatment. Special attention is given to an elder's lack of decision-making capacity in an abusing situation. In such cases appropriate use of guardians should be reviewed. Elders may be inappropriately labeled confused when they choose to return to an abusing situation. For example, a mother may prefer to live with an abusing daughter rather than face the prospect of an unknown caregiver. Overzealous protection of a competent elder is a form of ageism that infantilizes the older individual and takes away his or her autonomy. Each state has elder mistreatment reporting laws or requirements, which professional nurses should become familiar with. A key practice implication in this field is the inclusion of a family violence question in the history and attention to any signs or symptoms in the physical exam that might appropriate follow-up in suspected cases.

Terry Fulmer

See also:
ALZHEIMER'S DISEASE
CAREGIVING
COGNITIVE DISORDERS
COGNITIVE IMPAIRMENT
PHYSICAL RESTRAINTS

EXERCISE

The benefits of regular exercise in promoting health and preventing disease have been widely accepted. The overwhelming evidence of the positive effects of exercise has led the Department of Health and Human Services to develop within its program, *Healthy People 2000*, national objectives for increasing the numbers of adults who exercise regularly (U.S. Department of Health & Human Services, 1990). The American College of Sports Medicine (ACSM) has made specific recommendations for exercise in the adult population (ACSM,1995). As life expectancy increases in the United States and the population over the age of 65 grows, it is especially important to explore ways to maintain functional independence and the general health and well-being of older adults.

An investigation of older adults in industrialized countries reveals that the amount of physical exercise performed declines with age (Stephens & Caspersen, 1994). Although exercise tends to decrease in this age group, no physiological or psychological explanation has been found to explain such a decline (Dishman, 1994). Normal changes of aging, pathological conditions, and environmental deterrents do not prevent older adults from exercising.

Walking is broadly reported to be the most accepted form of exercise among older adults. Siegel, Brackbill, and Heath (1995) found that 35.6% of the sample they tested revealed that they were walkers. Walking is an exercise that can take place in both the community setting and health-care facilities. A study by Lacroix, Leveille, Hecht, Grothaus, and Wagner (1996) indicated that walking more than 4 hours a week correlated with a significantly decreased risk of cardiovascular-disease hospitalization. Krall and Dawson-Huges (1994), in a study of 239 white, postmenopausal female walkers, found that women who walk 7.5 miles or more per week had higher bone density throughout their body.

Other popular exercises for older adults include aquatic and weight-bearing exercises. Recent research shows that resistance or strength training improves strength and functional mobility in older adults (Fiatarone et al., 1994). Weight-bearing and muscle-building exercises help to maintain functional mobility, promote independence, and prevent falls (Connelly & Vandervoort, 1995, 1996). Weight-bearing exercises are shown to be highly effective in reducing the amount of bone-wasting which is common to osteoporosis (Katz & Sherman, 1998) Older individuals who suffer from arthritis find water exercise to be a painless way of promoting their health and increasing their functional ability. Exercises in the water are also an effective and enjoyable form of exercise for older adults without arthritis (Stamford, 1994).

Numerous studies have described the physiologic and structural effects of exercise. In the younger population, exercise has been shown to increase high-density lipoprotein levels, decrease blood pressure, enhance insulin sensitivity, improve bone-mineral density, and facilitate weight loss and weight maintenance. The effects of exercise are so impressive that it has become an accepted therapeutic modality in the treatment of many risk factors related to coronary-artery disease, hypertension, diabetes, and osteoporosis (ACSM, 1995; Kannel & Wilson, 1995). Similarly, studies have demonstrated the physiologic changes that may occur with exercise in the older population.

Chronic endurance exercise (6 months) at an intensity level of up to 85% of heart-rate reserve was shown to significantly increase maximal oxygen uptake, peak workload, resting end-diastolic volume, resting stroke volume, and was shown to decrease resting heart rate (Stratton, Levy, Cerqueira, Schwartz, & Abrass, 1994). The exercise regime used in this study was shown to contribute to a more efficient cardiovascular system in the older population. However these subjects consisted of healthy older men who were motivated to participate in a high-intensity program that met 5 times per week. Many older people could not participate in exercise of this intensity level. Other studies have demonstrated that greater levels of exercise participation over a 1-year period resulted in higher ratings of physical health, regardless of exercise intensity level (Spelman, Pate, Macera, & Ward, 1993; Stewart, King, & Haskell, 1993).

An exercise and health-promotion program established for older veterans prescribed exercise at 65%–75% of patients' measured maximal or nonischemic heart-rate reserve. This group met 3 times per week, and the mode of exercise was individualized according to the patients preexisting limitations, assuring that the exercise was a positive experience. The patients demonstrated improved fitness and general well-being, after 5 years (Morey, Crowley, Robbins, Cowper, & Sullivan, 1994).

Little nursing research is available describing the effects of exercise in older adults. One study by Dawe and Moore-Orr (1995) examined the effect of a single session of mild exercise on a group of cognitively intact, older institutionalized residents aged 70 and up, on cognitive performance. The data revealed that even mild exercise such as range-of-motion improved the recall ability of the resident, and that the effect remained for at least half an hour. The researchers recommend mild exercise programs as a practical and low-cost nursing intervention that may be used to enhance memory and independence.

Connelly and Vandervoort (1995) conducted a study to determine if simple resistance exercise at moderate intensity improved the quadriceps muscle strength of frail older women. The sample included 10 female, nursing home residents with a mean age of 81.6. Subjects completed an 8-week strengthening program consisting of 3 sets of 10 repetitions per leg at the rate of 3 group sessions per week. The exercises were held at a constant intensity between 30% and 50% of their one repetition maximum. Significant improvement was seen in strength and self-paced walking speed. The researchers recommended further investigation into the clinical implications of this type of exercise for both functional rehabilitation and fall prevention.

Another study by Jirovec (1991) examined the impact of daily exercise on the mobility, balance, and urine control of 15 cognitively impaired, incontinent nursing-home residents. A quasiexperimental pretest-posttest design was used. Outcome measures included: walking distance, speed of walking, balance ability, ability to rise from a chair unassisted, ability to walk unassisted, and incidence of urinary incontinence both before and after a month of daily assisted walking. The results showed that the older adults were walking significantly greater distances after the exercise regimen than before.

The benefits of regular exercise are well accepted and widely documented in numerous studies. As the population of the United States shifts to include a higher proportion of older adults, emphasis needs to be placed on research that will enhance independent living and improve quality-of-life. Despite the large amount of medical literature supporting the role and benefits of exercise among older adults, little nursing research on exercise in aging could be found.

Further descriptive and intervention research is needed on the types of exercise that are most effective in achieving optimal health and well-being outcomes in the older population. Adherence to exercise regimes presents a large barrier to effective outcomes, and presents an area ripe for nursing research. Dishman (1994) reports that only 50% of people who begin an exercise program will continue the program past 3 months. The best tools currently available to encourage continued exercise among our older adult population are communicating the role of exercise in maintaining quality-of-life and helping to choose exercises that older adults enjoy and to which they have easy access.

Teaching effective exercise regimes to older adults is another area in need of further nursing research. As one of the primary interventions necessary in assisting older adults to participate in exercise programs, instruction on the benefit of exercise remains the first factor in motivating the older adult to participate. Subsequently, individual counseling will help the nurse to identify exercises that the older adult will enjoy and will continue. Further research is needed on the variables influencing patients' adherence to a successful exercise program. Currently, the nurse should assist the patient to design an appropriate exercise program that maintains strength, flexibility, and balance.

MEREDITH WALLACE

See also:
ADHERENCE/COMPLIANCE
STRESS MANAGEMENT

GRANDPARENTS RAISING GRANDCHILDREN

Nurses, practicing in a variety of settings, are likely to encounter clients who are the full-time caregivers of their grandchildren. During the past decade there has been a tremendous increase in the prevalence of grandparents raising grandchildren in parent-absent households. The number of children in grandparent-headed households increased from 4.9% in 1992 to 5.5% in 1997 (U.S. Census Bureau, 1999). Thus, there were 4.1 million children raised by grandparents in approximately two million homes in 1997. Although this phenomenon impacts all racial and economic groups, the most significant rises have been among African Americans (Feig, 1997). Although there are numerous reasons for grandparents having to assume the responsibility of parenting their grandchildren, studies consistently report maternal substance abuse as the major factor (Burton, 1992; Dowdell, 1995; Dressel & Barnhill, 1994; Kelley, 1993; Minkler & Roe, 1993). Other antecedents to grandparents raising grandchildren include severe psychiatric disorders, AIDS, incarceration, and death related to homicide or illness.

Research conducted to date suggests that grandparents raising grandchildren are at increased risk for poor health and increased psychological distress. Thus, it is imperative that nurses are informed of the emerging body of research on this phenomenon, especially the research regarding the impact on the caregivers' physical and emotional health.

Impact on Caregivers

Physical health.   Studies that have examined the health status of grandparents raising grandchildren suggest that their health is often compromised. In a study examining caregiver burden in grandparents raising grandchildren, Dowdell (1995) found that 45% of grandmothers identified themselves as having a physical problem or illness that seriously affected their health, with single grandmothers reporting more health problems than married grandmothers. Those who indicated their health had worsened after assuming parenting responsibilities also reported financial problems and lack of family support. In another study, over one-third of participants reported heightened health problems since assuming full-time caregiving responsibilities for grandchildren (Burton, 1992). And when Kelley (1993) examined caregiver stress in grandparents raising grandchildren, 22% of grandparent participants scored in what is considered the clinical range on the health problem scale of the Parenting Stress Index (Abidin, 1990).

In a study of African American women raising grandchildren and great-grandchildren, Minkler and Roe (1993) found that 38% reported that their health had worsened since assuming full-time parenting responsibilities for grandchildren. Women who were married or had a partner, as well as those who were employed, were more likely to report themselves as physically healthy compared to others. Half reported breaking a medical appointment in the past year due to child care responsibilities. Approximately half reported that they had current concerns regarding their health, yet one-third had not been to a doctor in 3 years or more.

Because advanced aging is often associated with an increase in healthcare problems, it may play a factor in the health status of grandparents who are parenting for the second time around. Consistently, across available studies, the reported average age of grandparent caregivers is 55 to 57 years (Dowdell, 1995; Roy, Gordon, & Cohen, 1997; Kelley, 1993; Minkler, Roe, & Robertson-Beckley, 1994). A national study of kinship caretakers, of which 66% were grandmothers, found that 57% were aged 50 or higher, including 29% over age 60 and almost 10% over age 70 (Feig, 1997). Undoubtedly, if the age of grandparent caregivers was reported separately, the mean age of this subgroup of caregivers would be even higher.

Poor physical health in this population is of concern given that poor physical health contributes to psychological stress. For instance, fair to poor health has been found to be a powerful risk factor for major depression in African Americans (Brown, Ahmed, Gary, & Milburn, 1995). Undoubtedly, poor physical health negatively impacts parenting abilities, both emotionally and in the physical demands of parenting.

Psychological distress.   Numerous studies have found that assuming full-time parenting responsibilities for grandchildren is associated with increased psychological distress in the grandparent caregivers (Burton, 1992; Dowdell, 1995; Kelley, 1993; Kelley & Damato, 1995; Minkler & Roe, 1993). In a study conducted by Kelley (1993), grandparent caregivers scored significantly higher than a normative group on psychological distress as measured by the Symptom Checklist-90-Revised (SCL-90-R) Inventory (Derogatis, 1983). More revealing is the finding that 44% of grandparents scored above the 90th percentile or what is considered to be in the clinical range, e.g., psychological stress levels considered high enough to warrant professional mental health intervention. Social isolation and the restriction inherent in the parenting role, as measured by the Parenting Stress Index (PSI) (Abidin, 1990), were found to be predictors of increased psychological distress. Thirty-seven percent of grandparent caregivers scored above the 80th percentile on the PSI, which is considered in the clinical range. According to Abidin (1990), parenting stress refers to the stress a parent experiences that is a function of certain salient child characteristics, parental characteristics, and situational variables which are directly related to the role of being a parent.

Dowdell (1995) found a significant relationship between perceived caregiver burden and high levels of psychological distress. When Minkler and Roe (1993) queried grandparents regarding their psychological health,

37% reported their psychological health had worsened since assuming full-time caregiving of grandchildren. And the vast majority (72%) reported feeling "depressed" in the week prior to data collection.

In a study examining predictors of psychological distress in 102 grandmothers raising grandchildren, physical health, family resources, and social support affected psychological distress (Kelley, Whitley, Sipe, & Yorker, in press). Grandmothers who reported fewer resources, less social support, and poorer physical health tended to experience higher levels of psychological distress. Almost 30% of participants scored in the clinical range in psychological distress on a standardized measure.

A variety of factors may contribute to increased psychological distress in grandparent caregivers. As previously discussed, the majority of children in the care of grandmothers have been abandoned, abused, and/or neglected by biological parents. Because a substantial body of empirical literature has demonstrated that abused and neglected children are at increased risk for behavioral problems (Claussen & Crittenden, 1991; Famularo, Kinscherff, Bunshaft, Spivak, & Fenton, 1989; Kelley, 1992), children raised by grandparents are clearly at increased risk for emotional and behavioral problems. Thus, parenting children with behavior problems is most likely one of several stressors experienced by these grandparents. Other stressors experienced by grandparents raising grandchildren include concern regarding their own longevity, that is living long enough to raise their grandchildren; concern over their adult children who are often incapacitated by drugs; financial difficulties, social isolation, poor health, and the fact that most are raising multiple grandchildren (Burton, 1992; Kelley, 1993; Minkler & Roe, 1993). Grandparents raising grandchildren often experience feelings of anger and resentment related to their parenting role which are likely to contribute to psychological distress (Burton, 1992; Kelley, 1993; Kelley & Damato, 1995; Minkler & Roe, 1993).

The studies described above suggest the need for developing and testing interventions targeting this population. Kelley, Whitley, Yorker, and Sipe (in press) pilot tested a home-based nursing and social service intervention aimed at improving the well-being of 25 urban, African American grandparents raising grandchildren. The purpose of the intervention was to reduce psychological distress, improve physical and mental health, and improve the social support and resources of the grandparent. The 6-month intervention included home visitation by registered nurses and social workers, legal assistance, and support groups. Results included improved mental health scores, decreased psychological stress scores, and improved scores in social support. The investigators have extended the intervention from 6 months to 1 year in duration and are currently testing it with 150 families in a federally funded study.

In summary, while much attention has been given to the well-being of caregivers of spouses and parents, the emotional and physical status of grandparents raising grandchildren has only recently been examined. Further research on the physical and emotional health of this population is needed. There are limitations to the studies conducted to date. Many of the studies cited did not employ standardized measures of physical and emotional health and lacked comparison groups. Furthermore, the samples tended to be small to moderate in size, homogeneous, and nonrandomly selected. Future research should address these methodological limitations.

SUSAN J. KELLEY

See also:
CARING
CAREGIVER
RETIREMENT

NONTRADITIONAL THERAPIES

Definitions

Nontraditional therapies encompass a broad spectrum of practices and beliefs. Consequently, descriptions and definitions of the collective philosophy vary according to one's professional or occupational perspective. Historically, and from the point of view of some within the biomedical community, nontraditional therapies are defined as practices that are not correct, proper, or appropriate or are not in conformity with the beliefs and standards of the dominant group of health care practitioners in a society. To this definition others add that nontraditional therapies collectively are those interventions that are neither taught widely in schools of nursing and medicine nor provided generally by hospitals. In some cultures, alternative modalities refers to therapies that are offered in place of orthodox health care practices, some of which are far outside of the realm of accepted health care theory and practices in the United States.

Complementary medicine/therapies, a term introduced in 1976 in the United Kingdom, encompasses many of the modalities categorized as nontraditional and in that country refers to linking the most appropriate modalities to serve the patient physically, mentally, emotionally, and spiritually. A recent and similar definition for nontraditional therapies is "those interventions for improving, maintaining and promoting health and well-being, preventing disease, or treating illness" (Jacobs, 1995).

One problem that arises with the terms *nontraditional, complementary,* and *alternative* is that these are judgmental terms that inhibit dialogue about the therapies, and they are in conflict with the nursing perspective and tradition of providing care that includes noninvasive and naturalistic therapies (Watson, 1995). Therapies that have traditionally been an integral part of nursing have begun to appear within the newly emerging field of alternative and complementary medicine. Nursing does not consider therapies related to caring, comfort, pain reduction or relief, and other means of symptom control as alternative but rather as therapies that nurses have traditionally provided and that are considered the foundation of caring, holistic nursing practice. Consequently, the terms *nontraditional, alternative,* and *complementary* are controversial within the field of nursing today.

Societal Value of Nontraditional Therapies

Today's emphasis on health promotion mandates education, personal responsibilities, and empowerment of individuals, which encourages use of these therapies. There are those in society who desire nontraditional therapies as adjuncts to conventional care or, in some instances, in place of invasive, painful, or unsuccessful therapies that lead to pain, suffering, and lengthy hospital stays.

One in three adult Americans in 1990 reportedly used some kind of nontraditional therapy and paid for them mostly out-of-pocket (Eisenberg et al., 1993). Most often these individuals were searching for modalities that could fight the major chronic diseases and conditions that were reducing their quality of life.

In response to the increase in the public's interest in nontraditional therapies, Congress, in late 1992, established the Office of Alternative Medicine (OAM) within the Director's Office of the National Institutes of Health (NIH). Reorganization in 1996 placed the OAM within the Office of Disease Prevention. The OAM's classification scheme of alternative therapies includes more than 200 modalities with more than 10,000 uses and categorizes these under the headings of diet, nutrition, lifestyle changes, mind-body control, manual healing, pharmacological and biological treatments, bioelectromagnetic applications, and herbal medicine. The OAM (1992) fosters research on nontraditional therapies and seeks to reduce barriers that keep promising therapies from emerging. To promote research in nontraditional therapies, OAM established 10 research centers across the country, one of which is directed by a nurse. A Public Information Clearinghouse Database and Evaluations Section of the OAM is scheduled to be operational in 1998. It will be a resource to interested persons seeking state-of-the-science information on selected nontraditional therapies.

Researching Nontraditional Therapies From the Nursing Perspective

Theory-based nursing practices and the emerging "holistic nursing movement" (Watson, 1995) reflect a body of knowledge that includes therapies developed from the distinctive perspective of the nursing discipline. It is from the nursing perspective that nurse scholars and their students select from the phenomena of interest to the discipline those specific phenomena needing further development. Therapies such as aromatherapy, guided imagery and other forms of visualization, therapeutic touch, massage, acupressure, music listening, meditation and relaxation techniques, yoga, and support groups, although labeled nontraditional therapies, are and have been within the domain of nursing practice and research.

Good programs of research involving any of these therapies can begin with very basic questions: What's going on with a particular therapy in the investigator's target population? How do individual differences, as assessed by a given measurement tool, influence what happens or does not happen in the use of a particular therapy for management of a specified symptom? From general questions such as these, coupled with extensive literature reviews and consultation with experts, more specific questions about the use of these therapies in patient care evolve to guide the investigator's research.

Because nursing takes the position that patients' perceptions, thoughts, and feelings are an important part of their reality, these influence the nature of inquiry and the choice of outcome measures. Focusing on individual differences among patients when assessing use, efficacy, and effectiveness of nontraditional therapies permits the investigator to analyze disparate patient care findings and synthesize them into questions that will add to the body of knowledge about these therapies. Findings resulting from research studies testing the efficacy of nontraditional therapies may lead to knowledge that can be useful in making reliable predictions and linking appropriate therapies to a person for promotion of health or symptom management.

Certain problems may arise when researchers try to use conventional research techniques without adaptation for the evaluation of some nontraditional therapies. For example, use of placebo controls and double blinding may not be feasible in testing therapies such as massage, therapeutic touch, and acupressure. A variety of different study designs are appropriate to answer questions important to the evaluation of particular therapies. Existing nursing literature provides numerous examples of rigorous qualitative research as well as examples of studies without blinding or an active control. Solving methodological problems in testing nontraditional therapies is a matter of following simple guidelines that take into account the special features of the nontraditional therapy and research question being investigated. Each question raised by the researcher and the type of research implemented can play a role in developing a fuller understanding of the efficacy, effectiveness, and safety of nontraditional therapies within professional nursing practice.

Significant Issues for Future Research

Nursing knowledge development is driven by new questions and new conceptual frameworks. Reconceptualizing research problems with a new paradigm or framework may provide new insights into these therapies. Research efforts on nontraditional therapies should include additional efficacy and effectiveness studies, cost-effectiveness studies, and replication of existing studies. Research is needed to answer relevant questions about the use of complementary and nontraditional therapies in the nursing care of all persons. Attention should be given to the following:

- Outcome measures that are reliable, valid, and standardized for each specific therapy so that studies can be compared and combined;
- Qualitative research studies to determine patients' experiences with using particular nontraditional therapies in the management of their specific conditions;
- Research that includes examination of consequences or outcomes of not integrating a potentially useful nontraditional therapy as part of the treatment regimen for a condition or symptom and treating a symptom or condition with a combination of pharmacological and nontraditional therapy;
- Investigations that build on advances in neurobiological sciences and psychoneuroimmunology to understand mechanisms of action of the less understood nontraditional therapies;
- Research that assesses individual differences in outcomes for nontraditional therapies, including cross-cultural applicability and efficacy;
- Research that examines nontraditional therapies for different populations and conditions, giving consideration to the influence of age, race, gender, religious beliefs, and socioeconomic status on the treatment efficacy; and

- The most effective timing for the introduction of a nontraditional therapy in the course of conventional treatment.

Conclusions

Some therapies referred to as nontraditional are integral to professional nursing practice, and others are seen as important to emerging holistic care developments. These therapies have been studied less than other nursing phenomena, yet there is research to support the effectiveness of selected nontraditional therapies, such as the use of relaxation techniques, as well as to provide a foundation for further research. The challenge and crucial step toward recognition and acceptance by the biomedical community is to continue to engage in conceptual work toward explanatory theories and to investigate these therapies in the context of the nursing perspective.

ANN GILL TAYLOR

See also:
  MUSIC THERAPY

OLDER DRIVERS

Although older adults drive fewer miles than younger ones, drivers over the age of 69 are more likely to be involved in fatal automobile crashes than are individuals in any other age group, except those between 16 and 24 years of age (Persson, 1993). Fatal crashes are the most prevalent cause of accidental death in adults between the ages of 65 and 74, and they are the second leading cause in those over the age of 75. After the age of 86, there are 40 deaths per one hundred million vehicle miles traveled (Graham, 1995). Older women have a 35% higher accident rate than do men of the same age (Stamatiadis, 1996).

Crashes caused by older drivers are most likely to occur during daylight hours, at urban intersections, and to involve multiple vehicles (Graham, 1995). Nonfatal driving errors are also more prevalent among older drivers. The most frequent citations received by older adults are for traffic light, right-of-way, and turn violations. These figures are more telling when placed within the context of the fact that older adults tend to avoid driving at night, during rush hour, in hazardous weather conditions, and in unfamiliar areas.

It is predicted that traffic fatalities in older adults, particularly women, will show a dramatic increase in the future unless strict driving regulations are enforced (Crane, 1999). Yet, most older drivers believe they are safe, and equate driving with autonomy, independence, and convenience (Persson, 1993).

The physical abilities that are needed to drive safely begin to decline at about the age of 55, and significantly deteriorate after the age of 75 (Graham, 1995; Marottoli, Ostfeld, Merrill, Perlman, Foley, & Cooney, 1993; Persson, 1993; Reuben, Silliman, & Traines, 1988). Many older adults also exhibit a decline in cognitive function that negatively impacts their ability to drive safely.

Vision accounts for over 90% of the information needed to drive safely (Reuben et al., 1988). Declines in binocular and distance vision, as well as in color sensitivity, contribute to higher traffic morbidity and mortality rates for older adults. Nighttime driving poses a particular hazard due to an increased sensitivity to glare and a decreased ability to read road signs under poor lighting conditions. Age-related eye diseases, such as cataracts, macular degeneration, and glaucoma, can hinder further the driving ability of elders.

Recent evidence suggests that the useful field-of-view test, which measures visual processing speed, visual sensory function, and visual attention skills, may be an accurate predictor of automobile accidents involving older adults (Owsley et al., 1998). In a prospective cohort study of 294 drivers between the ages of 55 and 87, subjects were tested using the useful field-of-view test, and were then monitored for 3 years to determine their automobile crash rates. Subjects who exhibited a reduction rate of greater than 40% in their useful field-of-view were more than twice as likely to become involved in an automobile accident. The most common errors made were missed stop signs, the misjudgment of distance, and a failure to yield right-of-way.

There is a lack of evidence regarding the relationship between age-related decreases in other sensory functions and driving safety, and also between delayed classical reaction time and driving safety (Reuben et al., 1988). Hearing-impaired individuals tend to compensate by paying more attention to the visual cues needed for safe driving, and thus are assumed not to pose a significant crash risk. Perception-response time (the difference between the time a barrier first becomes visible and the time that the brake is applied) is a more accurate measure of the responses needed to drive safely than is classical reaction time. Older drivers demonstrate a perception-response time that is similar to that of younger adults.

Evidence also suggests that a large number of cognitively impaired older adults continue to drive, and that they make a significant contribution to the total number of fatal crashes and traffic violations by elders (Dobbs, Heller, & Schopflocher, 1998). Retrospective studies, using self-reports to collect data, show that 77% of older drivers with dementia of the Alzheimer's type exhibit changes in driving performance, and are involved in 5 times as many crashes as are noncognitively impaired drivers (Friedland et al., 1988; Lucas-Blaustein, Filipp, Dungan, & Tune, 1988). Over 58% of the cognitively impaired stopped driving only after being involved in a crash.

The few prospective studies investigating the actual driving performance of those with Alzheimer's disease suggest that driving ability is significantly reduced in even the mildly cognitively impaired. Although they drove slower, about 41% failed the on-the-road driving assessment test (Dobbs, Heller, & Schopflocher, 1998; Duchek, Hunt, Ball, Buckles, & Morris, 1998; Hunt, Carr, Duchek, Grant, Buckles, & Morris, 1997; Hunt, Morris, Edwards, & Wilson, 1993).

A study of 66 healthy and 70 cognitively impaired older adults examined their ability to accurately label 10 traffic signs that appear on the Traffic Sign Naming Test (Carr, LaBarge, Dunnigan, & Storandt, 1998). The results indicated that the test correctly differentiated between cognitively impaired and healthy drivers 74% of the time. This suggests that the Traffic Sign Naming Test is a short, and reliable, way to screen older adults for cognitive impairment that would adversely affect their driving.

Other illnesses, and the use of certain medications, are also thought to be risk factors associated with impaired driving in older adults (Campbell, M. K., Bush, & Hale, 1993; Reuben et al., 1988). These include cardiovascular disease, diabetes mellitus, stroke, Parkinson's disease, seizures, sleep apnea, and arthritis. The use of alcohol and/or tranquilizers also increases the risk of automobile accidents. The relationship between safe driving and other prescription (and nonprescription) drugs requires further investigation.

Despite the fact that nurses are in an ideal position to identify and counsel unsafe older drivers, little nursing research has been conducted in this area. Using triangulated methods, the decision to stop driving and forfeit one's driver's license was examined in convenience samples of 75 rural (Johnson, J. E., 1995) and 285 urban elders (Johnson, J. E., in press). In both studies, most of the participants had been involved in a car crash. Most of the rural elders indicated that involvement in an accident led to feelings of insecurity behind the wheel, and was a significant factor in their decision to stop driving. In contrast, the majority of urban elders maintained that they were safe drivers, and had no concerns about their driving ability. Seventy-five percent of the older urban drivers had their licenses involuntarily revoked by the state. None of their rural counterparts had been subjected to this. In both samples, the psychological consequences of no longer being able to drive included intense loneliness, brought on by increased isolation, and a profound regret at having lost a significant amount of independence. The lack of safe, reliable, and affordable public transportation was an issue for urban elders, but not for their rural counterparts.

Findings from three qualitative studies (Johnson, J. E., in press; Johnson, J. E., 1998b; Johnson, J. E., 1995) suggest that social support plays a significant role in the decision of older drivers to forfeit their license. Both urban and rural elders feel that friends are more important than family regarding this decision because they are more likely to understand its impact on their quality of life. However, rural family members are more reliable than their urban counterparts in assisting with transportation needs once older adults can no longer drive.

Very few nurses assess their clients for the sensory, cognitive, and motor functions needed to drive safely (Johnson, J. E., 1998a). Data from 50 randomly selected nurses who participated in semistructured interviews revealed that they lack confidence in their own assessment and communication skills—skills that would be needed to determine driving ability, and to even discuss such a sensitive topic. Interviews with a random sample of 25 nurse practitioners (Johnson, J. E., 1999) showed that the majority unintentionally assess their older clients for the functional abilities related to safe driving. The client's presenting complaint just happens to involve a system that is related to driving ability. Many of the nurse practitioners felt that it was not their place to discuss driving cessation with their older clients, or felt that they did not have the time needed to do so in the current healthcare environment.

Future research should examine the best ways to differentiate safe and unsafe older drivers, the efficacy of senior driver education programs, acceptable forms of alternate transportation, and the changes needed in license renewal requirements. It is imperative that the psychological and social consequences of driving cessation be investigated, as well as potential interventions to mediate them. The role of nurses in identifying and counseling unsafe older drivers, and the ethical and legal dilemmas involved in reporting them, must also be studied.

JULIE E. JOHNSON

See also:
COGNITIVE DISORDERS
COGNITIVE IMPAIRMENT

QUALITY OF LIFE

Quality of life research is an extensive field, with scholars who have thought carefully about the parameters, indicators, diversity, and variability of the dimensions of quality of life (Benner, 1985; Spilker, Simpson, & Tilson, 1991). However, there is no universally accepted definition of quality of life. A consensus among researchers seems to be that its components should include a person's satisfaction with his or health and function, economic status, family life, and spiritual, occupational, and psychosocial well-being. The scope of the research typically includes a general assessment of perceived well-being and subsets of health-related components of quality of life. General overall assessment of quality of life typically gauges the health and functional abilities of the person; the health-related aspects are often measured as symptom experiences, disease management, economic effect of disease and treatment, and level of wellness.

Definitions of quality of life vary greatly. Early studies measured patient functional capacity, illness status, and longevity. Currently, components measured include impact of an illness and its treatment, socioeconomic status, and cultural or personal characteristics influencing a person's ability to have a fulfilling life. Many researchers now use a health-related framework that defines quality of life as measures of rehabilitation following disease or disability. Rehabilitation indexes often use measures of a person's ability to carry out routines of daily living and roles of life (e.g., homemaker, employee, student).

Numerous measures that represent quality of life have been developed, and many of the early definitions were unidimensional. Early definitions of quality of life were often measures or ratings of physical function made by the physician. Both the unidimensional and the outside rater approaches to measurement of quality of life have been criticized as too simplistic as well as inaccurate. Nurse researchers indicate that qualitative methods are preferable to questionnaires. However, the ability to follow changes over time by using quantitative methods is important for researchers (Jalowiec, 1992). Utilizing quantitative methods is also appropriate with large sample sizes. Discussions about the validity of using subjective versus objective measures of quality of life have ended in the notion that both are available but must be discussed in relation to the purpose of the research study.

In the 1980s the Adjusted Quality of Life Years Utility Index was developed (Torrance, 1987). This formula-oriented definition of quality of life included the cost of medical treatments over the expected number of years survival and patients' preferences for living with the treatment. This approach and definition added the economic factor and the individual's opinions to quality of life measures. The World Health Organization's 1995 position paper on quality of life assessment broadens the view of quality of life beyond health without illness.

The current regulations by the Food and Drug Administration requiring quality of life to be a component of drug studies have resulted in numerous specific and narrow measures of medication efficacy, commonly using single-item indicators and linear analog scales. Many instruments have been developed for specific populations of patients, resulting in illness-, functions-, and symptom-oriented measures that reflect treatment outcomes (Smith, 1993).

Nurse researchers and others have expanded the definitions of quality of life to include a person's satisfaction with health and function, economic status, family life, occupation, and psychosocial well-being (Padilla et al., 1983). In 1989 the Institute of Medicine staff published a monograph on the quality of life measures they recommended for use. Padilla's quality of life instrument for cancer patients was the only nurse-authored questionnaire in the monograph. Medical studies and clinical trials have often employed health-rating scales. Judgment analysis also has been used in assessing quality of life (McGee, O'Boyle, Hickey, Olley, & Joyce, 1991).

In a unique instrument, Ferrans and Powers (1992) measured not only a person's satisfaction with health, family, economic status, and psychospiritual well-being but also measured the importance of each of those areas to the person. This comparison between importance and satisfaction ratings by the person better reflects quality of life unique to each individual's life goals. Self-comparison of importance versus satisfaction also allows for following changes in a patient's quality of life over time. One conclusion common to all researchers, in the past and currently, is that quality of life for individuals with incomes below the poverty line will be low, regardless of health and family status or self-perceived well-being.

The paradigm has shifted to a multifactoral basis of measurement: multiple variables which obtain a variety of subjective perceptions of each patient that go beyond the physical aspects of life. There are differences in a single-person quality of life measure, which measures personal function, and a community-oriented concept, which reflects the person's ability to have an effect on the greater society. Nurses have also expanded the notion of quality of life beyond the individual and his or her disease state. Research with family caregivers and discussion of family and community quality of life are being formulated for further study by the authors.

Carol E. Smith
Carol Gaskamp

See also:
CHRONIC ILLNESS
WELLNESS

RETIREMENT

The increased birth rate of the mid-1900s and longer life expectancies have resulted in an increase in the number of persons who are, or are soon going to be, retired (Anderson & Weber, 1993). In addition, the concept of retirement has changed. While retirement may simply mean the cessation of employment at a given age, the term is generally considered to be much more complex. Following "retirement," many people reenter the workforce, begin new careers, or work part-time (Myers, 1991). As a result, determining what retirement is and who is "retired" can be difficult, and the numbers can be equally misleading. The *Social Security Bulletin* (Social Security Administration, 1998) provides an estimate of 27,274,572 retirees in December 1997, based on the number of people receiving retired-worker benefits. This is indeed a substantial population. Another indicator of the number of retirees is the number of people in the civilian workforce by age group. In 1996, out of a total of 26,397,000 employed persons, 19.7% of the total work force was between the ages of 45 and 54; and 3,828,000 (2.9%) were 65 years or older (Bureau of Labor Statistics, 1999).

This is particularly important when examining the overall characteristics of older citizens, as well as the changes that have occurred over the last several decades. In *A Profile of Older Americans: 1998* (Administration on Aging, 1998), it is reported that in 1997 there were 34.1 million Americans who were 65 years or older, and they represented 12.7% of the U.S. population. In the same year, the 65–74 age group (18.5 million) was eight times larger than it was in 1900, and the 75–84 (11.7 million) group was 16 times larger. Nearly one-half (46%) of all older women in 1997 were widows and there were four times as many widows as widowers. The American Association of Retired Persons (AARP, 1999a, p. 1) reports, "Outliving men by an average of seven years, women typically have to finance those longer lives with lower wages, fewer benefits, and no pensions. The result? Three-quarters of the older Americans living in poverty are women." In 1997 approximately 1 in 7 (14.2%) households that had an elderly head of the family had an income of less than $15,000, and in 1995 older citizens accounted for approximately 40% of all hospital stays (Administration on Aging, 1998). These data have major implications not only for retirees and their families and friends, but also for the healthcare delivery system and the rising costs of health care.

Several theories of aging have been used to better understand retirement, and as frameworks for retirement research. The major ones include continuity theory, activity theory, role theory, disengagement theory, and political economy theory. Each has it own set of criticisms—as well as contributions—to the overall understanding of the retirement phenomenon. Continuity theory suggests that people develop habits and preferences that become an integral part of them, and that persist into their retirement years (Atchley, 1977). According to activity theory, people adjust most effectively in older age when they maintain previously established activities (Friedman & Havighurst, 1954). Role theories suggest that society is structured around various roles that provide both norms and expectations regarding a person's attitudes and behavior (Richardson, 1993). Disengagement theory is based on the premise that people tend to withdraw from some of the roles and activities as they age and enter retirement (Cumming & Henry, 1961). Political economy theory (Estes, Linkins, & Binney, 1996) posits that retirement is the result of decisions on the part of business and industry to reduce the workforce; as a result, retirement adjustment would depend on the personal resources of the individual.

Retirement marks a transition into the later stages of life (Floyd et al., 1992), and as a part of the Normative Aging Study, researchers suggest that retirement is now a normative event, not the unplanned occurrence it used to be (Bossé, Aldwin, Levenson, Spiro, & Mroczek, 1993). Increased longevity and a greater number of healthy older adults have changed expectations for retirement. Retirement may be a time for new recreational pursuits, such as travel, and presents an opportunity to develop new routines (Watts, 1987). However, economic constraints may place limits on these activities, and changes in the health of the retiree or significant other may interfere with previous plans.

Upon retirement, relationships with co-workers are terminated (van Tilburg, 1992), and this has an impact on the life of the retiree. As noted earlier, some retirees continue working after their initial retirement. In fact, eight out of ten "baby boomers" report that they plan to work at least part-time after retirement (AARP, 1999b). Myers (1991) found that having employer pensions reduced the probability of future employment, while having Social Security benefits alone increased the probability that a retiree would continue to work. Retirement can also have an impact on marital relationships. The retirement of one partner in a marriage suggests a reorganization of roles as the couple begins the transition to full-time retirement (Henretta, O'Rand, & Chan, 1993), and differences have been found in the division of household tasks among retirees and nonretirees (Szinovacz & Harpster, 1994). During retirement, spouses have been found to become increasingly aware of their partners' faults (Johnston, 1990), and women may have problems of infringement when husbands spend more time at home (Vinick & Ekerdt, 1989). Lee and Shehan (1989) found no beneficial effects of retirement on marital satisfaction among husbands and wives.

In recent years there have been a number of studies on retirement among women (Slevin & Wingrove, 1995). "Because of the prevailing 'myth' among women that they will be cared for in old age and women's fear of growing old, women often do not aggressively plan for their retirement" (Perkins, 1992, p. 526). Some studies suggest that women who have had recent employment are healthier in their later years than women who have not been employed (Hibbard, 1995). Keddy and Singleton (1991) found that among the women they studied, the primary concerns related to finances, the use of leisure time, and keeping a positive attitude in retirement. Women's adaptation to retirement may be more affected by life events than men's (Szinovacz & Washo, 1992). Daly and Futrell (1989) concluded that retirement attitude was the variable most predictive of retired and preretired women's and men's emotional health.

Preparation for retirement has many facets, however. In American society it focuses primarily on financial planning, with little or no emphasis on retirement adjustment. Retirement is frequently treated as a point in time rather than a complex process (Siegel & Rees, 1992); yet planning for retirement was the second strongest predictor of retirement satisfaction among male respondents in a study by Dorfman (1989). Among the elderly, a leisure repertoire is of concern due to the abundance of free time that accompanies retirement (Mobily, Lemke, & Gisin, 1991). Differences have been noted across race. Allen and Chin-Sang (1990) used a qualitative research approach to study older black women, and found that they continued their history of self-reliance in the context of leisure experiences and service to others in old age.

Numerous psychosocial changes have been found to occur with retirement (Rosenkoetter & Garris, 1998), and depression is a factor for at least some retirees (Rosenkoetter, Garris, & Hendricksen, 1997). The effect of retirement on mental health and health behaviors was investigated in the Kaiser Permanente Retirement Study (Midanik, Soghikian, Ransom, & Tekawa, 1995). Atkinson (1990) found that problem drinking in the elderly is a public-health problem of moderate proportion, and that many geriatric cases are not properly identified.

Retirement is an important concept for both nursing practice and nursing research; yet it receives little emphasis in the nursing literature as a significant life event, a transition, a stressor, or as a component of routine nursing assessments and interventions. While marriage, divorce, childbearing, and the like have received much attention not only as events but as transitions, considerably less attention has been directed toward retirement. Greater emphasis is needed on the impact of retirement on health and health-care, and its implications for nursing. Nurses need to be attending to the issues of retirement when working with retirees and their significant others, as well as with those who are in the preretirement phase. Assuming that retirement is a positive experience may not be appropriate or in the best interests of clients and their families or friends.

MARLENE M. ROSENKOETTER

See also:
GRANDPARENTING
WELLNESS

SMOKING/TOBACCO AS CARDIOVASCULAR RISK FACTOR

Smoking is an addictive behavior that causes both physiological and psychological dependence. Nicotine, the drug component leading to addiction, appears to have both stimulating and tranquilizing effects. Smokers tend to regulate the amount of nicotine delivered to the brain by varying the intensity, frequency, and depth of each puff. Smoking is also an "overlearned" habit. Success with quitting is dependent on identifying what triggers a person to smoke. Smoking is most often associated with many aspects of daily life, including habits such as driving in a car, eating a meal, talking on the telephone, or drinking coffee. Finally, smoking is used as a coping mechanism. Individuals smoke to deal with stress, boredom, anxiety, and many other emotions. Successful interventions must be directed to managing the complexity of the behavior, including nicotine addiction, the psychosocial influences, and the habit.

Prevalence in the United States

It is estimated that 49 million people, or at least one quarter of all Americans, are currently smoking. The prevalence of smoking in men is 28.2% and in women 23.1%. Smoking is highest in Black men (33.9%) and lowest in Hispanic and Asian women (15.2% and 7%, respectively). A strong relationship exists between smoking and level of education, the prevalence being several times higher among those with less than 12 years of education than among those with more than 16 years of education. Although smoking has declined by about 40% since 1965, recent data indicate that this downward trend may have leveled off. In fact, no decline has been seen in the number of cigarettes smoked since 1993 (American Heart Association, 1997).

According to the Centers for Disease Control and Prevention, 75% of all smokers begin smoking before the age of 18 and 90% before the age of 21 (American Heart Association, 1997). Approximately 3,000 teenagers begin smoking each day. The percentage of high school seniors now smoking is 22%, the highest since 1979. Teen smoking has not dropped since 1980, due heavily to the tobacco companies' targeting of minors through advertising. According to the U.S. Department of Health and Human Services, smokeless tobacco among youth also has increased, with about 1 million adolescents, including 20% of all high school boys, using this substance.

Economic Burden

Tobacco is an extremely important public health problem; smoking-related diseases cost the United States about $50 billion annually in medical care (American Heart Association, 1997). Smokers average $6,000 more in lifetime medical costs than do nonsmokers, are absent 6.5 more days per year from work, and make on average six more health care visits annually (MacKenzie, Bartecchi, & Schrier, 1994). The burden is compounded by the lack of work productivity associated with smoking. Approximately 50,000 additional fatalities from burns, pediatric diseases, and secondhand smoke are also attributed to smoking.

Health Effects

One in every five deaths in the United States is smoking-related. Almost every organ and tissue is damaged from smoking, the most common diseases being lung cancer, cardiovascular disease, and chronic obstructive pulmonary disease. On average, smokers will die 7 years earlier than nonsmokers, often suffering chronic debilitating conditions in the years prior to death. Although smokers are at risk for almost all diseases, the health benefits of smoking cessation are immediate and substantial for all individuals regardless of age, gender, disease state, and smoking history. For example, smokers who quit smoking at the time of a myocardial infarction (MI) decrease their chances of a recurrent MI by 50% within the first year of quitting. Within 10 years this risk drops to only slightly above that of a nonsmoker.

Nonsmokers also are at risk from tobacco smoke. Cigarettes contain more than 4,000 chemicals and carcinogens, which are found in high concentrations in sidestream smoke. The risk of death from cardiovascular disease increases by about 30% in those who are exposed to environmental tobacco smoke (American Heart Association, 1997).

Smoking Interventions

Many interventions have been undertaken to help smokers quit: strong physician advice, hypnosis, acupuncture, use of medications such as nicotine replacement therapy, self-help materials, and smoking cessation behavioral counseling groups. Based on a meta-analysis of 39 studies conducted in clinical practice from the late 1970s to the early mid-1980s, Kottke, Battista, DeFriese, and Brekke (1988) found that, irrespective of the intervention or delivery system, smoking cessation is most often achieved by increasing reinforcement. That is, increasing the number of contacts made to the smoker who is trying to quit or remain abstinent after quitting, the type of contacts, and the number of people making contacts offers the greatest success.

Multiple components (i.e., strong physician advice, nicotine replacement therapy, counseling) and multiple methods of delivery (videotape, audiotapes, telephone follow-up) are more successful than a single intervention. This is reinforced in the recently released *Clinical Practice Guideline on Smoking Cessation* published by the Agency for Health Care Policy and Research (AHCPR) of the U.S. Department of Health and Human Services (1996). All health care professionals can help people to stop smoking by (a) identifying them as smokers at every encounter; (b) asking if they are willing to make a quit attempt; (c) aiding them to quit by using such interventions as self-help materials, strong advice, nicotine replacement therapy; and (d) arranging for follow-up, which should include at least two contacts in the month after quitting. Telephone contacts offer a convenient, effective, and inexpensive method of follow-up.

Pharmacological Therapy

The most effective pharmacological aid to help highly addicted smokers quit smoking is nicotine replacement therapy. Both nicotine chewing gum and the transdermal nicotine patch are now available over the counter and are highly beneficial in helping individuals to quit smoking. The patch is the preferred pharmacological aid; however, some people benefit from nicotine gum because of the oral stimulation the gum provides. Studies indicate that treatment with the patch for 8 weeks or less is as efficacious as longer treatment periods. The patch is very well tolerated, minor local skin reaction being the main side effect. Nicotine chewing gum requires appropriate instruction about administration and caution about the use of acidic beverages, which interfere with absorption. The gum is more effective if prescribed on a fixed-dose schedule. Little evidence exists about the value of nicotine replacement therapy in light smokers (< 15 cigarettes per day). For these individuals, starting at a lower dose may be appropriate (AHCPR, 1996).

Nursing Practice and Research

As the largest group of health care professionals, nurses can play a major role in helping smokers to think about quitting. The hospital has become a unique setting to help smokers because bans on smoking prevent patients from continuing their habit. Smokers experience the worst of withdrawal effects during this time of enforced cessation. Interventions that focus on identification of patients, strong physician advice, and use of nurses to provide behavioral counseling at the bedside, with telephone follow-up, have proved highly efficacious in getting smokers to remain abstinent (Miller, Smith, DeBusk, Sobel, & Taylor, 1997; Taylor, Houston Miller, Killen, & DeBusk, 1990). Nursing research offers opportunities to improve interventions for smoking cessation. Nurses within community settings, schools, and clinics play a role in prevention, educating and counseling teenagers about not adopting the most addictive habit in the United States today.

NANCY HOUSTON MILLER

See also:
   ADHERENCE/COMPLIANCE
   PULMONARY CHANGES
   WELLNESS

STRESS MANAGEMENT

Stress management involves strategies to both decrease stress and prevent stress. Actions taken to decrease stress or alleviate it once experienced are commonly referred to as coping strategies or behaviors. Some of the coping strategies frequently used by nurses include taking action, drawing on past experiences, using problem-solving techniques, using humor, talking over problems with co-workers, accepting the situation, taking breaks (escaping from the situation), using diversions, using relaxation, and exercise (Lewis & Robinson, 1986; Petermann, Springer, & Farnsworth, 1995). Actions taken to prevent stress involve balancing demands and resources, focusing on the positive in difficult situations, maintaining perceived choice and sense of personal control, building social support, and viewing difficult situations as challenges that can bring gain or benefit through learning (Dionne-Proulz & Pepin, 1993; Lyon, 1996).

In addition to the research conducted on stress management strategies used by nurses, nurse researchers also have studied the effects of stress management interventions with various patient and client population groups. Snyder (1993) critically reviewed all 54 stress-related intervention studies appearing in the nursing literature from 1980 through 1990. The types of stress management interventions used included relaxation strategies (e.g., progressive muscle relaxation, imagery, meditation, breathing techniques, massage, music), educational strategies, and use of social support groups. A major flaw of most of the intervention studies was an inadequate description of the intervention used, and there was a lack of attempts to explain the theoretical link between the intervention and outcome measures. Manipulation checks as a way to assure that subjects mastered the intervention and to verify that subjects actually used the intervention also were lacking in the intervention studies. Studies using sensation information (e.g., Johnson, Rice, Fuller, & Endress, 1978) and studies using progressive relaxation techniques (e.g., Pender, 1985) have demonstrated positive effects on health-related outcomes such as less anxiety and an increased sense of well-being.

Future directions for nursing research should focus on the effectiveness of stress management interventions for both nurses and patients or clients. For meaningful results, however, it will be imperative that the researcher clearly define and delineate interventions and offer testable theoretical formulations that explain how the intervention affects outcome variables. It is also essential that the researcher incorporate manipulation checks into the methodology to verify that subjects have implemented a strategy correctly and that the intervention actually altered the target variable as proposed in the theoretical formulation.

Brenda L. Lyon

See also:
WELLNESS

WELLNESS

Definition

Wellness is an integrated method of functioning directed toward maximizing the potential of which an individual is capable within the environment where functioning occurs. Wellness is both a process and a goal that can be chosen by anyone of any age, in any setting, and with any condition of illness or disability. As a process, wellness is a movement toward greater awareness and satisfaction derived from engaging in activities that move the whole person toward fitness, positive nutrition, positive relationships, stress management, clear life purpose, consistent belief systems, commitment to self-care, and environmental comfort. The goal of wellness is the actualization of the person that results from learning how to remain healthy and the personal assumption of health-promoting behaviors.

Relevance to Nursing

Nursing is concerned with the phenomena of human responses to illness and health. Although it has been difficult to move nursing language systems such as that of the North American Nursing Diagnosis Association (NANDA) to descriptors of wellness and its maintenance and promotion, progress has been made. The wellness model focuses on what is "right" with the person; quality of life is more important that just being alive. The integration of body, mind, and spirit is the orientation of wellness. Nurses in all arenas of practice are in strategic positions to assist patients in making positive lifestyle changes directed toward wellness.

Nursing pioneers in the wellness movement adopted a holistic approach and promoted wellness through self-care and self-responsibility. Dimensions of a health-promoting lifestyle, encompassing behaviors that serve to maintain or enhance the wellness and fulfillment of the individual, were identified and scientifically validated. Those dimensions include health responsibility, nutrition, exercise, stress management, interpersonal support, and self-actualization. Later, wellness practitioners developed this theme into wellness practices. Promotion of health is an appropriate term for the wellness model because it emphasizes improving one's general state of health.

Historical Perspective

Dunn (1961) was the first to use the term *wellness* nearly two decades before the concept of high-level wellness and holistic health were popularized by

Ardell, Travis, and others in the late 1970s and early 1980s. Dunn's writings reflect and acknowledge the ideas of thinkers such as Eric Fromm, Carl Rogers, Abraham Maslow, and Hans Selye, who were also concerned about how individuals might achieve their full potential within their world. Dunn equated health with the integration of person-mind-body-spirit and maintained that what people feel, believe, and think affects their physical capabilities, and vice versa.

The wellness and holistic health movement of the 1970s evolved outside the traditional health professions. Major threads throughout the movement today continue to reflect the integration of body, mind, and spirit; the ethic of self-responsibility and choice; and the interdependence of individual, social, and environmental wellness originally conceptualized. These terms have become popularized and used by lay persons and health professionals alike, often without clear conceptual understanding of what the concepts really mean. The dichotomy between the characteristics of the medical model and the wellness model creates dissonance and makes the use of wellness language inaccurate and confusing in the context of a medically driven system of illness care.

Major Studies

Smith (1983) described distinctive models of health, which include a clinical orientation, a role-performance or functional definition of health, a eudaemonistic definition of health as exuberant well-being or high-level wellness, and an adaptive definition of health. The Laffrey Health Conception Scale (Laffrey, 1986), based on Smith's work, was developed to measure the perception of health held by individuals. The Health Promoting Lifestyle Profile, the work of Walker, Sechrist, and Pender (1987), contributed further to the development of the science of wellness and its defining variables.

Relationship to Nursing Practice

Well persons who want to learn to maintain and improve their health will not find answers to their questions in the medical system, which is characterized by diagnosis and cure of disease. Well persons are often unrecognizable in medical systems. They are, however, increasingly recognized in nursing systems of care, where health promotion and wellness diagnoses are commonly made and where interventions designed to assist clients to greater levels of wellness are based on rapidly accumulating evidence.

MARION M. HEMSTROM

See also:
FUNCTIONAL HEALTH
QUALITY OF LIFE
STRESS MANAGEMENT

Part II

NORMALCY THROUGHOUT THE LIFE SPAN

INTRODUCTION

What constitutes normalcy in aging? What is the "gold standard" associated with becoming older? Each gerontologist and each healthcare professional will discuss and debate the answer to this question differently. Each will offer a unique perspective relative to the respective frame of reference embraced by practice and interactions with older people. Each will paint a special complex picture of the parameters of what it means, to them, to be a normal older and aging person.

Phrases such as "age-related decline," "aging process," "typical aging," and "successful aging," all reflect viewpoints representing underpinnings of what is normal and abnormal in growing old. "Normal" depicts that which is the norm or standard, that which is typical. According to Taber's medical dictionary, aging is defined as "growing old, maturing. Progressive changes related to the passage of time. There is no precise method for determining the rate or degree of aging" (Taber's, 1989, p. 51).

This definition implies that as living things age, they change. But exactly how do they change and why? Scientists have attempted to make sense and order of the aging process by examining patterns associated with such changes. In addition, they have attempted to identify how older people react to disease states and respond to concurrent treatment. The phrase "atypical presentation" has come to define this response; that is, the older person reacts and responds to disease and treatment "atypically" or unusually compared to middle-aged people. Their presentation and reaction does not reflect the norm. The symptoms of pneumonia such as pleuritic pain, fever, and shortness of breath normally seen in middle-aged people, for example, may not be visible in older people. Instead, the older person may experience an increase in falls and change in baseline mental status. Fever may or may not be present and cough may be suppressed or absent. Our frame of diagnostic reference therefore needs to spur examination of that which is "atypical" so that the practitioner does not miss treatment and interventions necessary to return the person to "normal" or baseline functioning.

The answer to precisely why humans age remains a matter of theory yet to be fully supported by researchers. Some feel that DNA is the key to aging. As persons age, DNA, the building block of life, deteriorates and even mutates, accounting for increased incidence rates of cancers in older people as well as physiological and organ breakdown. Some contend that living things have a "biological clock," somewhat preset, predetermined. Others blame aging on environmental elements such as radiation, chemicals, and varying changes in air composition affecting the human system.

Perhaps aging happens because of simple wear and tear of the body and mind, as another school of thought purports.

The practical key endpoint is that humans *change* as they age. The speed of this change and method of change are often unknown variables, especially in terms of older people. Why does one 70-year-old appear robust and more vibrant than his counterpart who presents as debilitated? The transformation of aging holds dimensions of uniqueness and commonality. It is these commonalties which are discussed as "age-related changes," "normal aging," "age-related decline," and, sometimes, "successful aging." Differentiation between disease and normal aging is sometimes a fine line and becomes the challenge in understanding and caring for older people.

The following section of the digest describes the current research on functional aspects of normalcy and deviations in normalcy within the aging process.

Functional ability is revered and valued in society. To be functional is to have the means to be able to live. Waking up in the morning, getting out of bed, donning a robe, and putting on a pot of coffee or tea are sacred activities often taken for granted. And if your bedroom is upstairs and you must traverse down one or two flights of stairs to enter your kitchen, then the challenge, for some, becomes even greater. Those simple activities of daily living may be compromised in some older adults, resulting in an inability to attain the simple joys in life, the dimensions unique to habits of human living. Regardless of categorizing persons by medical diagnoses and physiological function, if these simple functions of human living can be carried out, the older person—or any person, for that matter—has the foundation for living life.

On the other hand, some older people have the functional capacity to perform all functions to drive their life, but elect not to. Motivation and desire to "do" fuels daily existence. No matter how capable a person is to take care of self, without the spark to live, the person will become nonfunctional. Depression in older people is a common cause of antifunctional syndrome, despite physical capability.

Minimally, functionality comprises carrying out ADLs, IADLs, including bathing, dressing, feeding, and providing nutrition and hydration for self, and elimination control. Furthermore, sexual expression contributes to normalcy, as it is integral to being human. All are upheld by adequate cognitive function and motivation or the will to live.

In reading the research and current information on essential functional aspects of aging, the reader must be mindful of two major over-arching issues, as follows.

First, do not read into research. Each piece of research has its limitations; it contributes one small piece to the puzzle of aging. Research is not the never-ending truth to be applied to all older people in all settings. Differentiate research on pathologies associated with aging and normal age-related changes; the two are distinct. Early research on older people was conducted on those with underlying diseases and thus did not depict healthy aging. A good example is the early research on cardiovascular age-related changes. Indeed, atherosclerosis is not part of healthy aging. Nor is immobility. Sexual dysfunction is never normal. Incontinence is never normal. Currently, there are better studies on healthy older adults, which are beginning to set a norm for healthy aging.

Second, variations of normalcy in aging may vary from culture to culture. The "gold standard" of achievement may differ. For example, some cultures do not promote independence in their elders. Old age is a time when dependence becomes a reward and has been earned after years of contributing to family and society. In old age, the younger generation gives help and assistance to grandfather or grandmother. All accept this standard as the norm. Therefore, it may be concluded that research is culture-specific and should be carefully examined before generalizing to other cultures as "truth."

The following section offers a snapshot picture on what we currently consider characteristics of aging and pathologies associated with some older people. Generally, functional living as defined by a culture is the means to support all dimensions of successful aging.

CORA D. ZEMBRZUSKI

ACTIVITIES OF DAILY LIVING

Measures of physical functional status such as activities of daily living (ADLs) and instrumental activities of daily (IADLs) have evolved over the past 40 years as important indicators of health status and disability. Disability refers to how an impairment or organic pathological change limits activities and functioning. As a measure of disability, ADLs refer to the basic tasks of everyday life, such as eating, bathing, dressing, toileting, and transferring. IADLs encompass the performance of a range of life activities more complex than those included in most ADL scales. They include activities necessary for independent function in the community, such as meal preparation, shopping, doing housework, traveling, and financial management.

Assessment of ADLs originated in clinical practice in rehabilitation as one way to measure performance, first for disability determination and later as an integral part of clinical management. These measures have been widely applied in clinical settings and population-based studies to define functional status and care needs and guide health policy for aging and chronically ill populations. They have also been used as outcome measures to evaluate treatment effectiveness and to monitor the effects of disease on patients' day-to-day activities.

Nurse researchers have described the impact of illness on patients' physical functioning and tested interventions to improve ADLs and IADLs in populations with cardiac disease, AIDS, Alzheimer's disease, cancer, and numerous other conditions. In nursing research these measures of physical functioning are frequently evaluated as one dimension of functional status, quality of life, or broader measures of health status that also incorporate mental and social function.

Many different methods have been developed to rate individual ADLs or IADLs. Standard tests of an individual's performance conducted by a trained observer and questioning the individual about current level of functioning are two general approaches. Three standard forms of rating include (1) the degree of difficulty in performing certain activities, that is, how hard it is to perform an activity; (2) the degree of assistance or dependency, for instance, whether or not a person uses or needs assistance to perform an activity; and (3) whether or not an activity is performed (Jette, 1994). Another distinction in the measurement of ADLs and IADLs is whether the items on the scale ask what a person can do (person's physical capacity) or what a person does do (actual performance). An index asking what a patient can do may exaggerate the healthiness of the respondent by as much as 15% to 20% (McDowell & Newell, 1996). Most recent ADL indices utilize the performance approach for ADL items, using wording to assess the health reasons that a person did not do an activity. The choice of which rating scale to use depends on the researcher's conceptual definition of physical functioning and objectives of the research and can have a profound impact on the estimates of disability within and across studies.

Katz's Index of Activities of Daily Living was the first scale published in the 1950s. It was developed to study the effects of treatment on the elderly and chronically ill and has been widely used. As with all ADL scales, it is appropriate only when measuring severe levels of disability. Other well-known instruments of ADL indices include the PULSES, Barthel, Kenny, and the Medical Outcomes Study. IADL scales are commonly used with less severely handicapped populations; they have been more thoroughly tested for validity and reliability and may be more sensitive to minor changes in a patient's condition. IADL scales are often combined with ADL scales in one instrument to broaden the definition of disability. McDowell and Newell (1996) and Frank-Stromborg and Olsen (1997) have published descriptions of ADL and IADL scales along with their conceptual basis and psychometric properties.

As the proportion of our elderly population with chronic diseases increases, knowledge is needed about how to keep these individuals functionally independent and satisfied with their quality of life. Nurse researchers are in key positions to broaden and strengthen this line of research. Instruments must be refined or new ones developed, with sensitivity to the small but clinically meaningful changes observed as outcomes of nursing interventions. Most ADL and IADL scales were developed to rate a patient's condition at a single point in time. To determine change over time or after some therapeutic intervention, investigators frequently compare the difference noted in two or more repeated values of the single-state ratings. The sensitivity of existing instruments to small but clinically important changes has been largely untested.

Another direction for future nursing research is to determine what factors predict physical functioning and satisfaction with physical functional status in different populations. Research using measures of ADLs and IADLs has often overlooked the personal perspectives of patients and what changes in the particular disabilities are most important to them. A better understanding of predictive factors and personal preferences could lead to more effective planning and evaluation of therapeutic interventions. Future use of physiological indicators such as ADLs and IADLs may also include monitoring quality of care. Nurse researchers should be positioned to conduct these investigations and to assist clinicians to utilize research findings to improve quality of care.

JERILYN K. ALLEN

See also:
COGNITIVE DISORDERS
COGNITIVE IMPAIRMENT
COGNITIVE INTERVENTIONS
FUNCTIONAL HEALTH

BOWEL FUNCTION

In all healthcare environments, bowel elimination in the older adult should be examined very closely because of the effects of age-related changes. A careful assessment will provide the necessary foundation for preventing bowel problems and disabilities in the future. Bowel elimination is the end process of digestion. This is the result of the interaction of the central nervous system, autonomic nervous system, endocrine system, gastrointestinal tract, and musculoskeletal system (Matteson, McConnell, & Linton, 1997b).

A study by D. G. Ross (1995) reviewed bowel-elimination patterns (BEP) among hospitalized older adult and middle-aged patients. Data was collected via interviews, diaries, questionnaires, and chart reviews. The Nagley Visual Analog Scale for Confusion (Nagley, 1984) was used to assess cognitive status; the Katz Index of Activities of Daily Living (ADL) was used to measure functional status (Katz, 1983); and the Medical Illness Severity Grouping System (MEDISGRPS) was used to determine the severity of a given illness (Brewster et al., 1985). Validity and reliability were supported in all instruments. Again both of the groups showed changes in BEP, but there was no significant difference between the two age groups. Cognitive, functional, and severity-of-illness status were more predictive of BEP changes in the older age group. Multiple regression analysis was employed, demonstrating that a relationship exists between diet and activity in the BEP of hospitalized elders.

Three major bowel-elimination problems consistently have been shown to affect the older adult population. They include constipation (Hogstel & Nelson, 1992; Vogelzang, 1999), incontinence (Hogstel & Nelson, 1992), and colorectal cancer (American Cancer Society, 1999).

Constipation is the most common complaint among older adults. Often it is due to a misconception of normal bowel function, and the need to have a bowel movement daily. This creates a potential overuse of laxatives, as is evidenced by the 30% of older adults who use laxatives on a weekly basis (Rodrigues-Fisher, Bourguignon, & Good 1993; Matteson et al., 1997b). One percent of physician prescriptions are for laxatives, not counting the 700 over-the-counter medication preparations (Rodrigues-Fisher et al., 1993).

In Rodrigues-Fisher, Bourguignon, and Good's study (1993), increased dietary fiber and fluid were used as nursing interventions, and their affect on the maintenance of bowel movements and elimination aid was evaluated. Bowel movements were maintained, while the use of both laxatives and stool softeners decreased. Statistical findings showed that the use of fiber and fluid significantly lessened the need for pharmacological interventions.

Vogelzang (1999) cited seven reasons for constipation in the elderly. Multiple medications (polypharmacy) had been identified as a primary reason for constipation—especially in nursing home residents. Six or more medications have been shown to adversely effect the motility of the digestive tract. Older adults living at home may be at an even higher risk for overdoses related to self-medication with over-the-counter drugs. In addition, having a limited income influences the quality of food purchased, and the amount of fiber-rich foods in the older adult's diet. The annual income of 40% of older Americans is less than \$6,000, leaving limited funds for groceries. Most do not take advantage of funded food programs available to them. Selection of the same foods is common, leading to a poorly balanced diet. Unhealthy snacking throughout the day adversely affects appetite, as well as bowel regularity. A lack of social interaction and physical inactivity, nausea (caused by contaminated food due to unclean food preparation), and inadequate cooking skills have all been identified as other factors that contribute to an increased risk for constipation (Vogelzang, 1999). Constipation can be controlled by a well-balanced diet that is high in fiber, adequate hydration (at least eight to ten 8-oz.glasses of water/day), along with increased activity (Doughty & Jackson, 1993).

Fecal incontinence has been shown to contribute to decreased social activity (Giebel, Lefering, Troidl, & Blochl, 1998; Wald, 1997). Older adults are embarrassed that incontinence may occur in public, so they tend to limit their outdoor activity. There is a strong correlation between urinary and fecal incontinence (Chassagne et al., 1999; Nelson, Furner, & Jesudason, 1998).

In a survey conducted in Germany by Giebel, Lefering, Troidal, and Blochl (1998), 500 randomly selected older adults responded to a questionnaire about their bowel habits. It was found that 4.8% were unable to control solid stool, whereas 19.6% experienced at least one type of incontinence. Women had more of a problem with pasty or liquid stools. They also experienced an urgency sensation to quickly reach the toilet. Men described soiling their underwear as very problematic and controlling flatus was also a concern. Findings suggest that the lack of control associated with bowel habits, plus the resulting reduction in activities, necessitate educational interventions aimed at better intestinal health and dietary change.

Another study done on fecal incontinence that enrolled 1,186 adults 60 years of age and older, in a long-term care setting, identified five risk factors associated with fecal incontinence: (a) A history of urinary incontinence; (b) neurological disease; (c) poor mobility; (d) severe cognitive decline; and (e) an age higher than 70 (Chassagne et al., 1999).

Fecal incontinence associated with impaction and diarrhea occurred in 234 (20%) of the sample. The study showed an association between permanent fecal incontinence and overall poor health in older adults. The researchers stated that increasing an older adult's mobility could aid in the prevention of fecal incontinence (Chassagne et al., 1999).

Treating fecal incontinence is based on the etiology of the incontinence, such as impaction, diarrhea, loss of muscle tone in the anal sphincter, and loss of daily living activities. The assumption that fecal incontinence is a way of life for older adults, and that it is part of normal aging, encourages a lack of aggressiveness in providing effective treatment measures (Matteson et al., 1997b).

Approximately 90% of individuals with colorectal cancer are over 50 years of age (American Cancer Society, 1998). This leads to the question of how colorectal cancer can be prevented in older adults. The United States Preventive Task Force recommends that individuals over 50 be screened for colorectal cancer (Donovan & Syngal, 1998). Numerous studies support annual testing for occult blood in stool, and flexible sigmoidoscopy every 5 to 7 years, which will reduce the risk by up to 75% (Donovan & Syngal, 1998).

A study by Borum (1998) evaluated the relationship of age to screening for colorectal cancer. A retrospective chart review of 200 patients over 50 years old who were in an ambulatory clinic showed that more rectal exams were done on 50–60-year-olds, than 60–70-year-olds. These results indicate that less screening is done in the older elderly population than is done in the younger elderly population. As aggressive screening diminishes, the risk for colorectal cancer increases (Borum, 1998).

Diet plays an important role in the prevention of colorectal cancer. Negri, Franceschi, Parpinel, and La Vecchia (1998) researched fiber intake and the risk of colorectal cancer. An investigation of the dietary habits of patients (1,225 with colon cancer, 728 with rectal cancer, and 4,154 with no history of cancer) were studied. They filled out a validated food-frequency questionnaire. The data indicated that dietary fiber has a protective affect against colorectal cancer. High-fiber diets may protect against colorectal cancer by allowing only brief mucosal exposure to carcinogens (Held-Warmkessel, 1998). The longer stool is forced to remain in the intestine, the more likely the chance of cancer.

Caygill, Charlett, and Hill (1998) investigated the relationship between the intake of high fiber and the risk of breast and bowel cancer. The study showed that cereal and vegetables protect against both colorectal and breast cancer while fruit had no protective effect on colorectal or breast cancer. However, fruit was shown to be more protective against cancers of the upper digestive tract (Caygill et al., 1998). In summary, older adults are at risk for developing bowel elimination complications, which may be associated with the physiological changes that occur with advancing age. A comprehensive assessment of bowel elimination is essential to optimum bowel health. Screening for cancer needs to be performed on all elderly, regardless of age. Diets high in fiber, adequate hydration, increased activity, and educational programs facilitate the prevention of complications. Accurate research-based information on bowel-elimination patterns would enable nurses to better assess and prevent potential complications, and to promote a better quality of life for older adults.

CORA D. ZEMBRZUSKI

See also:
EXERCISE

**CHRONIC GASTROINTESTINAL SYMPTOMS
GASTROESOPHAGEAL REFLUX DISEASE**

HEALTHCARE COMMUNICATION

Communication is a crucial medium for healthcare interactions between elders, nurses, and other healthcare providers. Effective verbal and nonverbal communication by both elders and healthcare providers could improve healthcare outcomes for elders. Verbal communication includes "all behavior conveying messages with language" (Caris-Verhallen, Kerkstra, & Bensing, 1997, p. 916). Nonverbal communication includes "all behavior which convey messages without the use of verbal language and consists of vocal nonverbal communication and non-vocal nonverbal communication. Vocal nonverbal contains all the voice qualities which accompany the transmission of words. . . . Non-vocal nonverbal communication includes body movement, physical appearance, the timing of conversations, personal space, and touch" (Oliver & Redfern, 1991, p. 31).

Nurses can promote more effective communication with elders by (a) better understanding the elder's perspective in healthcare communication; (b) enhancing facilitators, and avoiding barriers to communication; and (c) using interventions that promote more effective communication by elders. The following examines research findings in these three areas, and suggests areas for future research on the subject. Caris-Verhallen et al. (1997) recently reviewed research that focused on observational studies involving communication between nurses and elders.

Some elders may deliberately behave in a socially desirable manner when communicating with the healthcare provider. Elders living in a continuing-care retirement community said that being nice and patient increased the likelihood of a positive encounter with their healthcare provider. Elders who perceived a healthcare provider as being unwilling or not genuine did not seek him or her out for healthcare (Russell, 1994). Elders most favorably evaluated caregivers who were affectionate, had warm personalities, or did more than required for the elder (Russell, 1996). Shared laughter during an office visit with a physician correlated positively with satisfaction regarding the visit (Greene, Adelman, Friedmann, & Charon, 1994).

Elders may use a variety of different strategies to communicate their need for assistance to caregivers. Verbal strategies used by elders in a continuing-care retirement community included statements, complaints, expressions of preferences, and directives. The nonverbal strategies included movements, such as raising eyebrows; or volitional noises, such as sighing; or using the call light (Russell, 1996).

Several barriers to elders' healthcare communication have been identified. The barriers are grouped into four main areas: acute or chronic confusion; pain; sensory deficits; and healthcare system barriers. Acutely confused and chronically confused elderly women on a geriatric ward interacted significantly less with the healthcare staff (Armstrong-Esther & Browne, 1986). Lucid, acutely confused, and chronically confused elders on a general acute ward, a geriatric medical ward, and in a psychiatric unit demonstrated greater interaction with others than with staff. Lucid elders spent 84% of their interactions with others, compared to 7% with staff. Acutely confused elders spent 71% with others, compared to 14% with staff. Chronically confused elders spent 34% of their interaction time with others, and only 21% with staff. The researchers noted a deficit in social interaction between the staff and the elders (Armstrong-Esther, Browne, & McAfee, 1994).

Two studies with elderly dementia patients supported meaningful communication ability on the part of the elders. Twenty community-residing elders with dementia were interviewed about their life stories and their current stresses. More than 50% of the elders were aware of their cognitive impairment, made positive statements about their family caregiver and their past, expressed the need to be useful, and mentioned the importance of humor. All of the chronically confused elders managed to engage in some meaningful communication during their interview, and also laughed during the interview (Acton, Mayhew, Hopkins, & Yauk, 1999).

Acutely or chronically confused elders living in skilled nursing homes were interviewed and evaluated for pain. Of these, 62% reported pain, with 40% describing more than one pain location; 21% were unable to make any of their needs known. At least one of five pain scales was completed by 83% of the elders, and 32% completed all of the scales. Significant correlations among the pain scales supported consistent use of the scales by the confused elders. The Present Pain Scale of the McGill pain questionnaire produced the highest completion rate—65%. A large number of the elders had difficulty with the visual analog scale. Some elders (17%) answered appropriately to yes or no questions about their pain but were unable to complete any of the pain scales (Ferrell, Ferrell, & Rivera, 1995).

Increased aggressive behavior may be one means by which confused elders communicate pain. Confused elders demonstrating aggression, and residing in one of three nursing homes, were examined for a relationship between aggressive behaviors and pain. Elders with two or more pain-related diagnoses were significantly more aggressive than elders with one or no pain-related diagnoses (Feldt, Warne, & Ryden, 1998).

Further evidence regarding barriers to elders' communication may be found in two pain studies of lucid elders. Some frail, hospitalized, postoperative elderly women did not ask for analgesics, expecting nurses to know when analgesics were needed. Five of sixteen women experienced clouded perception that affected their response to pain. Other women asked for analgesics only for intolerable pain (Zalon, 1997). Well elders without chronic pain and living in the community described what they would do if they experienced acute pain while hospitalized. Some 53% stated that they would request analgesics from their healthcare provider. Only 13% planned to talk with healthcare providers about their pain (McDonald & Sterling, 1998).

Sensory deficits are another potential barrier to healthcare communication by elders. Thirty-two Australian healthcare providers, including 6 registered nurses and 16 nursing assistants, estimated that 62% of their nursing home residents had some hearing loss (Kato, Hickson, & Worrall, 1996). Legally blind elders were evaluated with one hearing test and two communication tests (Test of Adolescent and Adult Language and Self-assessment of Communication). Of these, 94% failed one test, 64% failed two tests, and 36% failed all three tests (Bennett & Dancer, 1997). A Comparison of elder women who used a hearing aid, versus those who rejected advice to use a hearing aid, revealed that those who used a hearing aid reported less difficulty communicating under average conditions. These women also reported a greater likelihood of employing verbal strategies to assist communication. A comparison of elderly men and women using hearing aids revealed that the women were more likely to use nonverbal strategies (such as watching the person's face), placed greater importance on communicating effectively in social situations, reported more distress about their hearing loss, and experienced more negative feelings in everyday communication (Garstecki & Erler, 1998). These findings must be interpreted with caution, due to the potential type I error from multiple t-tests in the analyses.

Healthcare system barriers to communication with the elderly have also been identified. There have been conflicting findings about communication patterns between nursing staff and elders in nursing homes. A Canadian study videotaped elders over two peak nursing care hours for each elder. During the total 72 hours, only 850 words were spoken to the 36 elders. Conversations consisted of task-oriented content with only one social interaction (Jones & van Amelsvoort Jones, 1986). A more recent study in the Netherlands suggests that health provider communication may contain more socioemotional content. Nineteen nurses, 28 nursing assistants, and 109 elders living either in the community or in a nursing home were videotaped, for a total of 181 nursing encounters. Using Roter's interactional analysis system to score the interactions, 44%–72% of the communication was classified as socioemotional. The majority of elders in the study had been receiving care for a year or more, which may account for an increase in the interpersonal nature of the communication (Caris-Verhallen, Kerkstra, van der Heijden, & Bensing, 1998). Affective touch was used in 40% of these nursing encounters, comprising 1.5% of the observation time (Caris-Verhallen, Kerkstra, & Bensing, 1999).

Three additional studies have examined different aspects of elder communication in the nursing home setting. Healthcare providers in an Australian nursing home estimated that 56% of the elderly residents understood what was said to them, and that the providers in turn understood about 55% of the elders' communication. The providers further estimated that 57% of the elders would like more chances to talk, but that only 34% could hold a normal adult conversation (Kato et al., 1996).

Baby talk with elderly nursing home residents was examined by having elderly adults view videotaped simulations of a nurse talking with an elderly patient. The elders rated the nurses using baby talk as less respectful and less competent than the nurses using neutral speech (Ryan, Hamilton, & See, 1994). Elder residents in two Finnish nursing homes described their need to discuss issues such as their fear of dying. They were unsure whom they should talk to about such things, and felt that the nursing staff was too hurried to talk with them (Liukkonen, 1995).

Type of nursing practice and staff may affect communication with hospitalized elders. An English study compared primary, team, and functional nursing, as well as nurses and nursing assistants. Ten categories of verbal communication were measured, including teaching, simple explanations, detailed explanations, and questions. The percentage of time spent communicating with the elders ranged from a low of 3.7% for team nurses in the afternoon to a high of 7.7% for primary nursing assistants in the morning. Primary nursing staff spent the most time communicating with the elders, and functional staff the least. Staff on primary units provided significantly more choice and general care explanations during morning care. The nurses spent significantly more time providing detailed explanations to the elders than the nursing assistants. Nursing assistants spent significantly more time engaging in social talk with the elders (Thomas, L., 1994).

Interventions promoting elder communication with healthcare providers enable elders to seek and obtain more effective healthcare. McCormick, Inui, and Roter (1996) conducted an extensive review of the literature pertaining to physician and elder healthcare encounters. Three additional studies relate the effect of communication interventions to assist elders during healthcare interactions. Diabetic elders were randomly assigned to a control or treatment group. The treatment consisted of an interview using the Patient Problem Survey to help elders identify problems they planned to discuss with their physician. The elders who received the previsit interview brought up a mean of 9.2 problems, compared to 7.6 for elders in the control group. Elders given a previsit interview raised an average of 7.6 more problems, ones not on their original agenda. An average of 2.4

(27%) problems were not addressed during the office visit, with 56% not raising important medical problems with the physician. Some 70% of the elders who had identified their most important problem raised that problem as their third problem, on the average, during their visit (Rost & Frankel, 1993).

Two intervention studies that included teaching elders aspects of communicating their pain resulted in significantly less pain for elders. Clotfelter (1999), working with elderly cancer patients, provided an educational intervention that included a consumer version of the video Managing Cancer Pain and a booklet. The video included specific pain-management content, and stressed the patient's responsibility to communicate pain and pain management effectiveness, to his/her healthcare provider. McDonald, Freeland, Thomas, and Moore (1999) provided an educational intervention for preoperative elders awaiting total joint-replacement surgery. The intervention consisted of a narrated slide show and pamphlet. The slide show contained general postoperative pain-management information, as well as communication skills to use when talking with their healthcare providers after surgery. These communication skills were derived from Communication Accommodation Theory, which describes perception, evaluation, and subsequent communication behaviors during communication (Coupland, Coupland, Giles, & Henwood, 1988). Neither Clotfelter (1999) nor McDonald et al. (1999) provided direct evidence that teaching elders to communicate with healthcare providers decreased pain; the decreased pain may have been entirely a result of the general pain-management information contained in both interventions.

Some barriers to elder communication have been identified. Higher risks for elder communication problems appear to be associated with confusion, pain, sensory deficits, and healthcare organization issues. Helpful suggestions emerged from several of these studies—for example, trying the Present Pain Scale, or another pain scale, while avoiding the Visual Analogue Scale, when assessing pain in the confused elder (Ferrell et al., 1995). Continued research is needed to further clarify facilitators and barriers, as well as additional high-risk groups of elders.

Some evidence suggests that interventions involving support for communication have resulted in better outcomes for elders. However, two of the three studies did not separately test the communication component. Communication Accommodation Theory (CAT) provides one helpful guide for developing communication interventions to support elders. Further research, using theory-based communication interventions that directly test communication interventions, will help to clarify the effectiveness of those interventions.

Effective communication between elders and healthcare providers increases the likelihood of successful health outcomes for elders. But much of the communication research with elders in healthcare has taken place in nursing home settings, whereas the majority of elders live in their own homes. Elders also comprise a large portion of acute-care patients. Research in these two settings deserves a high priority. The impact of effective communication will take on greater significance as the number of elders requiring healthcare continues to grow.

DEBORAH DILLON McDONALD

See also:
PAIN ASSESSMENT

FUNCTIONAL HEALTH

Functional health has been viewed as a requirement for independent living and is the ability to engage in daily activities related to personal care, socially defined roles, and recreational activities. Performance of these activities is integral to quality of life and to living independently and safely, particularly for elderly adults with adverse effects of aging and disease. Functional health is one dimension of health in the metaparadigm of nursing.

Although functional health represents well-being, most nomenclature used in research and clinical practice reflects its deficits. Researchers and clinicians have used different terms for deficits in functional health, including disability (Nagi, 1991), frailty (Lawton, 1991), functional limitation (Johnson & Wolinsky, 1993), and handicap (World Health Organization, 1980). Researchers and clinicians add to the confusion in nomenclature and theoretical definitions by using these terms to label other concepts.

The inconsistency in the nomenclature and theoretical definitions have limited the development of a theory of functional health. Several theories have been used to guide research on deficits in functional health. The World Health Organization (1980) model lacks conceptual clarity and theoretical consistency, and this makes operationalization and establishing relationships difficult. In the model by Johnson and Wolinsky (1993), functional limitations are sometimes confused with factors affecting these limitations, and perceived health is used as a proxy for functional limitations. In a proposed model of functional status, Leidy (1994) recommended nomenclature and definitions of this concept and others related to functional status that added to the conceptual confusion in this area.

Models of Functional Health

Three models, useful to guide research because they are theoretically clear and consistent, have been used in many research studies, and they add concepts and relationship that provide direction for future research. Hogue's (1984) model of functional health depicts the interplay between the environment and personal competencies (physical and psychological) and the influence on health. A strength of this model is the inclusion of cognitive appraisals of the environment and personal competencies as evaluative judgments that can be used in decisions about what activities to participate in and how. Cognitive appraisal is related to coping and adaptation, strategies to maintain the fit between the environment and personal competencies necessary to maintain functional health.

Nagi's (1991) model of disability is conceptually clear, logically consistent, and useful in interpreting current and past research. Disability (poor functional health) is the result of a sequence of temporal relationships. Pathology or lifestyle contributes to impairments that are anatomic, physiological, and psychological, causing functional limitations at the level of the whole person (e.g., poor memory or inability to get up from a chair). Functional limitations then lead to disability, that is, the inability to perform daily tasks or roles independently. Unique in this model is the notion of thresholds where a certain amount of change must occur before change in a subsequent concept is observed. There is potential for nurses to use thresholds to identify persons at risk for functional limitation or disability. Although poorly developed in this model, the definition of the situation is conceptualized as affecting these relationships and is consistent with cognitive appraisal from Hogue's (1984) model.

An extension of Nagi's (1991) model of disability is the model of the disablement process (Verbrugge & Jette, 1994). This process describes the interplay between the extraindividual factors and intraindividual factors that is consistent with person-environment fit found in Hogue's (1984) model of functional health. Aspects of these two factors are more developed than in the models previously described.

Activities of Daily Living

Because functional health is the ability to engage in everyday activities, a plethora of research has focused on daily activities related to personal care (ADLs) and tasks related to providing food and shelter and caring for the home (IADLs). ADLs are hierarchically structured by the complexity of the motor skills required. IADLs are dependent on the same motor skills but are more dependent on cognitive capabilities (Johnson & Wolinsky, 1993). Johnson and Wolinsky also determined that ADLs and IADLs are highly related and may represent a continuum of the same construct.

The theoretical definitions of ADLs and IADLs are well established. First, empirical indicators were obtained by self-report. Many researchers noted that the accuracy of these responses could not be verified and could be adversely affected by cognitive impairment, social desirability, or minimization of dependency. Thus, observational indicators were developed to address the inadequacies of self-report. Although they may reflect what the person is able to do, observational measures may not reflect what a person actually does. Hence, both types of measures have limitations and provide different types of information.

A significant amount of research has focused on physical and psychological factors contributing to independence in ADLs and IADLs. Characteristics of gait, dynamic and static postural stability, and muscle strength were physical factors affecting these activities. Moreover, upper body function (e.g., muscle strength and range of motion of the arms used in reaching) has been related to ADLs, whereas lower body function (e.g., muscle strength of the legs used in ambulation and transfers) have been associated with IADLs (Lawrence & Jette, 1996). Relevant psychological factors included cognitive impairment and depression. Certain types of social support were factors contributing to dependency in daily activities; however, men and women used different types of social support in response to limitations in ADLs and IADLs (Roberts, Anthony, Matejczyk, & Moore, 1994). The role of the environment has not been well established except for the increase in dependency noted during hospitalization and long-term residence in a nursing home. Although there is beginning to be evidence that the relationship between actual abilities and perceptions of them is low, how these perceptions influence decisions people make about what activities to perform and how have not been well studied.

More nursing research is needed to identify thresholds in factors related to declines in functional health and to identify factors and processes by which people make decisions about performing daily activities. This knowledge could provide directions for assessment in populations at risk for poor functional health and might lead to more sensitive assessment strategies. A greater understanding of the interplay between environmental and personal factors affecting functional health may lead to multidimensional interventions that are more effective than single interventions targeted to one factor.

BEVERLY L. ROBERTS

See also:
  ACTIVITIES OF DAILY LIVING
  COGNITIVE DISORDERS
  DEPRESSION AMONG OLDER ADULTS
  FAMILY CARE

HYDRATION

Hydration is defined as "the chemical combination of a substance with water; the addition of water to a substance or tissue" (Taber's, 1989). The percentage of water in older adults is approximately 60%, relative to electrolytes in the human body. Water is essential to sustain cellular function and metabolism, to cleanse and transport toxins and nutrients, and to facilitate medication absorption, distribution, metabolism, and elimination (Gilmour & Penny, 1991; Matteson, McConnell, & Linton, 1997). Clinicians contend that by promoting a sufficient quantity and quality of fluid intake, extracellular and intracellular fluid balance will more likely be achieved, thus maximizing the body's ability to function effectively and efficiently.

No healthcare environment is invulnerable to the issue of hydration in older adults. The concern becomes prominent when dehydration—and consequential hospitalization—are impending. According to Warren et al. (1994), the annual cost of hospitalization due to dehydration was estimated to be over $446 million. The researchers accessed national data from 1991 Medicare files, and examined the number of hospital admissions due to a diagnosis (or associated diagnoses) of dehydration. They found that related diagnoses included pneumonia and urinary-tract infections, and they discovered that, in the age group of 65 and over, males and Blacks had the highest number of hospitalizations for dehydration. Hospitalization for dehydration, as well as being quite common, is usually expensive.

The prevalence of dehydration in nursing home residents is not easily tracked, but it is hypothesized to be high based on the older adult's risk for fever and infection, for age-related and end-stage diseases that require subcutaneous, parenteral, or hypodermoclysis for fluid administration; and cognitive and functional decline (Ellershaw, Sutcliffe, & Saunders, 1995; Hussain & Warshaw, 1996; Noble-Adams, 1995). Access to treatment in different settings influences the researcher's ability to accurately measure and portray the incidence and frequency of episodes of dehydration (Weinberg & Minaker, 1995). No data was found on the rate of the occurrence of dehydration in home-care and assisted-living settings.

Older adults are at risk for dehydration and fluid-volume deficit for four major reasons:

(a)   Dehydration is more severe in older adults because of their lower *baseline* TBW (total body water). Episodic illnesses such as diarrhea and nausea—accompanied by vomiting and fever—result in an even lower TBW. As little of a depletion as of 1–2 liters of water can create a state of dehydration in an older adult (Kleiner, 1999). With a decreased TBW, hypernatremia or hyponatremia becomes a potential electrolyte problem (Ayus & Arieff, 1996).

(b)   Thirst response is diminished in older adults, suggesting that when their TBW drops below safe levels (1–2 liters), there is nothing to prompt them to drink, perhaps due to deterioration of antidiuretic hormone (ADH) and hypothalamus osmoreceptors (Kositzke, 1990). Stachenfeld, DiPietro, Nadel, and Mack (1997) suggest that the effects of central blood-volume expansion on thirst response are diminished in elders. After creating circumstances of rigorous exercise in younger and older adults, their thirst ratings were measured. Ratings were significantly lower for older adults. In a smaller study, Stachenfeld, Mack, Takamata, DiPietro, and Nadel (1996) compared six elders' to six younger adults' thirst perception. The study showed that thirst was unaffected by age during and after the administration of a hypertonic saline solution. The small sample size may have accounted for these results. The majority of studies and textbooks affirm a diminished thirst response in elders.

Some researchers feel that the thirst mechanism functions differently in dying individuals. Ellershaw, Sutcliffe, and Saunders (1995) showed that there was no relationship between the level of hydration, dry mouth, and thirst symptoms in their study of 82 individuals who were actively dying of a malignant disease. Michaelsson, Norberg, and Samuelsson (1987) interviewed nurses who described how they assessed thirst in dying patients with severe dementia. They used intuition, empathy, observation of patient behavior and of their state of hydration. Alleviating thirst was emphasized as an important aspect of patients' quality of life, and it has been identified as a goal of palliative care. However, Vullo-Navich et al. (1998) studied the comfort levels of 31 terminally-ill patients in need of clysis or intravenous fluids. They found no differences in patients' comfort scores before and after the dehydration episode. These results support the questionable role that hydration plays in the overall comfort level of patients experiencing end-stage disease.

The signs and symptoms of dehydration may be absent or misleading in older adults (Weinberg & Minaker, 1995). Signs and symptoms include changes in mental status, confusion, lethargy, tachycardia, and syncope. Assessing skin turgor and dry mouth—standard diagnostic indicators of dehydration in adults—are unreliable detectors of dehydration in older adults due to normal age-related changes. For example, if skin turgor is already poor, it becomes an unreliable predictor of dehydration (Weinberg & Minaker, 1995). Gilmour and Penny (1991) suggest assessing skin turgor over the forehead or sternum. Dry mouth is an unreliable indicator because of numerous associated causes.

(c)   An overall decreased reserve capacity and body-organ deterioration (especially in renal function and creatinine clearance) creates a more delicate homeostatic balance (Erkert, 1988; Andreucci, Russo, Cianciaruso, & Andreucci, 1996). Thus, it will take a lesser body stressor to fuel a crisis in an elder than would be necessary to similarly affect a younger adult. In addition, the older adult's ability to recover is also extended beyond that which would be expected in a younger adult.

(d)   It is hypothesized that older adults control and limit their fluid intake for convenience, especially if incontinence is present. For some individuals, the embarrassment of incontinence may outweigh the health benefit of drinking water or other fluids. In addition, concurrent disease states, such as diabetes or congestive heart failure, could put the older adult's fluid balance over the edge (Weinberg & Minaker, 1995).

Dehydration is consistently identified as a nutritional issue in nursing home care (Alford, 1991; Armstrong-Ester, Browne, & McAfee, 1996; Chernoff, 1995; Chidester & Spangler, 1997; Gaspar, 1988; Morley & Silver, 1995; Pals et al., 1995; Yen, 1998). Gaspar (1988) studied variables that determine adequate fluid intake in nursing home residents (n = 67). Statistically significant factors associated with inadequate hydration included the age of the resident, gender (fluid intake for females was significantly lower than for males), and speaking disability. Less speaking ability correlated with an increased water intake. An interesting finding was that residents who were fully dependent or independent met their water intake more than those who were semidependent (cognitively impaired yet mobile). Similarly, Armstrong-Esther et al. (1996) demonstrated that cognitive impairment in nursing home residents (n = 57) was associated with reduced fluid intake. Likewise, Holstein, Chatellier, Piette, and Moulias (1994) analyzed 3,447 records of nursing home residents and demonstrated that those with dementia, especially in conjunction with Parkinson's disease, had higher incidences of complications including dehydration. In another study, Adams compared the fluid intake of 30 institutionalized- and 30 noninstitutionalized older adults (Adams, 1988). Fluid-intake records demonstrated that the intake of noninstitutionalized older adults was statistically higher than that of institutionalized older adults. None of the institutionalized older adults complained of thirst—even after 15 hours without fluids—confirming that thirst is an inadequate measure of fluid status. In a subsequent study of 40 nursing home residents it was demonstrated that they received adequate fluid intake (1,500–2,000 ml), although it was mainly influenced by the frequency of medication administration (Chidester & Spangler, 1997).

Weinberg, Pals, Levesque et al. (1994) investigated the association between febrile episodes and dehydration in nursing home residents. Results from 48 episodes, when compared with a control group, showed elevated BUN and serum-sodium levels. Abnormal I&Os also correlated with the lab values, implying the importance of monitoring the intake and output of fluids.

Another study of Weinberg, Pals, McGlinchey-Berroth, and Minaker (1994) studied the lab values of 15 nursing home residents over a period of 6 months. Their findings demonstrated that clinical symptoms did not correlate with lab values. A high-to-normal range of serum osmolality was present in the absence of signs and symptoms of dehydration.

The research consistently recommends further investigation of assessment instruments, prevention, and fluid-intake programs for older adults who are prone to dehydration. A detailed hydration program for the nursing home and an assessment tool were developed, but the tool has not been psychometrically tested (Zembrzuski, 1997). Reliable and valid instruments are needed. Furthermore, the importance of the interdisciplinary team in all aspects of treatment, education, and prevention of dehydration is critical to keep elders healthy (Weinberg & Minaker, 1995).

CORA ZEMBRZUSKI

See also:
NUTRITION

MEDICATIONS IN THE ELDERLY

More than 35% of all prescriptions written in the United States are for older adults. On average, an adult over the age of 65 has 3–5 chronic health conditions and takes 5–10 medications daily. While there are exceptional people who take no medications, the likelihood is very high that an older person will need teaching and management guidance regarding his or her medications. Nursing research that examines the way in which elderly individuals take their medications is extremely important given the fact that professional nurses are responsible for medication teaching and follow-up. Further, nurse practitioners who prescribe medications for the elderly have a firsthand opportunity to observe the manner in which medications are taken, and to analyze the concomitant results.

An intervention study was conducted to enhance the degree of medication compliance in community-dwelling elderly individuals with congestive heart failure (Fulmer et al., 1999). The study's objective was to determine whether daily video-phone or telephone reminders would increase the proportion of prescribed cardiac medications taken in a sample of elderly individuals. Using medication-event-monitoring-system caps (MEMS), the elderly subjects were recruited from a major urban area to determine whether daily phone call reminders—or daily video-phone reminders—could make a difference in medication compliance. There was a significant time effect during the course of the study, which showed enhanced medication compliance relative to the control group. Those in the control group had a significant falloff in medication compliance during the course of the study—dropping from 81% at time logged MEMS cap placement, to 57% at the end of the study. These data indicate that with the assistance of technology, daily calls from a nurse can make an important difference in the way in which homebound elders take their medications.

In another study, De Geest and colleagues described the diagnostic value of structured interviews in assessing noncompliance with immunosuppressive therapy in heart-transplant recipients (De Geest, Abraham, Moons, Dunbar-Jacob, & Vanhaecke, 1998). In this study—again mostly using MEMS caps—interviews were used in order to discern reasons for the noncompliance of individuals with heart transplants. In this study MEMS was superior to structured interviews in detecting noncompliant patients. Moreover, as MEM-methodology is currently the most sensitive and valuable method of measuring the medication-taking dynamics in chronic-patient populations, the researchers were able to assess the link between noncompliance and clinical outcomes (De Geest, Abraham, Moons, Vandeputte, et al., 1998; De Geest et al., 1995).

Noncompliance with immunosuppressive medications was shown to be a major risk factor of negative outcomes (i.e., acute rejections and graft loss), which indicates the importance of investing in compliance interventions in the transplant population (De Geest, Abraham, Moons, Vandeputte et al., 1998; De Geest et al., 1995).

Wolfe and colleagues also have demonstrated the importance of medication counseling for the elderly in terms of the effect such counseling has on knowledge and compliance after hospitalization (Wolfe & Schirm, 1992). Additionally, exploratory studies have been conducted to examine the role of community mental-health nurses in medication management. In one study, 14 community mental-health nurses took a pharmacology module, and were compared to a sample of 7 that did not (Jordan, Hardy, & Coleman, 1999).

Noncompliance (or nonadherence) is a serious issue, with estimates suggesting that from 5%–60% of all medications are taken incorrectly, or are not taken at all (Fulmer et al., 1999). It has also been noted that, of all prescriptions written, only half will ever actually be filled, and only half of those will be taken correctly (Alliance for Aging Research, 1998). Clearly, medication noncompliance is a serious and costly issue. Undermedication, overmedication, pill sharing, medication-dosing changes implemented without the prescriber's knowledge, and the mixing of medications with nontraditional remedies all make for a confusing picture. Yet this is the table that is set for nurses as they try to avoid patients' readmission to acute-care facilities for symptom exacerbation brought about by the absence of medications. Thus, the area of medication compliance is prime for continued research.

TERRY FULMER
SABINA DE GEEST

See also:
ADHERENCE/COMPLIANCE

MINORITY POPULATIONS: ASIAN AMERICANS

Although nursing service should be based on knowledge developed through culturally sensitive research, there is a dearth of studies on Asian Americans. In recent years there has been increased interest in the study of health behaviors and health problems of minority populations; however, Asian Americans have received limited attention. Thus, there is little information on the prevalent health problems among Asian Americans and how they practice health care. Asian Americans share a core of common values and behaviors, including family values, views of health and illness, and attitudes and interaction styles with health care professionals. However, they are markedly different in their languages, religions, national history, epidemiological risk factors, health practices, and treatment of illness, as well as degree of acculturation. Most beliefs about Asian Americans are drawn from data on the general Asian population or the Japanese American population. Most studies are done in nonnursing disciplines—that is, medicine and sociology—and may represent data from one specific ethnic group of Asians that have been generalized to all Asian Americans. A MEDLINE search of journals in nursing and other relevant journals published since 1969 revealed 105 articles based on the identifying words *Asian, nursing,*

Pacific Islander, and Asian country names (Cambodia, China, the Philippines, Indochina, Japan, Korea, Laos, Southeast Asia, Thailand, and Vietnam). Studies reported by nursing institutions or nurse researchers in the United States were reviewed.

Asian American Population

Asian Pacific Islanders are defined by the U.S. census (1992) as a set of U.S. population subgroups whose origins are in "the Far East, Southeast Asia or the Pacific Islands," and they are the fastest-growing ethnic groups as a result of immigration and fertility. The population increased from 3.7 million to 7.3 million during the 1980s, with most residing on the Pacific Coast. Among the diverse ethnic groups included in the Asian Americans category, the Chinese (1.6 M) are the most numerous and Filipinos (1.4 M), Japanese (.87 M), Koreans (.8 M), Asian Indian (.79 M) and Vietnamese (.6 M) follow. Although the Chinese, Filipino, Korean, and Vietnamese population in the U.S. has doubled in recent years, the Japanese American population grew only 20% (U.S. Bureau of the Census, 1992).

Historical Background and Research

The Asian Pacific Islanders population consists of 60 ethnic groups and subgroups. Within these groups there exist both commonalities and a wide range of differences. The history of immigration of each ethnic group is different; therefore the level of acculturation and language barriers also differ. The Japanese and Chinese immigration started in 1910, Filipinos and Koreans began to enter the U.S. in the 1940s, while the others came in the 1960s. The Southeast Asians, also known as Indochinese (Cambodians, Laotians, and Vietnamese), are the largest refugee group in the U.S., and they came to the U.S. soon after the fall of Saigon in 1975. Fewer than 20% of Japanese but over 81% of Cambodians speak a language other than English at home.

Of the 105 articles reviewed, 12 were categorized as clinical reports, 27 tutorials, and 56 were data based articles. Educational and clinical reports emphasized the importance of understanding the health beliefs and practices of Asian Americans. Along with an increased East Asian immigration, a massive influx of Southeast Asian refugees occurred in the 1980s and the majority of these refugees were relocated in low-income inner cities in California and Massachusetts. These settlers required special attention for their health problems which challenged nurse researchers and practitioners to understand and utilize cultural themes in intervening with these highly traumatized immigrants.

Research Topics

Migration and Stress. The majority of descriptive studies were comparative; Asian Americans' health problems were compared with those of Blacks, Whites, and Hispanic Americans. These studies revealed that Cambodians, Koreans, and Vietnamese often suffered from psychiatric problems, and researchers interpreted this phenomenon in light of acculturative and socioeconomic stress in the host country. Culture-specific somatic symptoms of psychiatric illness were reported in Koreans and Cambodians, and perhaps this is due to the negative attitude toward psychiatry in their cultures.

Culture, Health, and Illness. The majority of Asian Americans, especially those who were foreign born, use both Western medicine and traditional treatment. Educational and clinical reports indicated that although Asian Americans generally believe in and use Western medicine, especially for diagnostic purposes or acute illness treatment, they also use traditional treatments and home remedies like acupuncture, acupressure, herb medicines, massage or amma, moxibustion, cupping, and Qi-gong (medication). Evaluation of the treatment is based on the quality of the pulse, restoration of appetite, healthy appearance and voice, and the disappearance of symptoms. Studies indicated that Korean (Choi, 1986) and Vietnamese (Wadd, 1983) mothers have continued their cultural practices related to pregnancy, birth, and the postpartum period; for example, they avoid cold (drafts and showers), sexual intercourse, and activity, and encourage bed rest. One departure from traditional birth practices was related to infant feeding with the bottle rather than breast feeding. Jambunathan and Stewart (1995) reported that Laotian women delayed prenatal visits because of fear of miscarriage when touched by doctors and nurses.

A few articles examined the aging population of Japanese and Chinese, reflecting the immigration history of Asian Americans. Several studies revealed that the majority of Asian Americans (except for the Japanese), have language barriers that cause problems in health-seeking behavior and actual treatment. D'Avanzo's (1992) study of Vietnamese revealed that concern about not having a translator in health care facilities ranked as the top barrier to seeking treatment.

Administration and Management. Because of the shortage of nurses in the late 1980s and early 1990s, many foreign nurses were recruited to work in this country. Filipino nurses represent over 75% of these foreign nurses. Articles related to Filipinos have emphasized the importance of well-developed hospital orientation programs for newly recruited Filipino nurses and staff education about Philippine culture and nursing practices. Parallel with international trends in many disciplines, articles about nursing management and administration for Japan were often published after the middle of the 1980s.

Summary

Although the Asian American population doubled during the 1980s, far exceeding the increases seen in other ethnic groups, there is little data to document the physiopsycholgical conditions, health-seeking behaviors, and health barriers of various Asian Americans. Stereotypes of Asian Americans are pervasive; however, it is critical for nurses who care for Asian Americans to understand their diversity in culture, native language and ability to speak English, time and condition of immigration, educational and socioeconomic levels, and health beliefs. However, for most, knowledge of the health beliefs and practices and issues and problems in health care for Asian Americans was derived from educational reports, clinical experience, or other disciplines rather than from research. Moreover, the data that exist are often skewed in favor of more socioeconomically established Asian Americans or in favor of more traumatized Asian American communities. Because the level of acculturation and socioeconomic status influences differently the barriers and access to health care as well as interactions with health care professionals, these variations should be studied and compared among Asian Americans, Blacks, Whites, and Hispanics.

HAE-OK LEE

See also:
  NONTRADITIONAL THERAPIES

MINORITY POPULATIONS: HISPANIC AMERICANS

Hispanics historically have been and will continue to be an important population group in the United States. Currently, Hispanics comprise 9% (22.4 million) of the U.S. population, and because of high fertility rates among certain Hispanic subgroups and continued migration, the Hispanic presence in the United States will continue to grow. Between 1980 and 1990, Hispanics accounted for 35% of the U.S. population growth and are expected to account for 57% of the growth between 2030 and 2050 (U.S. Bureau of the Census, 1993a).

Hispanics are not a monolithic group. The term *Hispanic* was derived by the U.S. Census Bureau to categorize persons of Spanish descent, including those from Mexico, Puerto Rico, Cuba, Spain, and Central and South America. Although Hispanics share many common elements, such as the Spanish language, core values of family, respect, a strong sense of spirituality, and explicit gender differentiation, each subgroup has unique characteristics. As an example, Hispanic subgroups have both a shared and unique history with the United States. The shared history consists of one of migration and conquered nation status. Migration into the United States has been fueled by U.S. labor needs and political and economic unrest in Latin America. The degree to which Hispanics are welcome in the United States is tenuously tied to economic prosperity in this country. It is important to recognize that Hispanics have not only "crossed the border" but, as in the case of Puerto Rico, Cuba, and Mexico, also have had the U.S. border cross over them. Differences in citizenship and refugee status among Hispanic groups are linked to differences in social, economic, political, and health outcomes.

Demographic Characteristics

There are several demographic characteristics of Hispanics that are important to consider. First, Hispanics are younger than the U.S. population, with a median age of 26 years, compared to 34 years among non-Hispanic persons (U.S. Bureau of the Census, 1993a). Second, the importance of the family is evident in family structure. Although the proportion of female-headed households among Hispanic families continues to increase, two-parent families still comprise the largest percentage of family structure type. Further, Hispanic families of all types are more likely to have their own children living at home than are non-Hispanic families (U.S. Bureau of the Census, 1993a). Third, indicators of income consistently show that Hispanics have a lower level of income than that of non-Hispanic families.

Of special significance is that two out of every five Hispanic children under the age of 18 (39.9%) are currently living in poverty, a rate that is two times higher than for non-Hispanic youth (19.5%) (U.S. Bureau of the Census, 1993b). Puerto Rican children living on the mainland have the highest proportion of children living in poverty (57.9%) among all Hispanic children (U.S. Bureau of the Census, 1993a). Unemployment and underemployment are major factors contributing to poverty among Hispanics; they have higher rates of unemployment and, when working in full-time yearlong jobs, are more likely to be living in poverty. Fourth, Hispanics continue to lag behind the U.S. population in educational attainment at all levels. Only 52.6% Hispanics, compared with 81.6% of non-Hispanics, reported that they had at least a high school diploma (U.S. Bureau of the Census, 1993a). A characteristic common to many Hispanics is language; Spanish speakers comprise 54% of all non-English speakers in the United States, with 8.3 million reporting that they do not speak English well or at all.

Health Issues and Priorities

Despite high rates of poverty, limited educational opportunities, and cultural and linguistic barriers to health care, the health issues and priorities of Hispanics are similar in many respects to that of the U.S. population generally. The development of acute and chronic health conditions and causes of death across the life span are similar to those of non-Hispanic Whites.

However, because of high rates of poverty and unemployment, Hispanics are vulnerable to health conditions associated with unsafe environments as well as having limited access to care. For example, there is a higher prevalence of asthma among Puerto Rican youth (Mendoza et al., 1991) and a homicide rate among Hispanic youth that is nearly five times as high as that of non-Hispanic White youth. Also, Mexican-Americans and Puerto Ricans in the United States have increased morbidity and mortality from non-insulin-dependent diabetes mellitus (Maurer, Rosenberg, & Keemer, 1990). Similarly, for some diseases, as in the case of cancer, the incidence of certain cancers may be similar to that of the general population; however, morbidity is higher among Hispanics because of barriers to early detection and treatment.

The incidence of AIDS has disproportionately affected all Hispanics but particularly women and children. The annual rate for AIDS among Hispanic women was 61.9/100,000, compared with 18.5/100,000 among White women, and the cumulative rate of pediatric AIDS cases was three times higher among Hispanic children than among White children (Centers for Disease Control, 1996). Differential modes of transmission of HIV, as well as rates of infection among Hispanic subgroups, illustrate the importance of considering the unique characteristics, health needs, and resources of each Hispanic subgroup in order to design effective care.

To address the health issue and priorities of this emerging majority, a landmark work group was convened as part of the Surgeon General's National Workshop on Hispanic/Latino Health (1992). Areas identified in which critical action is needed include (a) health data, (b) development of a comprehensive research agenda, (c) access to culturally and linguistically appropriate care, and (d) parity of Hispanic representation in all the health professions.

In relation to data on Hispanic health there is a significant lack, and existing data are insufficient to examine differences among subgroups of Hispanics. For example, in a recent survey of 21 major national data systems of the U.S. Department of Health and Human Services (DHHS), only the U.S. vital statistics system is designed to provide data on all four of the major Hispanic subpopulation groups (Delgado & Estrada, 1993). Furthermore, six of the data systems do not contain sufficient data on Hispanics to permit adequate and meaningful analysis. The development of a comprehensive research agenda is concerned with devising strategies to ensure that research with Hispanics is conducted in a culturally competent manner and, further, that there is an infrastructure in place to develop and support Hispanic researchers. The lack of data on Hispanic health is a major reason Hispanics are omitted from significant health policy initiatives.

A common issue and priority among Hispanics is access to culturally and linguistically appropriate health care. Lack of insurance coverage, whether public or private, is a major barrier in accessing health care. The high proportion of working poor among Hispanics limits access to public or private health insurance. But health insurance is only one component of access. The lack of culturally sensitive and competent providers, lack of access to transportation, lack of linguistic access, and lack of community-based health services have been identified as significant barriers to health promotion and maintenance services. Another priority in improving access to health care concerns is increasing the number of bilingual and bicultural Hispanic health providers. As an example, less than 2% of the registered nurse population is of Hispanic origin, with no significant increase in the number of Hispanics employed in nursing in the past 10 years (*National Sample Survey of Registered Nurses,* 1997).

Implications for Nursing Research and Practice

Nursing has only tangentially begun to examine the health care needs of this growing population. First, nurses must first recognize and understand the political, historical, economic, and social contexts that affect the health of Hispanics. Second, descriptive research must be conducted in nearly all health areas, not only to understand disparities in health outcomes but to recognize the strength and protective factors employed by this population in the areas of health promotion and management of symptoms and disease.

Finally, nurses must develop and test interventions that are culturally acceptable and effective.

ANTONIA M. VILLARRUEL

See also:
DIABETES MELLITUS

MOBILITY

In the gerontological literature, mobility is viewed as essential to human
function; the absence of which adversely affects quality of life. In some
nursing theories, mobility is conceptualized as a functional entity (Henderson & Nite, 1978; Roy & Andrews, 1991; Roper, Logan, & Tierney, 1996)
while in others it is approached from a holistic perspective involving movement in time and space (Newman, 1994; Fitzpatrick & Whall, 1996). However, the functional perspective is predominant in nursing as is evident in
current research.

The functional orientation has influenced knowledge development of
mobility in two major ways. First, the research has tended to focus on
specific components of mobility such as gait, balance, mobility tasks, and
joint movement (Galindo-Ciocon, Ciocon, & Galindo, 1995; Hogue, Studenski, & Duncan, 1990; Ring, Nayak, & Isaacs, 1988; Tinetti & Ginter,
1988). Much of this research has been conducted within the context of
fall prevention in individuals with mobility challenges resulting from either
aging or disease.

Second, nursing's functional view of mobility has yielded approaches to
concept measurement that have generated tools for evaluating specific
mobility components for use primarily with older adults (Hogue et al.,
1990; Johnson & Maas, 1997; Spellbring & Ryan, 1997). Although this body
of research has contributed to an understanding of some of the physical
aspects of mobility, it has only minimally advanced nursing's understanding
of the concept. Moreover, research has tended to be fragmented due to
the lack of a common organizing framework.

Mobility-related research has generally been conducted using quantitative research methods. The results of such studies have frequently yielded
mobility interventions based on the views of nursing or other healthcare
professionals. Consequently, the client perspective, particularly that of the
older adult, has been overlooked. Added to this is a certain degree of
ambiguity surrounding the concept of mobility, and this ambiguity has
been reinforced by adherence to the quantitative paradigm. Thus, nursing's

shift away from the quantitative paradigm as the only paradigm for knowledge development has opened up new ways of looking at nursing concepts such as mobility. This has afforded an opportunity to reexamine and broaden mobility's conceptual base.

Integrative View of Mobility

In an attempt to advance nursing's understanding of mobility as a concept for nursing practice, research has been undertaken with the purpose of concept clarification. This work represents a departure from the traditional functional view of mobility. Instead, it includes a more integrated conceptualization of mobility. The work began with an analysis of the concept as a means of deriving attributes from the literature, tentatively arriving at a theoretical definition, and formulating research questions (Rush & Ouellet, 1993). To address the research questions and explore the meaning of mobility from client and nurse perspectives, a qualitative study was undertaken, guided by Schwartz-Barcott and Kim's Hybrid Model (1986). The fieldwork study involved interviews with two populations: older adults living in their own home environments, and their primary nurses.

Both older adults and nurses viewed mobility as extending beyond the physical dimension to include a social and a cognitive one (Ouellet & Rush, 1996; Rush & Ouellet, 1998). Moreover, these dimensions were interrelated, interdependent, and dynamic. This multidimensionality previously had not been captured in the nursing literature as part of the concept; rather, the cognitive and social dimensions were identified as consequences of a lack of mobility. In the 1973 NANDA nomenclature of nursing diagnosis, impaired mobility was initially proposed as having physical, social, emotional, intellectual, and developmental dimensions, but only the physical dimension has been retained (Gordon, 1994).

Older adults assigned more attributes to the mobility concept than did their primary nurses, reflecting variations between groups in the composite of life experiences, developmental stage of the participants, and perspectival lens. The attributes extracted from the older adult's descriptions of mobility also more closely approximated those derived from the concept analysis. This is not surprising given that the conceptual analysis drew from multiple disciplines to produce a more inclusive meaning of mobility that was captured by older adults' range of perspectives and their different walks of life. Nevertheless, conceptual discrepancies, although contributing to the evolution of the concept, should at some point be resolved.

For the purpose of analysis, the dimensions and attributes of mobility were treated as mutually exclusive categories, but conceptually the attributes were embedded in the dimensions. For example, ease and freedom of movement were evident as much in the cognitive and social dimensions as in the physical dimension. This suggests that the attributes underlie the dimensions and that together they constitute the mobility capacity of the person (Rush & Ouellet, 1998).

Mobility capacity was influenced by the presence or absence of forces. These forces, including person characteristics, human presence, environmental elements, personality facts, meaning of mobility resources, perceptions, and enhanced well-being (Ouellet & Rush, 1996), serve to form the context within which mobility may occur (Ouellet & Rush, 1998). Actuation of mobility—or putting the mobility capacity into motion—will occur in concert with the facilitating or impeding influence of these forces.

Ouellet and Rush (1998) proposed a model of mobility that incorporates older adult perspectives. It surpasses the traditional conceptualization of mobility by including multiple interactive dimensions and attributes and by making explicit that mobility is an actuated, everchanging phenomenon. The element of forces supports other work in the area of mobility, particularly that of Hogue (1984) and Tinetti (1986), who address perceptual, personal, and environmental factors and their interactions in fall prevention and mobility problems.

Ouellet and Rush's (1998) mobility model has a number of potential clinical and research applications. Since it is grounded in the views of older adults, it has the greatest application to this population. Clinically, the model could serve to guide and strengthen practice, particularly in the area of gerontological assessment, thus allowing practitioners to base their practice on research findings. Another potential application of the model is that it may provide a framework for integrating existing theoretical and empirical works. By serving as a rubric under which future research efforts may be examined, use of the model may prevent further fragmentation of research related to mobility in older adults.

Demographic data indicate that older adults are a fast-growing population, and that a large number of these older adults reside in the community. This projected trend will likely accelerate during the early part of the 21st century, and it has significant implications for the practice of nursing, as well as for nursing's research agenda. Nursing has a role in generating knowledge to improve both the quality of life of older adults and the quality of nursing practice. To fulfill this role, nursing must intensify its study of the concept of mobility from a broader perspective within a health context as it relates to the older adult. In so doing, the systematic examination of mobility cannot be divorced from practice, but must be grounded in it and inextricably linked to evolving theoretical formulations (Liehr & Smith, 1999).

Much of the work in the area of mobility rests on an unfounded assumption that a theory of mobility exists. In the absence of such a theory, the research undertaken by Ouellet and Rush may represent an early phase of theorization of mobility in older adults. However, further testing and refinement of the concept by examining mobility with diverse aging populations is necessary to reach the level of middle-range theory (Liehr & Smith, 1999). Meanwhile, this work may serve to close the research/theory gap by providing a stronger foundation for guiding mobility-related research.

A critical element that will drive the research agenda is nursing's ability to articulate its discipline-specific perspective on the mobility of older adults within the multidisciplinary healthcare milieu. Only when nursing becomes clear about its role in the area of mobility will the research agenda move ahead. This is a challenge that nursing must now confront.

KATHY RUSH
LOUISELLE OUELLET

See also:
ACTIVITIES OF DAILY LIVING
FALLS
FUNCTIONAL HEALTH
HIP FRACTURE
PHYSICAL RESTRAINTS

NUTRITION

Nutrition as a research area crosses a variety of disciplines, including biochemistry, pharmacology, nutrition science, public health, medicine, and nursing. From a nursing research perspective, nutrition has been studied for its role in health promotion and disease prevention and its use as a therapeutic intervention. In addition, nurse investigators have long been concerned with the impact of disease and therapeutic treatments (e.g., chemotherapy) on nutritional intake. Thus, nutrition studies run the spectrum, from studies of subcellular mechanisms to epidemiological surveys of large groups of individuals. Clinical nutrition studies have focused on patients at risk (e.g., the elderly, pregnant and lactating women, low-birthweight infants), those with specific diseases, and age-related nutritional needs.

There is a sizable body of data supporting the link between diet and common health problems, the most notable of which is coronary artery disease. This relationship is complicated by the addition of genetic factors that place the individual at risk for problems related to lipid metabolism and body fat accumulation. Nurse scientists have participated in the study of this relationship, from molecular bench research to epidemiological studies. These studies provide important insights into our understanding of the pathophysiological and sociocultural mechanisms linking diet to blood vessel changes. There is also a need to increase the number of individual and community-based intervention studies to reduce dietary fat intake and decrease the risk for coronary artery disease.

Specialized nutrition therapies, including total parenteral nutrition, enteral feedings, and supplemental oral feedings, also have been the focus of research for nurse scientists. In these studies, nurses have examined strategies for delivering nutrition, including amounts, constituents, and timing, as well as strategies to reduce adverse consequences (e.g., diarrhea, hyperglycemia, catheter infection). In the early to mid 1970s nurse scientists began to describe the current practice of enteral nutrition support as well as the frequency of complications associated with this therapy in the acute care setting. The ongoing improvements in patient assessment techniques, commercialized diets, and diet delivery technology such as tubes and surgical techniques require nurses to collect descriptive information on the frequency of complications and the adequacy of nutritional intake. In addition, nurses should continue to conduct intervention studies focused on reducing complications (e.g., aspiration). With the trend for more patients to receive total parenteral nutrition and enteral nutrition in the home setting, descriptive research related to types and frequency of complications is needed. Also, patient and family education strategies, as well as providing support for family members, must be examined.

Another important nutrition-related problem in the United States is obesity. Obesity, or excessive body fat, is a complex phenomenon involving a multitude of factors, including genetics, lifestyle, and nutrition. Research has informed the public about the adverse outcomes such as mortality and morbidity. Again, nurse researchers working with animal models have provided insights into the links between heredity and metabolism. Clinical therapeutic studies have focused on the role of exercise, diet counseling, and psychological support in weight reduction in adolescent and middle-aged groups. Issues of compliance, self-efficacy, cultural variations, and individual physiology variations are often considered in examining patient responses.

Undernutrition states can be produced by a number of conditions, including anorexia nervosa, anorexia, wasting diseases, and symptoms such as nausea, pain, and fatigue. Of recent importance are studies linking tumor growth and inflammation to suppression of appetite. Nurse scientists working with animal models have shown that specific cytokines—interleukin-1 (IL-1), interleukin-6 (IL-6), and tumor necrosis factor

(TNF-α)—decrease food intake. Such studies are likely to increase our ability to develop therapeutic strategies to enhance nutritional intake in select patient groups.

Other nurse scientists have focused on strategies to improve the caloric intake of patients undergoing chemotherapy for cancer treatment. Of particular significance is the previous work in instrument development and identification of patient groups most at risk for nausea and vomiting and thus for inadequate nutrition. Therapeutic interventions such as relaxation therapy, guided imagery, and music therapy have been tested to determine their utility in reducing nausea and vomiting with therapy. The results of these studies are, for the most part, inconclusive because of the heterogeneity of the small samples, but they do suggest that they may be useful adjunct therapies along with antiemetics. More work is needed to examine biobehavioral strategies to enhance nutrient intake in select patient groups. Similarly, dietary intervention studies are being conducted in patients with compromised immune function (e.g., AIDS patients). The role of high fiber and low dietary fat intake in reducing diarrhea and thus improving nutritional status also is being studied in dietary intervention research.

Lactose intolerance is another common nutritional problem that has received some investigation by nurse scientists. Individuals with lactose intolerance have a decrease in lactase enzyme, the small intestine enzyme that is necessary for the breakdown of milk sugar lactose. In these individuals the consumption of lactose results in symptoms of bloating, increased flatus, and abdominal discomforts. Nursing research has focused on identifying patients at risk and testing strategies to enhance compliance with a low-lactose diet.

Margaret Heitkemper
Eleanor Bond

See also:
HYDRATION
CHRONIC GASTROINTESTINAL SYMPTOMS

PULMONARY CHANGES IN ELDERS

Most of the pulmonary changes associated with aging are gradual, giving elders the opportunity to adapt (Stanley & Beare, 1999). The physiologic and functional consequences of age-related anatomic changes, altered gas exchange, ventilatory changes, and altered pulmonary-protective mechanisms are important considerations in the comprehensive assessment of the older adult. Clinicians need to thoroughly understand these changes in order to differentiate between normal alterations and disease, and to provide appropriate management.

Thoracic-cage compliance is decreased due to stiffness resulting from the calcification of the costal cartilages and costal vertebral junctions. There is also a decrease in the mass of respiratory muscles, and elastic recoil is diminished. These changes result in an increased elastic work of breathing, an increased residual volume, and an increase in the thoracic anterior-posterior diameter that gives the chest a rounded barrel shape. It has been shown that difficulties in breathing can increase by as much as 20% between the ages of 20 and 60 (Lonergan, 1996).

Anatomic changes result in an increased use of abdominal and diaphragmatic breathing (Stanley & Beare, 1999). As a result, the breathing patterns of elders are more dependent on intraabdominal pressure changes (Lueckenotte, 1996). Kyphosis, an exaggerated curvature of the thoracic spine, has been associated with postmenopausal osteoporosis (dowager's hump) in elderly women. However, this condition is common well before menopause, is related to physical fitness, and is less prevalent in women who maintain an adequate level of exercise (Cutler, Friedman, & Genovese-Stone, 1993). Elders with severe kyphosis often compensate by hyperextending their necks to maintain their level of vision. This condition affects mobility, impairs cardiopulmonary function, and causes significant back pain (Jarvis, 1996).

The lung's decreased elastic recoil causes the early closure of the airways, resulting in the trapping of air in the alveoli. The closing volume rises linearly with age and increases ventilation/perfusion mismatch (Estes, M., 1998; Lonergan, 1996). Supine positioning and shallow breathing also contribute to early closure of the airway. Interventions such as upright positioning and deep breathing diminish the chance of airway collapse (Lueckenotte, 1996). Other factors that contribute to an altered alveolar gas exchange are a decrease in the number of alveolar capillaries and a thickening of the capillary membrane. These changes result in a reduced surface area for gas exchange. Hemoglobin's affinity for oxygen also decreases with age (Estes, M., 1998). Increased ventilation/perfusion mismatch, structural changes, and loss of alveolar surface area lead to decreased PaO_2 values which should not be misconstrued as an indication of pulmonary disease in healthy elders. PaO_2 changes in elders can be expressed as $PaO_2 = 109 - .043$ (age) $+4$ (Lonergan, 1996).

The forced expiratory volume in one second (FEV_1), for a nonsmoker, begins to decrease by 30 ml/yr in the third decade of life. Height, weight, gender, age, race, temperature, and barometric pressure affect FEV_1 measurement (American Thoracic Society, 1991). Vital capacity (VC)—the volume of air that is exhaled after a maximal inhalation—decreases, while residual volume (RV)—the volume of air that is left in the lungs after a maximal exhalation—increases with age. However, total lung capacity (TLC) remains unchanged.

Maximum oxygen consumption decreases with age. This is due in part to deconditioning and age-related cardiovascular changes involving a decreased maximum heart rate and stroke volume. In elders without heart disease and/or lung disease, exercise capacity can be maintained by active physical conditioning, which can have many beneficial physiological and emotional effects (Karper & Boschen, 1993; Lonergan, 1996; Rowe & Kahn, 1998). While age-related lowered arterial oxygen tension and diminished ventilatory reserve can negatively affect exercise tolerance in elders, the changes in respiratory functioning can vary widely. Differences are largely dependent on fitness and activity levels in early life (McCance & Huether, 1990). Other factors to consider in an analysis of exercise tolerance include joint function, skeletal-muscle strength, coordination, and illness.

Despite the increase in the physiologic dead space seen in a healthy elder, the arterial pH remains within the normal range of 7.35 to 7.45 because of the ventilation/perfusion mismatch. The $PaCO_2$ does not increase with advancing age because of an increased respiratory rate (Kinzel, 1991). Respiratory rates in elders are generally higher, the normal range being 16–25 breaths per minute (Pierson & Kacmarek, 1992).

Smoking accelerates the age-related decline in pulmonary function. But unlike other risk factors, smoking can be eliminated. Smoking cessation, even after the age of 60, has been found to halt the progressive decline in pulmonary function (Higgins et al., 1993). Healthcare providers should ask patients about their smoking history and their prior attempts at quitting, and should gauge their interest in trying to quit again. Smoking cessation strategies for elders should encompass appropriate modalities including the use of nicotine patches, oral medications, and behavioral interventions. Smoking-cessation interventions must be planned, should consider any medications being taken concurrently, and should be sensitive to the difficulties associated with a longstanding nicotine addiction.

Age-related neurochemical changes affect ventilatory function. In the elder adult the medulla is less sensitive to changes in the levels of carbon dioxide and oxygen, and both the peripheral and central chemoreceptors are blunted (Estes, 1998). This blunted ventilatory response of elders to hypoxemia or hypercapnia is due to a reduced sympathetic nervous system response. Ventilatory responses may be diminished by as much as 50% when compared to those of adults in their 20s (Pierson & Kacmarek, 1992). A thorough knowledge of changes in ventilatory response related to aging is essential for clinicians involved with ventilator-dependent elders (Thompson, 1996).

Dyspnea or shortness of breath is a frequently reported symptom associated with illnesses such as chronic obstructive pulmonary disease (COPD), asthma, lung cancer, and heart failure. Dyspnea is the most common reason for emergency department visits and increases the likelihood for hospital admission (Parshall, 1999). Studies have shown that self-report of dyspnea does not always correlate with pulmonary function testing. In a longitudinal study of elders with COPD, individual ratings of dyspnea were not directly linked to changes in lung impairment (Lareau, Meek, Press, Ansholm, & Roos, 1999). This blunted perception is thought to caused by physiologic adaptation over time (Barnes, 1992).

Assessment of dyspnea can be accomplished using several available scales. The use of a visual analogue scale (VAS) to measure dyspnea in elderly persons with COPD has been validated by Gift (1989). This type of measure provides a quick and reliable measure of dyspnea. The Pulmonary Functional Status and Dyspnea Questionnaire (PFSDQ) designed by Lareau, Carrieri-Kohlman, Janson-Bjerklie, and Roos (1994) is another reliable scale which has been used to measure dyspnea intensity and changes in functional ability in elderly persons with pulmonary disease.

Decreased t-lymphocyte function contributes to altered immune response, making elders more susceptible to pulmonary infections (Lonergan, 1996). Elders also show a decrease in IgA, an immunoglobulin found in the airways, making them more susceptible to viral infection. Alveolar macrophages, which protect the alveoli by phagocytosis of bacteria and foreign materials that reach the acinus, are deficient in older adults, particularly in smokers (Lueckennotte, 1996). Elders also exhibit impaired humoral immunity that can result in decreased antibody response. Elders can have false negative results to tuberculosis tests, and immunizations such as for flu or pneumonia may not be as efficacious. These age-related changes in immunity are further exaggerated in elders who are on long-term steroid therapy. These elders should be monitored for signs of masked infection due to their compromised immune response. There is also a decreased beta$_2$ receptor function which diminishes the response to inhaled beta$_2$ agonists such as albuterol. This can interfere with managing asthma in elder adults (Stanley & Beare, 1999).

Diminished cilia and less effective cough reflex compromise the pulmonary system in elders, making them more susceptible to pulmonary infection. Cilia beat in a wavelike motion, propelling the mucous blanket—and any entrapped particles—toward the oropharynx to be either swallowed or expectorated. Fewer cilia make the mucociliary escalator less effective in clearing secretions, infectious agents, or environmental pollutants (Blair, 1990; Estes, 1998; Lueckenotte, 1996; Stanley & Beare, 1999). The less efficient a cough is in terms of volume, force, and flow rate (most likely from weakened respiratory muscles), coupled with a less effective gag reflex, contribute to an increased risk of aspiration and potential pulmonary obstruction or infection. Decreased esophageal and gastric motility, along with decreased cardiac-sphincter tone, are both age-related factors that increase the risk of esophageal reflux and aspiration. Poor dental hygiene should also be considered a risk for potential pulmonary infection.

Elders who present pulmonary infection often do so atypically. Initial symptoms of pulmonary infection can be misdiagnosed as a pulmonary embolism or as heart failure (Blair, 1990). The classic triad of cough, fever, and pleuritic pain may not be present in elders. Instead, such subtle changes as increased respiration, increased sputum production, confusion, loss of appetite, and hypotension can be clues to possible pulmonary infection. Signs of sepsis may already be evident when elders present with a pulmonary infection (Stanley & Beare, 1999). Elders who have neurological illnesses such as Alzheimer's disease or Parkinson's disease, or who have sustained a CVA, are at risk for aspiration pneumonia and should be closely monitored for dysphagia. Interventions aimed at diminishing the risk for aspiration are critical.

Altered pulmonary-protective mechanisms have implications for elders undergoing surgery. In any given year about 25% of the 600,000 elders who undergo major abdominal or thoracic surgical procedures in the United States experience postoperative pulmonary complications. Common interventions aimed at preventing postoperative pulmonary complications include cessation of smoking, bronchial hygiene, and incentive spirometry. Prevention of venous thrombosis with possible pulmonary embolization is critical in the elder population undergoing abdominal, thoracic, or orthopedic surgery. This is best accomplished with low-dose heparin, administered subcutaneously every 12 hours, and with the use of pneumatic stockings. For elders at high risk for pulmonary embolism, more frequent subcutaneous dosing of heparin may be used or coumadin may be ordered.

ELIZABETH MCGANN

See also:
  DYSPNEA
  OSTEOPOROSIS
  SMOKING AS A CARDIOVASCULAR RISK FACTOR

SEXUALITY RESEARCH

Attitudes of American nurses toward sexuality have gone through many phases (Bullough & Bullough, 1997). Before they could do major research in the area, nurses had to feel that the subject matter was worth researching and then gain the expertise to do the research. Through at least the first 50 years of modern nursing, they neither felt that the topic was worth researching nor had the knowledge to do more than repeat the standard prejudices and misconceptions of their time. In the first phase, which coincided with the emergence of the Nightingale schools, the topic was ignored; nurses wrote nothing on it.

The second phase could be called a hortatory one; the duty of nurses was to educate their patients to the dangers inherent in sexual activity (Robb, 1907), and this was believed to require little special knowledge. Representative of this phase are the writings of Lavinia Dock (1910), which emphasized the dangers of masturbation in children and the importance of the nurse in bringing this message to the mother. She taught that the "reproductive rituals" should "only be performed in the sincerity of aspiration to bring a new being in the world." In her attitudes, Dock simply mirrored the assumptions of the period.

A step forward was taken in the 1917 *Standard Curriculum Guide* of the National League of Nursing Education, which specified that sexual hygiene be included in the subjects covered by students. This seems like a real effort to gain some expertise, but unfortunately the sexual material was to be covered in a 1-hour lecture. It was extended to a whole unit in the curriculum guide of 1927. Still, nursing education was more influenced by the prohibitions and dangers of sex than by promotion of any real understanding (Smiley, Gould, & Melby, 1931).

The third phase was somewhat a reorientation of nursing education to coincide with some of the ongoing research into sexuality. The National League of Nursing Education set up a Committee on Social Hygiene in 1931 to draft a curriculum to better prepare nurses for the sexual problems they were likely to encounter. The result of this was a special curriculum guide in social hygiene for nurses (McCorkle 1934), and gradually elements of this report were integrated into nursing education. Although sex education in nursing remained mainly hortatory, there was more real information being given.

Nurses Margaret Sanger and Emma Goldman pushed for a different type of sex education; and although neither did much research themselves, Sanger was a key figure in promoting sex research, particularly on reproductive issues. She was instrumental in stimulating the research that led to oral contraceptives, bringing researchers and potential donors together (Bullough, 1994).

The fourth phase coincided with the formation in 1964 of the Sex Information and Education Council of the United States, which was a major factor in changing the nature of sex education. School nurses participated in this phase, which led to new demands for sex research by nurses. In part, the development and distribution of the pill gave women a new view of sexuality, and this coincided with the changing attitudes and receptiveness within the feminist movement on the importance of female sexuality.

Major evidence of change did not appear until the early 1970s. One sign of a new official nursing interest was a compilation of articles on sexuality by Browning and Lewis (1973). Articles were grouped under subsections of "mind-body continuum" (i.e., masturbation, homosexuality, transsexualism), sex education (emphasizing the role of the nurse in the education of the young person), fertility regulation (including family planning, contraceptives, sterilization), abortion (stressing attitudes as well as the procedures), and sexually transmitted diseases (including incidence, types, tests, and treatment). The fact that the compilation was published by the *American Journal of Nursing* gave encouragement to nurses to think about the topic and even begin to do tentative research. Shortly afterward, in 1974, *Nursing Clinics of North America* published a symposium with articles on various aspects of sexual behavior.

Nursing textbooks rapidly followed the new lead, and sophisticated textbooks on the subject of human sexuality appeared; they were specifically designed for nurses and authored by nurses who were doing research in human sexuality. Nancy Fugate Woods (1979), well known for her research into menstruation, published a sexuality text. Many nurses began to examine sexual markers in women's lives, from menarche to menopause; and in the process, they entered the mainstream of sex research. Among the major researchers in various aspects of sexuality were Bonnie Bullough, Beverly Whipple, and Vern Bullough. Whipple's (1982) work in sexual physiology, particularly her work with the G spot, made her one of the better known U.S. nurses. Although the G spot remains somewhat controversial, Whipple has gone beyond the controversy to do major research.

As with many other subjects of pertinence to nursing, nurses researching sexuality have moved from being disseminators of information and misinformation gathered by others to becoming researchers in their own right, although few have so far achieved recognition outside the nursing profession.

Vern L. Bullough

SLEEP

The purpose of sleep is not well understood. Proposed theories to explain the role of sleep include: restoration, energy conservation, instinct, adaptation, and memory reinforcement (Chokroverty, 1994). In a classic 1933 study, a subject awake for 231 hours became both argumentative and disoriented and reported hallucinations. By the end of the study period the subject was unable to express his thoughts and exhibited paranoid behavior (Hales, 1981).

Sleep cycles consist of both quiet and active components. The quiet sleep component is popularly labeled nonrapid eye movement (NREM) sleep, and consists of four stages. The progression of stages results in slower frequency and higher amplitude wave patterns, with a concomitant slowing of physiologic processes. Active sleep, or rapid eye movement (REM) sleep follows, revealing an active EEG wave pattern that resembles wakefulness. Rapid, bilateral, synchronous eye movements occur in bursts, with a concomitant increase in physiological processes. Dreaming occurs during this stage of sleep.

The effects of aging on changes in sleep patterns are the subject of much descriptive nursing research. Researchers have associated changes in sleep patterns with circadian rhythm changes among older individuals (Bliwise, 1993; Czeisler et al., 1992). Webb (1987) reported that in a sample of 134 healthy subjects ranging from 50 to 70 years of age, 16% took longer than 30 minutes to fall asleep, 21% awoke for more than 30 minutes after sleep onset, and 8% had difficulty in both falling asleep and in awakening periods.

Libman et al. (1998) conducted a study to compare the quality of sleep between younger and older age cohorts. The study used data gathered both longitudinally and cross-sectionally over a 2-year period. The sample included 149 community-dwelling subjects over the age of 55. Subjects were sorted into three groups based on self-report of good, medium quality, or poor sleep at pretesting, and again for the 2-year follow-up. The sample was also divided into "young old" or "old old" (over the age of 70) groups. The results of the study showed that in each age group—and at both pretest and two year follow-up—the percentage of individuals in the three sleep status categories were similar. The researchers subsequently reported no evidence for age-related increases in sleep complaints.

Minors, Atkinson, Bent, Rabbitt, and Waterhouse (1998) conducted a longitudinal study of 112 non-institutionalized subjects ranging from 53 to 82 years old for a period of 10 years. At specified points throughout the study period, subjects recorded in their diary their times of going to bed, awakening, and eating, and whether they lived alone or with another person(s), during a "typical week." The diaries were scored by the researchers to determine the effects of living alone on the subjects' lifestyle. The results indicated that age was correlated with changes in the sleep/wake cycle and mealtimes, and indicated a decrease in lifestyle variability. When the changes were examined between subjects living alone and those living with another person, an increase was found in the amount of time spent in bed, and a decrease was revealed in lifestyle variability among those living alone. The researchers concluded that both a deteriorating body clock and an increasingly inflexible lifestyle explain some of the variability in circadian rhythm that is seen in older adults.

Evans and Rogers (1994) conducted a study to examine the 24-hour sleep/wake patterns of healthy older adults. The sample included 14 elderly subjects. Subjects wore a wrist actigraph for 48 hours, and completed an activity log. The data indicated that although subjects spent more than 7.5 hours in bed at night, the total amount of time spent sleeping was just over 6 hours. Subjects did not experience difficulty falling asleep, but had trouble maintaining sleep. All subjects in the study took one or more naps during the study period.

In a study of 12 institutionalized, older, demented men, the influence of twice-daily exposure to sunlight on sleep was examined. Subjects' sleep/ wake patterns were observed and documented every hour for 3 consecutive weeks. The results showed statistically significant improvement in sleep-wake cycles. However, the effect of the sunlight was not sustained when subjects were returned to their normal routine. The researchers concluded that sunlight deprivation may be a factor in the altered sleep patterns of older, cognitively-impaired, institutionalized residents, but that further study is needed (Castor, Woods, Pigott, & Hemmes, 1991).

Several sleep disorders common to older adults have been the subject of nursing research studies. Periodic limb movements in sleep (PLMS), or nocturnal myoclonus, are defined as repetitive jerking movements of the extremities, occurring every 20 to 40 seconds at night and causing frequent, brief arousals. The prevalence of PLMS is thought to be high among the elderly. The effect of periodic limb movements (PLM) on sleep and daytime alertness was examined in a sample of 23 men with severe, stable congestive heart failure (CHF) and 9 healthy control subjects. Data were collected with polysomnography during the night, followed by standardized assessment of alertness the following day. The CHF subjects with moderately severe PLM showed significantly more arousals from sleep, more NREM sleep, and less daytime alertness than the control group and the CHF patients with fewer PLMs. The researchers concluded that PLMs are more common in CHF patients, and may contribute to sleep/wake complaints in this population (Hanly & Zuberi-Khokhar, 1996).

Obstructive sleep apnea syndromes have been the subject of much research literature (Dement et al., 1985; Hoch, Buysse, Monk, & Reynolds, 1992; McGinty, Littner, & Stern, 1987; Thorpy, 1994). Sleep-related breathing disorders, including apnea and hypopnea, have been thought to cause sleep arousal because of the hypoxemia resulting from decreased ventilation. Older adults with sleep apnea do not often report a sleep-related complaint because they do not know they have the disorder. The disorders may be associated with hypertension, cardiac arrhythmias, and cognitive complaints (Hoch et al., 1992; McGinty et al., 1987).

There are many sleep disorders associated with the cognitive decline in the older adult. Dementia is often thought to result in disrupted sleep and agitated behaviors. Pollak and Stokes (1997) conducted a study to compare the sleep and motor activity patterns between older adults and their caregivers. They had 25 cognitively-impaired and 18 noncognitively-impaired adult day-care participants and their paired caregivers keep daily sleep diaries, and they recorded wrist-motor activity every one-half minute for 9 days. The data indicated that on the whole, older adult day-care participants were not significantly more active at night than their caregivers. The day-care participants were found to be significantly less active in the daytime than were their caregivers. Noncognitively impaired older adults were significantly more active at night than their caregivers, but the daytime activity of these two groups was the same. The rest-activity patterns between caregivers of cognitively impaired and noncognitively impaired older adults was similar. The researchers concluded that increased nighttime motor activity may cause decreased daytime activity. Alternatively, decreased daytime activity may have been a result of decreased stimulation or frailty. Frailty may also explain why the nighttime activity of the older, cognitively impaired sample was not higher than that of the noncognitively impaired group. Increased nighttime activity may also be attributed to depression, sleep-schedule disturbances, restless legs, or other sleep disorders.

A study by Matthews, Farrell, and Blackmore (1996) was conducted to determine the effect of a more client-centered care approach on both the level of agitation and 24-hour sleep patterns of 33 older, cognitively impaired nursing home residents. The levels of both dementia and sleep were measured 4 times over a 12-week period, using standardized instruments. When data gathered before the change of care delivery were compared to data after change of care approach, verbal agitation levels decreased significantly, and infrequent, agitated behaviors significantly increased. Daytime sleep initially increased, but then returned to baseline after 6 weeks. Further research is needed on the effects of care delivery on residents' sleep patterns.

Treatment for sleep-related disorders in the elderly include both pharmacologic and nonpharmacologic options. Little nursing research has been conducted on the pharmacologic interventions for sleep in older adults. The consensus of the research literature recommends pharmacologic intervention for older adults for a 2-week maximum time period, in order to avoid developing a dependence on these sleep aids. If pharmacological intervention is necessary, a benzodiazepine with a short or intermediate action is recommended. Temazepam and Triazolam are two drugs which are effective at low doses, and they result in fewer potential side effects than longer acting drugs.

Nonpharmacological sleep interventions are more commonly conducted by nurse researchers. A study by Richards (1993) was conducted to test the effect of muscle relaxation, mental imagery, relaxing music (MRMIM), or massage on the sleep and arousal of 69 older men in a critical care unit for cardiovascular disorders. Subjects were randomly assigned to a control group that received regular nursing care (N = 17), the MRMIM group (n = 28), or the massage group (N = 24). The results, comparing the three groups on level of arousal, revealed no significant differences. There were significant differences between the massage and the control group in sleep, but not between the MRMIM and the control group.

In another study of 55 randomly selected women over the age of 65, a pretest-posttest design was used to examine the effects of relaxation on sleep. Data were collected with polysomnography and a sleep instrument. Subjects spent 8 nights participating in the study. Relaxation was introduced to the subjects on the fourth and fifth days of the study. The results indicated that relaxation significantly improved the sleep of older women in the study. The researcher encouraged nurses to use relaxation with women who report sleep disturbances (Johnson, J. E., 1991).

PLM, sleep apnea, and cognitive disorders have been shown to cause sleep disturbances in older adults. In addition, pain producing diseases such as arthritis, fractures due to osteoporosis, or cancer may also contribute to sleep disorders in older adults. Symptoms of heart failure may worsen during the night, with nocturnal dyspnea contributing to sleep disruption. Nocturia, dementia, alcoholism, and depression are other examples of medical or psychiatric disorders which can cause sleep disturbances. A sleep-related complaint of an elderly person may be related to a treatable medical or psychiatric condition. Further research into the pathological causes of sleep disturbance in older adults is necessary in order to develop more effective treatment.

Despite the prevalence of sleep disorders among older adults, no sleep-assessment instrument has been identified as valid and reliable in the older population. Chokroverty (1994) indicates that there are four areas of assessment to be addressed concerning sleep disorders: sleep history, medical history, drug history, and psychiatric history. Further research is needed on the development and testing of an instrument, incorporating these components for the assessment of sleep in older adults. Further research into both pharmacological and nonpharmacological sleep interventions is also needed.

Meredith Wallace

See also:
  ALZHEIMER'S DISEASE
  COGNITIVE DISORDERS
  COGNITIVE INTERVENTIONS
  MEDICATIONS IN THE ELDERLY

SPIRITUALITY AND AGING

Recent scientific research has positively correlated the well-being of individuals with improvement in their health status. Thus, healthcare providers need to recognize and address the connection between spirituality and health (Ellis, Vinson, & Ewigman, 1999; O'Neill & Kenny, 1998; Summer, 1998). Nurses (and others caring for elderly patients) promote spiritual caregiving as older individuals grapple with social change (i.e., retirement, loss of friends or partners) (Brennan, 1994; Bauer & Barron, 1995), chronic or terminal illness (Fehring, Miller, & Shaw, 1997), and/or quality-of-life issues (Isaia, Parker, & Murrow, 1999).

Much of the research pertaining to spirituality and aging is descriptive. Zorn and Johnson (1997) described the role of spirituality in the lives of 114 noninstitutionalized rural elderly women (median age = 75) in their analysis of individuals' religious well-being. The authors reported a significant positive correlation between religious well-being and social support and hope. Respondents scored higher on religious well-being if they reported regular participation in religious activities, if they highly rated the value or influence of religious beliefs in their lives, and if they believed that religious beliefs were increasingly important with age.

Several studies examine "religion" (or "religiosity") and its relationship to health and illness in the elderly (Ainlay, Singleton, & Swingert, 1992). Young (1993) reported that spirituality enabled chronically ill elders to be more productive and adaptive than nonreligious elders. Forbes (1994) noted a significant correlation between spirituality and coping ability among older adult-care recipients and caregivers. Older black adults and women in the study tended to be more religious than white individuals and men. A study of 3,963 adults aged 65 and older revealed that individuals who attended weekly religious services, read the Bible regularly, and engaged in routine prayer were 40% less likely to have elevated blood pressure than their peers with little, limited, or infrequent religious activity (Koenig et al., 1998a). There are also numerous studies that examine the relationship between religion and mental health in various groups of older adults (Koenig, George, Blazer, Pritchett, & Meador, 1993; Koenig, George, & Peterson, 1998b; Morris, 1996; Musick, Koenig, Hays, & Cohen, 1998; Stolley & Koenig, 1997).

Other descriptive analyses of spirituality and aging utilize a broader definition of spirituality that includes religion, but does not assume that religion and spirituality are synonymous constructs. For example, Ross, L. A. (1997) questioned 10 hospitalized elderly patients about their perceptions of spiritual needs and care and noted that spirituality was expressed as religion, love and belonging, morality, and death and dying. Hungelmann, Kenkel-Rossi, Klassen, and Stollenwerk (1996) developed the JAREL Spiritual Well-Being Scale based upon the findings of 31 in-depth interviews with older subjects about spiritual well-being. They defined spirituality as a multidimensional construct that encompassed broad dimensions of relationships with oneself and others, with ties to past, present, and future events.

Other studies aim to quantify spirituality through the use of pretested instruments that measure various parameters of spirituality. Isaia, Parker, and Murrow (1999) measured spiritual well-being among 37 community-dwelling older adults (mean age = 74) using the Spiritual Well-Being Scale (Paloutzian & Ellison, 1982). The purpose of their study was to determine the effects of age, gender, ethnicity, and religious affiliation on patients' self-perceptions of spiritual well-being. Because the study participants were all Protestant, 68% Caucasian, and 57% women, little was gleaned about the effects of religious affiliation, racial/ethnic categorization, or gender. Moreover, the difference in scores between participants in the 56–74 age group (n = 19) and those over age 75 (n = 18) was insignificant. Nonetheless, the authors concluded that spirituality was important to most older adults, particularly to older women, and suggested that nurses include a spiritual assessment as a part of their routine practice.

Brush and McGee (1999) demonstrate how spiritual assessment can be operationalized in clinical practice. They studied a group of homeless men (mean age = 40.5) in recovery from substance addictions. Like Isaia, Parker, and Murrow (1999), they encourage nurse educators to teach future nurses to assess patient spirituality, agreeing with Millison (1995) that most nurses feel ill-equipped or unqualified to do so.

The chief reason for the lack of assessment of patient spirituality is the ambiguous meaning of spirituality. Definitions such as "a process and sacred journey" (Burkhardt, 1989), "a life relationship with mystery, higher power, God, or universe" (Narayanasamy, 1993), and "connectedness with oneself, others, nature, or God" (Meraviglia, 1999) are elusive and abstract. Leetun (1996), however, defines "wellness spirituality" in relationship to the care of older adults, along with a clinical protocol for assessing and managing wellness spirituality in older persons. This is an important first step in helping nurses move from spiritual-care theory to spiritual-care practice.

Despite increased attention to the spiritual dimension of caring for older patients, few nursing models operationalize spiritual assessment and care into clinical practice (Price, Stevens, & LaBarre, 1995). As a result, Millison (1988) noted, "many carers steer clear of spiritual material for fear they are unqualified and ill-equipped, or because they feel it is not a part of their job description" (p. 38). Lacking an understanding of the full dimension of patients' spirituality, most nurses are unable to offer adequate spiritual interventions in situations where they are most needed (Pilch, 1988). Future research in the area of spirituality and aging must measure outcomes of spiritual care, explore the meaning of spirituality across different racial, cultural, and socioeconomic groups of elders, and demonstrate clear educational and practice goals for nurses.

BARBARA L. BRUSH

See also:
QUALITY OF LIFE
WELLNESS

WIDOWS AND WIDOWERS

The review covers 39 studies concerning older widowed persons (OWP) that nurses authored or co-authored and published in periodicals between 1977 and 1998. The research designs included 26 predictive correlational studies, 11 descriptive studies, and 1 experimental study. Twenty-six of the studies used quantitative research methods, ten were qualitative, and the remaining three were both qualitative and quantitative. For the review of findings, studies were grouped into three categories: (1) bereavement as loss, crisis, or transition, (2) health of the widowed; or (3) living alone.

Bereavement as Loss, Crisis, or Transition

Most widowhood research has pertained to bereavement; common concepts include grief, stress, adaptation, coping, and social support. The work reflects four perspectives on bereavement: (a) as loss, (b) as crisis, (c) as both loss and crisis, and (d) as transition.

Loss. In 4 of 5 studies, qualitative methods were used. Anderson and Dimond (1995) analyzed twelve interviews to compare experiences of younger and OWP; these categories were described: feelings, physical symptoms, special hardships, and coping. The fifth category of support was discussed elsewhere (Rigdon, Clayton, & Dimond, 1987), and a theory of helpfulness for bereaved elders was presented. Jacob (1996) conducted a grounded theory study to generate a definition and theory of grief for 6 widows whose husbands had been hospice clients; core concepts were *being aware, experiencing distress, supporting, coping,* and *facing new realities.* In an ethnonursing study of older Greek-Canadian widows' grief, Rosenbaum (1991) relied on 12 key informants, concluding that their unique lifeways were inconsistent with professionals' typical bereavement advice (such as joining a self-help group). Alston, Small, and Whiteside (1992) compared loneliness scores of 35 older black widowed, married, and unmarried persons, finding that widows tended to rationalize their loneliness as a general feature of living or aging; loneliness scores were compared to qualitative data.

Crisis.   Vachon and colleagues reported a 2-year study grounded in crisis theory (Walker, K. N., MacBride, & Vachon, 1977). Vachon (1976) found that older widows reported less distress than did younger widows. At 1 month post-bereavement, psychological distress and the spouse's short final illness predicted distress 2 years later (Vachon, Rogers et al., 1982). Enduring high distress was linked to problems with social support, health, and finances (Vachon, Sheldon et al., 1982b). In an intervention study, 68 widows paired with a supportive contact person adapted more quickly than controls in the intrapersonal, interpersonal, and psychosocial realms (Vachon, Lyall, Rogers, Freedman-Letofsky, & Freeman, 1980).

Other crisis-based papers included a general report on problems and coping of 26 OWP (Hegge, 1991) and studies of coping resources and strategies. Owning a pet did not influence OWPs' ($N = 192$) psychosocial adjustment (Lund, Johnson, Baraki, & Dimond, 1984). Valanis, Yeaworth, and Mullis (1987) found that alcohol use was more prevalent among the 60 OWP studied, than among the 60 married elders in the study, although widowhood was not linked to problem-drinking.

Loss and Crisis.   Robinson (1995) studied 65 older widows' resources, grief, and coping; the path model explained 18% of the variance in grief. Kirschling and McBride's (1989) study of 72 OWP was based on stress and coping theory; grief was defined as "the stress experienced by the bereaved" (p. 208). Compared to younger widows, older widows reported more personal power (on an internal support scale) and less loss of control (on a grief scale). Coping did not vary by age or gender; no differences involving older widowers were reported. Kanacki, Jones, and Galbraith (1996) concluded that depression of OWP did not differ by gender during early bereavement.

Transition.   Dimond (1981), who viewed bereavement as a transition period rather than as a loss or crisis, developed a model of bereavement incorporating both grief and coping; the model was a basis for a 2-year study of 192 OWP. OWP who were coping 3 weeks after the death were likely to do so 1 year later; initially high stress levels did not moderate over time (Johnson, Lund, & Dimond, 1986). In gender-based analyses, there were no differences in bereavement processes, depression, or life satisfaction (Lund, Caserta, & Dimond, 1986). Qualitative aspects of social support influenced bereavement outcomes more than its structural parameters (Dimond, Lund, & Caserta, 1987). In the first 2 bereavement years, support networks were stable (Lund, Caserta, van Pelt, & Gass, 1990). Herth (1990) tested Dimond's model with 75 OWP, finding associations between grief resolution and hospice care for the dying spouse, no more than one concurrent loss, a high level of hope, and certain coping styles.

Health of the Widowed

In 8 correlational works, co-variates of health in the first bereavement year were reported. Valanis and Yeaworth (1982) correlated 60 OWP self-reports of physical and mental health with professional ratings, finding (a) differences in health self-reports and ratings only for the oldest persons (> 70 years); (b) no differences in mental health ratings; and (c) no gender-based differences. When 60 OWP were compared to 60 age-matched married persons at two time-points, they improved on all variables except social resources. At Time 2, OWP health and depression scores were lower than those of the married elders (Yeaworth & Valanis, 1985). Gass (1987a) reported qualitative data on 100 widows' helpful and less helpful coping strategies and correlations of ways of coping and measures of dysfunction. With that sample, Gass (1987b) also found that health was not associated with number of coping strategies, although it was linked to good mental health prior to bereavement and to more coping resources. For 159 OWP, Gass and Chang (1989) noted that gender directly influenced resource strength and contributed minimally to variance in psychosocial health; men reported more resource strength. When that sample's data were analyzed with gender as the independent variable (Gass, 1988), there were no differences in health, resource strength, or coping (except that widows used more mixed coping). For 339 OWP, Caserta, Lund, and Dimond (1990) found that 25% of the variance in perceived health status was explained by number of symptoms, but unresolved grief explained 1% of the variance. In interviews with 10 OWP whose depression scores were at the sample's high/low extremes, the 5 depressed OWP reported more illness, relocation, relationship changes, and deaths of friends or family (Dimond, Caserta, & Lund, 1994).

Just 2 studies focused on health of women widowed longer than one year. Aber (1992) found that the work history and attitude toward work of 157 widows were predictors of self-reported health status 2 years after bereavement. For 84 older widows (most of whom were Black), Rauckhorst (1987) noted an association between the practice of health habits and health locus of control (HLOC), although HLOC explained only 7% of the variance.

Living Alone

Several correlational studies focused on the older widow's life after the initial year of bereavement. In a secondary data analysis of 816 subjects, predicting life outlook, Hoeffer (1987b) found that compared to never-married women, widows' outlook was less positive. In this study, marital status was not a predictor of life outlook; the regression equation explained 29% of the variance. Using the same data, Hoeffer (1987a) tested a model of loneliness that explained 27% of the variance; widowhood was a predictor, but the perception of time passing slowly, health status, and living alone were much more significant. In Brock's (1984) study, younger and older widows differed in education, work history, and number of children, but age did not predict well-being.

To explore the essence of widows' experience of living alone, several scholars have used descriptive phenomenology. Porter's studies emanated from critical analyses of the literature (1994b; 1995a). Following lengthy interviews with 7 women, phenomena of living alone were described: *making aloneness acceptable, going my own way* (1994a), *reducing my risks* (1994a, 1994b), and *sustaining myself* (1994a); features of older widows' life-world were characterized (1995a). Porter found that widows sought to *keep the generations separate* by continuing to live alone and by trying not to burden their children (1998a). Nine, older rural widows' intention to *stay close to shore* for healthcare resulted in a new interpretation of access as familiarity (1998b). Letvak (1997) interviewed 8 rural Canadian older widows, reporting themes of connectedness and need for control and noting the importance of living at home alone.

Widowhood Research in Context: Demographics, Health, and Healthcare Use

Of persons over age 65 in 1990, 16% of men and 46% of women were widowed (U.S. Bureau of the Census, 1997). By age 75, 70% of women are widows (Keith, 1986); most widows live alone (Choi, 1991), facing an increasing risk of poverty (Barusch,1994). Widowhood has not been directly linked to chronic disease incidence or course (Kriegsman, Penninx, & van Eijk, 1995), but compared to married elders, older widows with breast cancer (Neale, Tilley, & Vernon, 1986) and older single men with cardiovascular disease (Williams et al.,1992) have poorer survival rates. For OWP, favorable chronic disease outcomes co-exist with positive family support (Kriegsman et al., 1995). With regard to mental health, older widowers' suicide risk is much higher than that of any other older group (Li, 1995). Most OWP have children (Keith, 1989) to rely upon (Dwyer & Coward, 1992), and they are also heavy users of healthcare, particularly home care (Freeman, 1995), with higher home care use rates linked to living alone (Choi, 1994), increasing age (Branch et al., 1988), and female gender (Wan & Arling, 1983).

Future Directions for Research: Attending to Heterogeneity

The salience of the critical trends affecting OWP is not particularly evident in the nursing research. Without neglecting the relatively short-term period of bereavement, scholars must develop the science of long-term issues affecting OWP—chronic health problems and living alone—by revealing the heterogeneity that exemplifies aging persons (Dannefer, 1988; Porter, 1995b). The predominant method in OWP research—conducting significance tests of hypotheses with small samples—has masked participants' diversity, in part by increasing the risk of Type II error. In the correlational studies reviewed, no more than a modest degree of variance was explained. OWP variation must be explored within *both* the explained and unexplained variance.

The trends affecting OWP suggest that exploration of aged heterogeneity is needed in three interrelated realms as a prelude to intervention studies. First, researchers must describe the unique experiences of demographic subgroups such as older widowed persons-of-color. The dearth of gerontological research on widowers (Horowitz, 1992) is echoed in the nursing literature; this must be corrected. Aside from the work of Rosenbaum (1991), there are no nursing ethnographies of OWP; there are no crosscultural nursing studies of OWP. Cross-cultural and cross-gender studies must be undertaken cautiously; if the genders experience widowhood differently (Lee, Willetts, & Seccombe, 1998; Hustins, 1993), nurses need to know this to plan and implement effective, sensitive care. The second crucial need is to ascertain the health-related needs of vulnerable OWP subgroups, such as widowers at risk for suicide and widows at risk for breast cancer, rather than comparing OWP on global well-being scales. Finally, because elders' heterogeneity presents a challenge to healthcare policy and service delivery (Brubaker & Brubaker, 1995), descriptive studies of

intergenerational support and elder care are needed to undergird individualized healthcare services for OWP.

EILEEN PORTER

See also:
DEATH & DYING
GRIEF

Part III

ISSUES IN ENVIRONMENTS OF CARE

INTRODUCTION

Changes in functional status, fluctuating acute and chronic illness, diminished economic resources, and alterations in family dynamics all impact upon the environment where an older adult resides. Environments of care range from an intensive care unit in an acute-care setting to a rural single-family dwelling. Changes in reimbursement and healthcare policy have a significant impact upon where older adults reside. Cutbacks in inpatient and outpatient long-term care contributes to the growing need for creative, innovative solutions including adult day care, continuing care communities, assisted and assistive living programs, and other support services provided in a variety of environments. As the acuity level of patients being cared for at home increases, so does the risk of environmental changes due to readmissions to the hospital or the nursing home. However, the relationship between environments of care, and health for the older adult is not well recognized (MacDonald, Remus, & Laing, 1994). The Ottawa Charter for Health Promotion states that "the inextricable links between people and their environment constitute the socio-ecological approach to health" and requests healthcare and related professionals to create supportive environments for health promotion (World Health Organization, 1992).

Nursing must take the lead to improve the continuum of care between settings. As new approaches to care are developed, including a variety of housing alternatives, maintaining the continuity of care is paramount. Nurses who work in different settings on the continuum can promote health in the older adult population in many ways. One consistent intervention that runs throughout the continuum of care is patient education. Weinrich and Boyd (1992) report increased educational needs of older adults based on the frequency and complexity of medical problems. They further report on various factors such as: lifestyle, developmental levels, role changes and body image, which may impact upon the education of older adults (Weinrich & Boyd, 1992). Therefore, a comprehensive nursing assessment of these factors, including an older adult's readiness to learn, is essential in creating an appropriate teaching plan.

Long-range and discharge planning, especially in environments of transition, such as the acute-care setting, are an essential component of any nursing care plan. From the acute-care setting through each stage of the continuum, until the client returns home, there are opportunities for nurses to introduce clients to community resources. The acute-care nurse is in an opportunistic position to initiate teaching and then communicate the educational plan across sites.

Maintaining continuity of care across settings can be achieved through the utilization of standardized practice protocols and models of care which can support the care of older adults in these settings. Models such as: (a) Nurses Improving Care to the Hospitalized Elderly (NICHE) Project (Abraham et al., 1999); (b) Geriatric Resource Nurse (GRN) model (Fulmer, 1991); (c) Acute Care of the Elderly Medical-Surgical Unit (ACE Unit) model (Landefeld, Palmer, Kresevic, Fortinsky, & Kowal, 1995); and (d) the Hospital-wide Educational model (The NICHE Project Faculty, 1994) all enable nurses in acute care to provide expert specialized geriatric care. Two models that specifically address continuous care are: (a) The Quality Cost Model of Transitional Care (Naylor et al., 1994) which targets elderly at high risk for poor discharge outcomes; and (b) The Multi-disciplinary Case Management Model (Cohen & Cesta, 1993) which provides outcome-oriented patient care, ensuring the appropriate use of resources through the use of patient care pathways.

Enabling a smooth transition into the nursing home for a new resident has always been challenging for nurses in long-term care. The proliferation of subacute and rehabilitation units in traditional inpatient, long-term care facilities, requires nurses in these settings to develop skills in discharge planning. Establishing collaborative relationships with nursing colleagues in home care and other community agencies promotes communication, which is essential to maintain continuity across settings. Additional community resources that may help the older adult discharged from a long-term care facility include support groups and medical resources, such as telephone information and referral services.

Nursing must advocate for interdisciplinary communication through the use of discharge summaries and standardized assessment tools to maintain continuity across sites. The communication of specific vital information, including advance directives and healthcare proxies are essential to maintaining high-quality care. The transition back to the community is facilitated when the community health provider is provided with a comprehensive assessment prior to making the initial home visit.

Community health nurses function as referral sources and provide healthcare information and services to both patients and their families (Keating, 1995). The resources available to community health nurses are often rich and enable them to draw on a variety of sources to assist them in promoting the health of community-dwelling older adults. Transportation procurement, home-delivered meals, assistance with housekeeping, socialization, exercise programs, and self-help groups are only a few of the resources available within the community.

Long-term care nurses are also challenged to create environments for residents which promote wellness, function, and the optimal quality of life. Innovative planning and creativity are evident with the use of walking tracks, gardens designed with Alzheimer's patients in mind, and the use of pets trained to prevent wandering (see pet therapy). Although a great deal of attention has been given toward developing specialized care units for dementia patients, most nursing homes do not have specialized services or environmental considerations for residents with special needs.

Environmental considerations have been an essential component to any falls-prevention program across settings. An environmental assessment enables the provider to develop a comprehensive falls-prevention plan, thereby reducing the number of falls caused by environmental factors. Alterations in environments are also necessary at times when reducing the use of physical restraints. Individual room assignment changes, low beds, and floor mats are but a few of the interventions utilized to facilitate restraint free environments (Capezuti, Evans, Strumf, & Maislin, 1996).

Rapid changes in healthcare delivery throughout all healthcare environments affects nursing care to older adults across the continuum. Changes in healthcare delivery, dictated by financial regulations, occur faster than providers can shift focus, leaving at times significant gaps in healthcare for older adults. Therefore, the need for a systematic approach to discharge planning, and case management, utilizing models and protocols aimed at maintaining communication and dialogue across sites, are essential. Nursing must recognize the need for additional research related to environments of care. Evidence-based nursing care provided in the acute-care hospital, the community, or in long-term care settings will enable nursing to continue to contribute to improving the care of older adults.

ELLEN FLAHERTY

ACUTE CARE

Older people have a greater prevalence of chronic diseases and disorders that lead to hospitalization. On average, people over 65 are hospitalized more than three times as often as younger individuals, and the length of their stay is estimated to be 50% longer than that of younger individuals. Nursing research that defines the evidence for practice interventions is needed for patients of all ages, and especially for the elderly. Nursing research that provides the basis for best practice for hospitalized elders is often embedded in interdisciplinary studies. For example, in one study, 244 patients aged 70 years and older were enrolled in a geriatric care program which used a geriatric resource-nurse intervention to improve the quality of care received by the hospitalized elderly. The intervention decreased patients' length of stay, and improved quality indicators (Inouye et al., 1993b). In another study, Kresevic and colleagues were able to demonstrate improved care through the use of an ACE (Acute Care of the Elderly) unit, in which protocols for skin care, urinary-incontinence management, and pressure-ulcer prevention were used (Palmer, Landefeld, Kresevic, & Kowal, 1994). This unit showed improved outcomes for the elderly.

Data for acute care are also found in research which looks at "nurse sensitive" indicators for patient outcomes. For example, hospital staff has been shown to make a difference in patient outcomes (Aiken, Sloane, Lake, Sochalski, & Weber, 1999; Kovner & Gergen, 1998). Nurse accountability and models of patient and nursing administration have also been examined (Mark, Salyer, Geddes, & Smith, 1998; Scherb, Rapp, Johnson, & Maas, 1998). These studies give us some information regarding outcomes for the elderly, but intensive effort needs to be focused on understanding the differences between outcomes for younger individuals versus older individuals in the case of hospital care. For example, do older adults have different cardiac output post-coronary artery bypass surgery than younger individuals when other variables are held constant, such as premorbid conditions? Such parameters are needed for the improvement of care for the elderly.

Historically, elders were not considered to be "suitable candidates" for surgeries and treatments that today are considered routine. In the early 1970s, individuals over the age of 65 were excluded from surgical intensive-care units, as it was felt that the cost-benefit was not going to be in the favor of the older patient. Today individuals in their 80s and 90s undergo open-heart surgery and require appropriate postoperative care that only a surgical intensive-care unit can provide.

Ethical issues abound regarding elders during a hospitalization. For example, if there is an insufficient number of beds in an intensive-care unit, should older individuals be sent out to the floor before younger individuals? Are scarce resources allocated to younger individuals before they are used to care for the elderly? Subjectively, many nurses will say these issues arise, and there are few supports (and little data) available to help them make decisions. Further, elder abuse, a serious and potentially fatal syndrome, is frequently overlooked when elders come into the hospital with severe symptoms, such as bilateral bruising, histories incompatible with injuries, and overt fear of caregivers. All of these issues are a part of acute care of the elderly, and need to be addressed with rigorous research studies. Replication of studies involving younger individuals need to be conducted in order to discern differences between the age cohorts.

TERRY FULMER

See also:
CARING

**CHRONIC ILLNESS
HEALTH CARE FINANCING ADMINISTRATION
HEALTH MAINTENANCE ORGANIZATION**

ADULT DAY CARE

Research strongly suggests adult day programs work well for their clients, are financially viable, and are a desired and accepted form of assistance (Strang & Neufeld, 1990; Reifler et al., 1997). Adult day programs have emerged slowly over the past four decades in the United States. The largest growth in programs occurred from 1970 to 1986 when numbers increased from 12 to 1200. The current financial, insurance, and healthcare climate demands that these programs objectively demonstrate positive financial and care outcomes (Eng, Pedulla, Eleazer, McCann, & Fox, 1997; Weinberger et al., 1993). Yet, the process of objective measurement remains a challenge.

An adult day program is a structured, community-based, group program designed to meet the assessed physical, emotional, and psychosocial needs of functionally limited older adults. These needs are met through individualized plans of care developed by an interdisciplinary team—e.g., nurse, social worker, therapist, recreation specialist, nutritionist, etc. Physicians function primarily as consultants to the team. Each client must have an identified physician for medical care, who is available to adult day staff for consultation and guidance. The nurse is in a position to coordinate, initiate, and implement complex plans of care with the other team members and to lead those activities.

Day programs are conducted in a variety of settings (freestanding, attached to a nursing home or hospital, community service agency or center, departments of aging, and area agencies on aging); each is uniquely designed depending upon its sponsorship, the composition and skills of its staff, and client need. Although many adult day centers began as safe places for older people to go during the day for socialization and activity, they have developed into places where health-care, in its broadest definition, is provided. In addition to providing physical nursing care to people, an activity that health professionals understand, can delineate and quantify, adult day programs have given people a sense of purpose, belonging, well-being, and improved self-esteem (Hunter, 1992). Nursing has a primary role in the development and operation of adult day care services. It is an excellent setting for the continued evolution of comprehensive geriatric nursing care.

A review of adult day-care literature reveals a paucity of research by nurses and other healthcare professionals in the field. The studies that have been conducted fall into several general categories: the economics of adult day care, e.g., entrepreneurial opportunities, cost of care; factors influencing usage of adult day care; structure of day programs; dementia care; and a few studies on the role of the nurse in adult day care. Since previous studies have demonstrated the difficulties of evaluating small day centers, which includes the majority of centers in the United States, coordination of large-scale, collaborative investigations supported by geriatric nursing research should be encouraged. Outcomes of care need to be defined and measured differently than they have been in the past in other healthcare settings. These new definitions will require broader thinking to insure a shift from traditional measurements of care to ones focusing on, for example, client function; client/caregiving satisfaction; and nutritional status.

Models of Adult Day Care

Three models of adult day programs have evolved in this country. They are: (a) the medical model serving individuals with high need for rehabilitative care due to serious illness and where the intensity of service may be time limited; (b) the long-term maintenance model focused on the mental and physical well-being of functionally limited older adults; and (c) the psychosocial model with less emphasis on physical health and more on psychosocial and emotional well-being. The core services in any adult day program include meals, transportation, activities, socialization opportunities, and supervision. The emphasis, focus, and/or expansion of these core services vary depending on the model and the particular program (Fulmer & Edelman, 1991).

Adult day programs serve individuals with a wide range of functional limitations due to dementia, mental and physical illness and developmental disabilities and assist families who are under enormous psychological and financial stress. Research has examined the role of the nurse practitioner in adult day care. According to Maddox (1992) the nurse practitioner can perform physical exams, complete comprehensive histories, evaluate and manage ongoing health problems, and provide acute episodic health care. The effect of exercise on function; quality-of-life issues; and assessment techniques have also been studied (Hunter, 1992; Rowe & Kahn, 1998).

Economics/Funding

The services provided in adult day programs and the definition of a program as a medical or social model have been influenced in large measure by the source and type of funding available. Initially, funds were provided by Title III of the 1965 Older Americans Act, social service block grants, and programs focused on social and recreational activities. In 1974, Medicaid funds became a source of revenue and adult day services became more medically oriented. In 1981, the Omnibus Budget Reconciliation Act encouraged community-based services for older adults and additional state Medicaid funds were used for adult day programs. Medicare monies have not and are not used for these services. Since public financing is limited, a multiplicity of grants, contributions, in kind services, and donations have supported adult day programs over the years. As the incidence of functional impairment, including dementia, has increased, research has focused on the cost of caring for people living in the community using adult day services versus those in long-term care facilities (Leon, Cheng, & Neumann, 1998). Capitated systems of care, such as the Program for All Inclusive Care of the Elderly (PACE), integrated health systems, and the introduction of long-term care insurance, will require continued study to determine the financial performance of adult day programs in a dynamic eldercare environment.

Future Directions

Adult day programs will continue to grow in size, diversity, and complexity in the years ahead. The provision of primary care services within them will increase. Consequently, new roles for the professional nurse will develop. Day centers will continue to define levels of care. The National Association of Adult Day Services (NADSA) Task Force began this process by delineating three levels of need. The programs that will survive and thrive will be those offering the broadest range of services from supportive to restorative care with attention to the social, emotional, physical, and spiritual needs of participants and caregivers.

Since nursing research should be guided by the problems or questions that occur in a particular healthcare setting, the potential for future research and its positive impact on nursing practice in the adult day setting is enormous (Resnick, 1999). Day programs allow for screening activities (hypertension, vision, hearing, cancer, dental, podiatry); prevention activities (immunization, nutrition assessment, exercise); evaluation of medications and treatments; education, support, guidance, and prompt attention to disease manifestations. Many unanswered questions may provide the basis for future nursing research: What are the effective methods for performing these activities? What is the cost benefit? What levels of nurse training are needed? How should nurses be educated? Which activities prevent unnecessary emergency department visits, contribute toward delay of institutionalization?

BARBARA W. ABRAHAM

See also:
   ACTIVITIES OF DAILY LIVING
   FUNCTIONAL HEALTH
   QUALITY OF LIFE
   RESPITE CARE

ADULT FOSTER CARE

In the past two decades, a proliferation of alternative housing options has occurred in the United States. Called by a variety of terms, these alternative settings provide varying degrees of assistance to the elder individual. One such setting, geriatric adult foster care, provides needed support services while allowing the older adult to remain in the community (Steinhauer, 1982). AFCs are the oldest form of alternative living arrangements, dating back to the Middle Ages (Braun, Horwitz, & Kaku, 1988; Linn, Klett, & Caffey, 1980; Sherman & Newman, 1977). Similar to assisted living facilities, regional variations exist regarding regulation and licensure. Depending upon the state, AFCs may be under the jurisdiction of none to several state agencies. Even in states that require licensing, variation exists in the minimum standards, delegated responsibility, and degree of enforcement (Steinhauer, 1982). Since most AFCs are private residences, it is unknown how many AFCs there currently are in the United States.

For the purposes of this review, the definition of an AFC home is a private home that is residentially zoned for a nonrelated, live-in caregiver. In general, AFCs limit the number of residents to no more than 5 individuals, although larger AFCs do exist. Often, an additional stipulation is that only one resident may be bedbound or require maximum assistance with care (Nyman, Finch, Kane, Kane, & Illson, 1997; Stark, Kane, Kane, & Finch, 1995; Steinhauer, 1982). A comprehensive literature search revealed 13 articles that were research-based, conducted in the United States, and met the definition of AFC homes. Most studies were descriptive designs or case reports.

Characteristics of Adult Foster Care Homes in the United States

Nine articles provided information on the characteristics of over 700 AFCs as either a primary or secondary aim (Braun, Horwitz, & Kaku, 1988;

Braun & Rose, 1986; Davis, 1982; Kane, Kane, Illston, Nyman, & Finch; 1991; Linn et al., 1980; Nyman et al., 1997; Oktay & Volland, 1987; Stark et al., 1995; Talmadge & Murphy, 1983). All of the AFCs were residential. Typically, most had fewer than 5 tenants, although upwards of 13 tenants were reported (Linn et al., 1980; Sherwood & Morris, 1983). Several programs designated that AFCs must provide a private bedroom (Davis, 1982; Oktay & Volladge, 1987) with access to a bathroom on the same floor as the bedroom (Davis, 1982). Depending upon the state, AFC caregivers could accept private pay, Medicaid payments, or both.

The basic service requirement of a live-in caregiver was a constant factor in the AFCs, regardless of where the AFC was located. Formal training of caregivers varied greatly, however. Kane and colleagues (1991) and Sherwood and Morris (1983) reported on foster home caregivers who participated in state programs from Oregon and Pennsylvania, respectively. Both reported that the majority of caregivers had no formal training. On the other hand, foster home caregivers who participated in programs linked to medical centers received formal training of up to 40 hours (Braun et al., 1988; Braun & Rose, 1986; Oktay & Volland, 1987; Talmadge & Murphy, 1983). This formal training included acquiring skills and knowledge related to personal care assistance, home health care, special diets, physical therapy, and psychosocial aspects of aging and illness. Additionally, some reported that up to 70% of the caregivers had some form of health-related employment (K. L. Braun et al., 1988; Braun & Rose, 1986).

Of interest, only two studies reported on children residing in the AFCs. Linn and colleagues (1980) reported that of the 191 individuals in 150 AFCs across five states, 43 (23%) lived in an AFC where children also resided. Braun and Rose (1986) reported that upwards of 78% of the individuals in Honolulu lived in an AFC with children.

As compared to nursing home facilities, Oregon AFCs provided more privacy in a homelike environment at a lower cost (Kane, Kane, Illston, Nyman, & Finch, 1991; Nyman et al., 1997). Unlike nursing home facilities, AFCs lacked physical rehabilitation services and organized activities.

Individual Preferences.   Physical, environmental, and social characteristics of a facility are important to older adults. Surveys of older adults from Oregon nursing homes and AFCs were conducted to determine factors influencing their choice of residence (Nyman et al., 1997). Significant characteristics influencing older adults' choice of an AFC were: homelike atmosphere, privacy, and flexibility in routines; whereas organized activities and the availability of physical rehabilitation were important to those who chose nursing homes.

Services Provided.   The articles reported a wide range of services, somewhat dependent on state versus medical center oriented programs (K. L. Braun et al., 1988; Braun & Rose, 1986; Hopp, 1999; Nyman et al., 1997; Oktay & Volland, 1987; Sherwood & Morris, 1983; Talmadge & Murphy, 1983). All provided room and board with 24-hour supervision. While all reported that formal caregivers provided personal care services, some described programs that trained caregivers to supervise medications including injections, provide special diets including tube feedings, bladder training, catheter irrigations, and dressing changes (Braun & Rose, 1986; Davis, 1982; Sherwood & Morris, 1983; Stark et al., 1995).

Characteristics of Individuals Served in Adult Foster Care

Seven articles described characteristics of individuals residing in AFCs as either a primary or secondary research aim (K. L. Braun et al., 1988; Braun & Rose, 1986; Davis, 1982; Hopp, 1999; Kane et al., 1991; Nyman et al., 1997; Oktay & Volland, 1987). Older adults in AFCs are typically older than 55 years with reported mean ages greater than 70 years (Davis, 1982; Oktay & Volland, 1987). AFC tenants were likely to be poor, single, living alone, and often rejected by family members (Oktay & Volland, 1987).

Tenants had fewer reported major health problems as compared to those in nursing homes, but this finding may reflect a reporting bias since nursing home personnel are more likely to have current medical histories of their residents (Kane et al., 1991). In spite of fewer reported health problems among those residing in AFCs, difficulties with managing IADL and ADL do exist. AFC residents requiring assistance with activities of daily living included 9%–78% requiring assistance with walking; 4%–58% requiring assistance with transferring; 12%–27% requiring assistance with dressing; 30%–51% requiring assistance with bathing; 4%–7% requiring assistance with eating; and 5%–70% requiring assistance with toileting (K. L. Braun et al., 1988; Braun & Rose, 1986; Hopp, 1999; Kane et al., 1991). Although a higher proportion of AFC residents as compared to nursing home residents are independent in ADL and IADL, significant overlap occurs. Not surprisingly, AFC residents are more likely to require assistance with IADL than ADL (Hopp, 1999). Last, it is not unusual for residents of AFCs to experience cognitive and/or behavioral deficits (Braun & Rose, 1986; Goodman, Pynoos, & Stevenson, 1988).

Outcomes of Those Served in AFCs

Several articles reported on outcomes of older adults residing in AFC facilities (Braun & Rose, 1986; K. L. Braun et al., 1988; Kane et al., 1991; Linn et al., 1980; Oktay & Volland, 1987; Sherwood & Morris, 1983; Stark et al., 1995). Reported outcomes included psychosocial well-being, functional abilities, and cost. AFCs affiliated with a medical center and formal caregiver training reported improved patient well-being, decreased anxiety, improvement in ADL function, and decreased cost compared to nursing homes (K. L. Braun et al., 1988; Braun & Rose, 1986; Braun & Rose, 1987; Oktay & Volland, 1987). Contrastingly, AFCs lacking affiliation with a medical center reported little to no improvement in ADL function (Kane et al., 1991; Sherwood & Morris, 1983; Stark et al., 1995). Moreover, Stark and colleagues (1995) reported that 49% of AFC residents had increased ADL dependency within the first year of admission to the AFC. Indeed, increasing personal care needs influenced whether residents could remain in an AFC (Goodman et al., 1988). Other personal factors influencing continued residency included whether the resident was likable and able to participate in the home; presence of family support; staff trained to provide services; and caregivers who felt that the care needed could legitimately be provided. AFC characteristics other than caregiver training found to be associated with positive outcomes included children residing in the AFC (Linn et al., 1980), caregivers who involved the older adults in activities (K. L. Braun et al., 1988; Linn et al., 1980), and caregivers who rated the variable "needed to work" as unimportant (Braun et al., 1988).

Future Directions

Review of the literature reveals that not only are there a variety of terms used to describe "adult foster care," but a standardized definition for adult foster care is lacking. Importantly, the lack of federal regulations impact the quality of care rendered and services provided. The articles reviewed demonstrated that regional variations exist among states regarding regulations, licensure, caregiver selection, and services provided. An aging population and longer life expectancies will put increased demands on alternative environments and caregivers to provide services to individuals with varying degrees of functional and cognitive impairments, as well as, psychosocial needs. Findings that older adults who reside in foster homes require personal assistance and have a significant decline within the first year of residency are troubling. The lack of knowledge and formal training of caregivers, the numerous terms and lack of a standardized definition of adult foster care including purpose and services provided, and the lack of federal regulations pose a number of issues. What is adult foster care and who would best benefit from this form of alternative living arrangement? What type of training should be required and resources made available to caregivers? What are the characteristics of caregivers that are associated with caregiver success and subsequent optimal resident outcomes? What types of services should be provided at a minimum by all adult foster care homes? Future research in these areas will assist policymakers and healthcare providers to best meet the needs of an aging population.

KATHLEEN A. ONDUS
LORRAINE C. MION

See also:
CAREGIVER
RESPITE CARE

ADVANCE DIRECTIVES: DECISION MAKING

Historically, nurses have played a crucial role in helping people and promoting patient choice. Patients and families look to "their" nurses for information, advice, and support when facing difficult health care decisions. This relationship offers unique privileges and responsibilities. The Code of Ethics of the American Nurses Association (ANA) states that nurses must support patient autonomy and provide care according to the patient's wishes (ANA, 1985). A survey of nurses conducted in 1994 by the ANA found that one of the most critical ethical issues facing nurses today is the end-of-life decision (ANA, 1997). Thus, advance directives are relevant to nurses. Advance directives, living wills, and the durable power of attorney for health care are mechanisms whereby individuals are able to exercise control over their bodies and direct the kind of care they want or do not want in the event that they lack decision-making capacity at the time a medical decision must be made. They affect nursing practice and have an impact on the ethical values of society at large.

A living will is a document that provides specific instructions to health care providers about the type of health care choices and treatment an individual would or would not want in order to prolong life. An individual may execute a living will to instruct health care professionals not to administer any "extraordinary treatment," "heroic treatment," "artificial treatment," or "life support" in the event of terminal illness. However, living wills also can be used to give instructions and/or directions about the kind of medical treatment an individual wants to have administered. Although most states recognize living wills, they are not recognized by statute in New York, Massachusetts, and Michigan.

A durable power of attorney for health care is a document that permits individuals to designate another person to make health care decisions for them should they lose decision-making capacity. The person appointed to make decisions is called a health care proxy, health care agent, attorney-in-fact, or surrogate.

Patient Self Determination Act

The Patient Self Determination Act (PSDA), a federal law effective December 1991, attempted to ensure that all patients are advised about their right to accept or refuse medical or surgical treatment and their right to execute an advance directive (Omnibus Budget Reconciliation Act of 1990, 1991). The intent of the act was to encourage early, full, and ongoing communication between health care professionals, patients, and families, when appropriate, about care at the end of life. All institutions that receive Medicare and Medicaid funding must advise patients about this right, document in the medical record whether the patient has an advance directive, implement advance directive policy, and provide staff and community education about advance directives. In addition, institutions are prohibited from refusing to provide care if an individual has not completed an advance directive.

Advance directives should become effective only when it is determined that the individual is incompetent and lacks decision-making capacity. As long as the patient retains decision-making capacity for the particular decision at hand, his or her decisions govern. When the patient is deemed to lack decision-making capacity, the surrogate decision maker is authorized to make all treatment decisions on behalf of the patient in accordance with the patient's stated wishes, whether rendered in writing or given verbally. However, in situations where the patient has never been competent and/or there is no clear and convincing evidence of what the person would have wanted, the surrogate decision maker will be called on to make decisions on the basis of what he or she believes is in the "best interest" of the patient.

Research to date on nurses' actions in facilitating patients' autonomous decision making and in implementing the PSDA is sparse. Mezey, Mitty, Rappaport, and Ramsey (1997) found that nurses are central to the implementation of the PSDA. Nurses disseminate advance directive materials, are responsible for asking whether the patient has an advance directive, and are involved in PSDA education to inform patients about their rights (Fleming & Scanlon, 1994; Wetle, Walker, & Blechner, 1994). A number of studies identified reasons that patients do or do not formulate advance directives (Berrio & Levesque, 1996; Cugliari, Miller, & Sobol, 1995; Mezey, Ramsey, Mitty, & Leitman, 1995). Reasons given by patient respondents for executing an advance directive are (a) wanting to make up their own mind, (b) feeling that it would help their families if they knew what was wanted, (c) having the peace of mind it would give, and (d) not wanting to be kept alive in a coma and with "tubes and wires." Reasons given by patients for not executing an advance directive were that (a) they needed more information, (b) their family would decide what to do, (c) their doctor would do what was right, (d) they never heard about advance directives, and (e) they want everything possible done.

Nursing research is needed on how nurses meet the letter and spirit of the PSDA to support patients' rights to make decisions about their health care. This research is necessary for informed ethical nursing practice. Important issues that should be explored include but are not limited to nurses' understanding about advance directives. What are the practical clinical implications for the use of living wills and durable powers of attorney for health care? What do these documents provide for and not provide for? How does this affect on the care of patients, particularly those who are terminally ill? What is the role of the nurse vis-á-vis the patient, family, and other members of the health care team? What is the role of the nurse in advance directive education for the surrogate decision makers?

Nurses play an important role in ongoing PSDA education, and part of the education should include the surrogate decision maker. This individual is thrust into the world of medical decision making and often is not provided with the information or is unable to comprehend—at that time—all that is necessary to make an informed choice. It is important to understand better how the nurse may further support surrogate decision makers. Further research is needed to determine how nurses might better assist patients, families, and surrogate decision makers to understand the medical and nursing treatments being proposed. It is imperative that individuals understand the language used and the treatments being proposed, to ensure that individuals are able to make informed decisions. Finally, further research is needed to determine the impact of race, culture, ethnicity, and religion on medical decision making of the patient, family, and nurse.

Today there are many more discussions about decision making and advance directives. Careful thinking, open communication, and further research are essential to foster a climate that is both supportive of and conducive to medical decision making. Nurses must continue to be part of this process, and nurse-based research, by and about nurses, will further that end.

Gloria C. Ramsey
Mathy Mezey

See also:
   AGEISM
   CHRONIC ILLNESS

END OF LIFE DECISION MAKING
QUALITY OF LIFE
TERMINAL ILLNESS

AGEISM

The majority of nurses will spend most of their careers caring for older adults in a variety of settings; nurses must continually examine their attitudes and role in the prevention of ageism. Older persons may be discriminated against because of the way they look, speak, or function in a society that values productivity, economic wealth, speed, youth, and beauty.

Ageism may be defined as a negative attitude or bias toward older people that can lead to a belief that older people cannot (or should not) participate in certain activities, or be given the same opportunities as younger persons (Holohan-Bell & Brummel-Smith, 1999). Ageism, according to geriatrician Robert Butler in his book, *Why Survive,* suggests that we have a deep and profound prejudice against older people (Butler, 1975).

This prejudice and stereotyping may lead to policies for rationing healthcare; withholding treatment based on age alone, a lack of qualified personnel to care for older adults, and the under-recognition of geriatric syndromes. Ageism may also be seen on a personal level when a nurse, or other healthcare worker, has low expectations of an older person's ability to perform a task. Ageism may lead staff to perceive that an older adult does not "know what is going on," and older individuals may be excluded from decision making regarding their own hospitalization and care.

Nursing research in ageism has centered on several main areas including education, student and practicing nurses' attitudes, sociopolitical issues, and clinical-care issues. Several early studies have highlighted the problems of student attitudes toward aging and care of the older adult, the lack of trained professionals in gerontology, and the need for more research in gerontology. These studies have utilized both qualitative and quantitative techniques including meta-analysis, survey research, cross-sectional studies, ethnographic research, and randomized clinical trials.

A 1981 review of geriatric nursing research articles (1977–1980) from the *Western Journal of Nursing Research, Research in Nursing and Health,* the *Journal of Gerontological Nursing,* and *Geriatric Nursing* found only 44 research articles. The author recommended several courses of action to increase nursing research and improve quality of care, including: increasing gerontological nursing curriculum in all schools of nursing, preparing nurse practitioners for leadership roles, and starting actions to make the salaries of nurses in nursing homes equal to the salaries of nurses in acute-care hospitals (Kayser-Jones, 1981a, p. 222). Mezey and others recommended strategies for attracting staff and faculty to work with older adults (Mezey, 1988; Johnson & Connelly, 1990; Yurchuck & Brower, 1994).

Brower and others have analyzed variables related to working with older adults and attitudes toward them (Brower, 1981; Kayser & Minnegerode, 1975; Tuckman & Lorge, 1976). In a study of 581 registered nurses, the investigator found that hospital nurses spent less time with the elderly than did RNs in nursing homes and home care, and among older nurses higher education (bachelor's and master's degrees) was associated with more favorable attitudes toward the elderly (Brower, 1985). Generally, studies have conflicted in their findings of whether age, length of time working with elders, and education influenced attitudes toward the elderly (Campbell, 1971; Futrell & Jones, 1977; Haight, Christ, & Diaz, 1994; Prevost, Wilson, & Gerber, 1991; Taylor & Harned, 1978; Smith, Jepson, & Perloff, 1982). However, studies have agreed that past experiences with the elderly, and faculty role models affect attitudes (Chaisson, 1980; Fox & Wold, 1996; Penner, Ludenia, & Mead, 1984; Whilhite & Johnson, 1976).

Both the availability of government funding for gerontological nurse traineeships and innovative teaching models in the early 1980s have increased the number of trained professionals and has influenced the attitudes of both student nurses and practicing nurses. A Delphi study with on-site interviews indicated one of the most important results of the Robert Wood Johnson Teaching Nursing Home Project (TNHP) was, "improving graduate and undergraduate students' attitudes toward the elderly and aging" (McCracken & Torgerson, 1994; Mezey, Lynaugh, & Cartier 1988, p. 286).

Kayser-Jones, who is both a nurse and medical anthropologist, has done much to advance our understanding of ageism, ranging from her early qualitative research on living conditions in nursing homes to her most recent studies on eating problems in nursing homes. In her first book, *Old, Alone, and Neglected,* she studied and compared conditions in nursing homes in the United States and Scotland, and focused on the three themes of depersonalization, dehumanization, and victimization. In her studies on the treatment of acute illness in nursing homes and on eating problems in nursing homes she again illustrates the danger of undertreating problems in the elderly, making judgments based on age alone, and stresses the importance of individualized care and adequate staffing in nursing homes (Kayser-Jones, 1996, 1997).

Other studies on ageism have focused on the prejudice against older women in our society (Bernard, 1998; Blair & White, 1998; Estes, 1979; McCracken, 1994). Bernard (1998) reported on the results of a questionnaire completed by 41 female nurses in the UK, and found that many professional caregivers of older adults feared growing older and looking and feeling older. She concluded that, as a predominantly female profession, we must be more involved in improving older women's lives, and in engaging in discussions with older women about what is important to them (Bernard, 1998, pp. 636–639).

Ageism is related to many other areas of clinical and health-services research. The older population that is at the greatest risk for prejudice and stereotyping are persons with mental illness, dementia, and mental retardation. The diagnosis of dementia often stigmatizes both the patient and the family. Research by Beck and others has helped to explain aggressive behaviors in persons with dementia by illustrating the need for individualized care and behavioral-systems theory to understand aggression in Alzheimer's disease patients, has promoted autonomy and personal control in the care of persons with dementia, and has highlighted the need for greater resources to care for older adults with mental illness (Beck et al., 1997; Buckwalter, Maas, & Reed, 1997; Rice, Beck, & Stevenson, 1997; Sherrell, Anderson, & Buckwalter, 1998).

Research on the prevalence and factors related to restraint use, the quality of life in persons with dementia, the quality of care of the frail and vulnerable older adult, and barriers to the recognition of delirium that are superimposed on dementia have recently advanced our understanding of persons with dementia, and have exposed myths often held about this population (Brod, Stewart, & Sands, 1999; Evans et al., 1997; Fick, 1997; Fick & Foreman, in press; Frengley & Mion, 1998; Mezey & Fulmer, 1998; Minnick, Mion, Leipzig, Lamb, & Palmer, 1998; Sherrell & Buckwalter, 1997; Strumpf & Evans, 1988; Volicer, Hurley, & Camberg, 1999). This research is important, as it forces us to reexamine stereotypes we have held about older persons with dementia, and influences both the care and treatment of older persons.

Despite the research on ageism, it is still prevalent in our society, and often leads to the stigmatizing and devaluing of older persons and those that work with and care for older adults. However, progress has been made in increasing both the number of trained faculty in gerontology, and the number of programs addressing care of and attitudes toward the elderly. A 1999 study of 480 baccalaureate nursing programs found that almost 40% of programs had at least one full-time faculty member with ANA certification in gerontology (Rosenfeld, Bottrell, Fulmer, & Mezey, 1999). In addition, there are presently several schools of nursing and granting agencies that are combining their efforts to advance the care of older adults in acute-care and community settings, and reverse stereotypes about caring for older adults and being old.

These programs are promoting positive attitudes toward older adults by showcasing geriatric nursing as a challenging and attractive specialty for practicing nurses, bringing national attention to nursing care of the elderly, reaching out to hospital, home-care, and nursing-home nurses, and illustrating the need for more advanced practice nurses, and more basic gerontology content in baccalaureate nursing programs (Abraham et al., 1999; Fulmer & Abraham, 1998; Titler & Mentes, 1999).

Ageism will continue to be important to almost every area of geriatric nursing research. Ageism will influence both the type of research that is done and the public dissemination of research. As researchers we must describe the relationship of ageism with qualitative and quantitative research in the areas of ethics, workplace studies, decision-making and informed consent research, genetics, health promotion and preventive screening, cancer, presentations of disease, symptom research, quality-of-life, barriers to treatment, nursing-home care and organizational studies, resource utilization in healthcare, dementia care, mental health, and the care of the disabled older adult.

Nursing has had a vital role in combating ageism, and continues to be in a key position to minimize ageist attitudes in the future. Nurses must be prominent in other related arenas that challenge the stereotypes of aging and promote appropriate views and care of older adults, including: (a) better pay for those who care for older adults in long-term and community settings; (b) better policies for caregivers in the workplace; (c) improved gerontological content in nursing and medical school programs; and (d) continued research funds for investigating the unique problems of aging and disease.

Donna Fick

See also:
ETHICAL DECISION MAKING
QUALITY OF LIFE

ALZHEIMER'S DISEASE: SPECIAL CARE UNITS IN LONG-TERM CARE

Following "transinstitutionalization" of persons with dementia from state mental hospitals to community nursing homes in the 1960s and 1970s, Coons (1983), Danford (1982), and Lawton (1975) pioneered the study of the effects of the environment on behavior among the demented. Their work influenced investigations of rehabilitative interventions (e.g., reality orientation, pet and music therapies, and behavioral and psychotherapies) designed to improve care for institutionalized persons with dementia. One result was the suggestion by nurses and others that integrating demented and nondemented residents may violate the rights of both parties and jeopardize quality of life and safety.

Special care units (SCU) in nursing homes for persons with Alzheimer's disease (AD) and related dementing disorders emerged rapidly in the 1980s. AD is the most prevalent type of dementia; however, the disease cannot be definitively diagnosed prior to autopsy. More than one cause of dementia often afflicts an individual, and persons with all types present many of the same care problems. For these reasons, SCUs usually serve persons with dementias of all types. Currently about 15% of nursing homes in the United States have an SCU. The number of SCUs may continue to increase for two or three decades because of growth in the number of elderly, the public's perception that SCU care is superior to traditional nursing home care, and the likelihood that SCUs will be profitable. However, other options for care, such as assisted living facilities, offer a lower cost advantage and may curtail the growth of SCUs.

Five key features are recognized as characterizing an SCU: (1) admission of residents with dementia, (2) special staff specification, selection, and training, (3) activity programming tailored to residents with dementia, (4) family programming and involvement, and (5) a segregated and modified physical and social environment. Although there is substantial consensus that these five features distinguish SCUs, there is disagreement about the specific nature of special programming, staffing, and services.

Care of persons with dementia and their families in all settings is an important aspect of gerontological and geropsychiatric nursing research as well as a National Institute for Nursing Research (NINR) priority. Leading nurse researchers in the care of persons with dementia on SCUs are Buckwalter, Maas, Hall, Matthew, and Ryden. Other researchers, primarily supported by NINR and the National Institute of Aging, also study SCUs.

Studies of Special Care Units

Hall and Buckwalter's (1987) progressively lowered stress threshold (PLST) model provided the conceptual framework for the development of many SCUs and for research to evaluate their effects. Descriptive studies have documented the characteristics of nursing homes that offer SCUs. State and regional surveys provide detailed information about the programs and practices of SCUs in particular geographic areas, and national surveys contribute information about structures, programming, and staffing that are characteristic of nursing facilities and SCUs nationwide. Survey results are limited by methodological differences that restrict comparisons.

Most early evaluative studies conducted by nurse researchers and others were single group efforts that assessed selected characteristics of residents with AD, family members, and staff at intervals before and after SCU admission. These studies documented some positive outcomes, including decreased nighttime wakefulness, improved hygiene, and weight gain in residents. Only half of the studies found improvement in resident physical function and behavioral symptoms. Confidence in these studies is compromised by small sample size, lack of rigor in design, potential researcher bias, and unclear outcome measure definitions.

Other studies compared outcomes for residents with dementia on a SCU with those in another setting, measuring selected characteristics of residents, family members, and staff caregivers at intervals. Only two studies revealed significant benefits for residents on the SCUs, contrasted with comparison residents, noting less functional decline (Rovner, Lucas-Blaustein, Folstein, & Smith, 1990), fewer catastrophic reactions, and increased social interaction (Maas & Buckwalter, 1990). Results for family members also were mixed, with one study finding significant decreases in feelings of depression, anxiety, guilt, and grief compared to family members in the control group (Wells & Jorm, 1987). Only one study found statistically significant reductions in staff stress and burnout and a statistically significant increase in job satisfaction (Maas & Buckwalter, 1990).

In 1991 the NIA Special Care Units Initiative supported 10 studies for 5 years to systematically study the characteristics and effects of SCUs. Preliminary results indicated few benefits for residents and family members or differences in costs of care in SCUs versus other settings. Staff caregivers, however, continue to report that persons with AD are better cared for and that staff can provide care more easily on SCUs (Work Group on Research and Evaluation of SCUs, 1996). Some investigators suggest that current instruments used in SCU research are inadequate to measure these staff perceptions.

Another group of studies measured specific interventions or modifications of SCUs rather than the SCU strategy as a whole. Nursing studies of pet therapy, music therapy, bathing, dressing, eating assistance, wandering deterrent strategies, specific environmental modifications, and staff training are among the interventions that have been systematically tested with positive effects for demented residents. Interventions to assist family members with their caregiving roles on SCUs also are being tested (Maas, Swanson, Reed, & Specht, 1996).

Large national nursing home data bases are now used to describe characteristics of facilities and SCUs and to study the cost of care on SCUs versus care on traditional nursing home units. Results support the findings from other studies that the cost of care on SCUs is comparable to costs on other units.

Issues in SCU Research

SCU field research is fraught with methodological problems that make achieving and maintaining rigorous study designs difficult. Potential sources of bias are inherent in the selection of study sites; resident, family, and staff subjects; and outcome measures. Overall better care in nonprofit versus for-profit homes, irrespective of the SCU, may explain results. Newer SCUs may have less impaired residents, and turnover of staff is greater. Differences in SCU size, nature of the environment, type of programming, admission and discharge policies, the nursing care delivery system, staff ratios and staff mix, and the type and amount of staff training are some additional variables that influence outcomes. Administrators, clinicians, and family members usually determine whether or not a resident is placed on an SCU and may disrupt randomization by transfer of residents or staff. Residents are seldom randomly assigned to treatment groups within facilities because of contamination issues. Family members are assigned to groups because of their relationships to residents and staff by administrative decision. Subject attrition is a huge problem. Most studies employ quasi-experimental designs with nonequivalent control groups at the outset or experiments become quasi-experiments due to subject attrition. The myriad of resident, family, and staff characteristics, such as comorbidity, type of dementia, health, or education, pose measurement challenges.

Although development of standardized resident, family, and staff outcome measures has progressed, measures that capture clinically meaningful change may not be available due to floor or ceiling effects or inadequate sensitivity and validity with ethnic minority populations.

Summary and Future Research Recommendations

To date, research by nurses and others has not clearly established the efficacy of SCUs for residents with dementia, family members, or staff caregivers. Efforts to systematically document the cost effectiveness of SCUs also have not yielded clear results. The few positive findings from studies are counter to the prevailing views of nursing home providers and consumers. Most staff members believe that SCUs benefit residents and families as well as staff, who find it easier to care for demented residents on SCUs. Future nursing research must focus on documenting what is special about SCU care; refining measures of the SCU environment and programming; developing more sensitive outcome measures for residents, families, and staff; conducting larger multisite studies; evaluating the SCU strategy with minority populations; and using existing national datasets to analyze cost effectiveness.

MERIDEAN L. MAAS
JANET P. SPECHT

See also:
ALZHEIMER'S DISEASE
DEMENTIA CARE
NEUROBEHAVIORAL DISTURBANCES OF THE OLDER ADULT:
  DELERIUM AND DEMENTIA
PHYSICAL RESTRAINTS FOR THE ELDERLY

ASSISTED LIVING FACILITIES

The philosophy of using the physical environment to normalize the function of the older adult was developed in the 1960s. One such environment, the assisted living facility (ALF), has experienced a phenomenal growth in the past two decades. Rarely found in the United States in 1980, there are now over 30,000 ALFs in the United States (Meyer, 1998). No federal regulatory body oversees ALFs, and degree of oversight varies from none to licensing and oversight by a state department of health.

Designed to promote or delay institutionalization, assisted living facilities have been called numerous other names including residential-care facilities, homes for the aged, continuing care retirement communities, and congregate-care homes. For the purposes of this review, an assisted living facility (ALF) is defined as a special combination of housing, supportive services, personalized assistance, and healthcare designed to respond to the individual needs of those who need help with activities of daily living (ADL) and instrumental activities of daily living (IADL) (Assisted Living Federation of America [ALFA], 1997).

The comprehensive review of the literature revealed 25 research-based articles that were conducted in the United States and met the ALFA (1997) definition, with two modifications. Facilities must have had 10 or more residents (to distinguish from adult foster care homes) and, for articles predating the 1997 definition, the criterion for 24-hour availability of supportive services was waived.

Characteristics of ALFs in the United States

Sixteen articles described the characteristics (type, environmental characteristics, service provision) as either a primary or secondary research aim.

Major findings are summarized below and citations provided only when the information presented is pertinent to one or two articles.

The majority of ALFs are for-profit facilities and chain ownership is not uncommon. Size of facility can vary greatly, accommodating as few as 10 tenants to over 350 tenants. ALFs also vary on physical layout; they can be freestanding facilities or attached to other complexes, such as nursing homes. Moreover, ALFs can be residential and homelike in nature or be multistoried apartment buildings that can have an institutional nature.

Surveys revealed that while basic services, such as meals, transportation, housekeeping, and laundry, were similarly available at ALFs, the degree to which these services were provided ranged considerably (Kalymun, 1990; Kane & Wilson, 1993). Although services beyond a basic package had additional costs, ALFs still offer a considerable savings when comparable costs were analyzed in the long-term care settings (Heumann, 1991). Few sites appeared to have medication management (Crutchfield, 1999; Williams et al., 1999) or specific programs for dementia care (Forbes, 1997). If provided, these additional services required additional staff and modification of the physical environmental features of the typical ALF.

Preferences for ALF characteristics did not differ among older adults residing in ALFs as compared to those residing in the community; these included safety features, such as a method to summon help, transportation services, and social activities (Brennan, Moos, & Lemke,1988). Interestingly, experts emphasized the desirability of physical environmental characteristics.

When examining physicians' knowledge of community geriatric services, Damron-Rodriguez and colleagues (1998) reported that few physicians understood ALF characteristics, such as that most ALFs require self-pay. Moreover, most surveyed physicians confused the level of care between ALFs and nursing homes.

Common Characteristics of Older Adults Residing in ALFs

Several articles described the characteristics of older adults residing in ALFs or compared them to those residing in the community or nursing home. Characteristics can be broadly categorized as sociodemographic, physical function, cognitive function, and psychosocial characteristics.

The assisted living resident is typically white (90%), female (75%), and 80 years old or older. Most are single, either widowed or never been married (90%), and were living alone before entering assisted living (85%). Since ALFs typically cost greater than $1,000 per month, most residents are in the middle to upper income bracket. The exception to this is in states, such as Oregon, that use public monies to support elderly residents. Many had been professionals (Kane & Wilson, 1993; Yee, Capitman, Leutz, & Sceigaj, 1999). Although most authors agreed that assisted living is for the frail elderly, these individuals were poorly or variably described. Yee and colleagues (1999) found that the assisted living residents needed assistance with an average of one ADL and four IADL. Kane and Wilson (1993) noted a higher level of disability in Oregon assisted living facilities where state policy encourages assisted living as an alternative to nursing home care. Most facilities reported that many of their residents have mild memory impairment and some have moderate impairment. Those residents which staff found most difficult were those with behavior problems. Indeed, Kane and Wilson (1993) reported that in 63 ALFs, 36 had tenants move out because of behavior problems.

Outcomes and Their Associated Characteristics of Older Adults Residing in ALFs

Several articles reported on outcomes of older adults residing in ALFs or examined characteristics of the facility and/or of the older adult associated with the outcome(s). Most of these articles examined the significant influences on the person's adjustment to relocation and/or satisfaction with the ALF. These influences can be categorized by resident characteristics or perspectives and by the ALF housing model characteristics. Residents who had greater choice in deciding their living arrangement, higher self-health ratings, or greater sense of control with their lives had better adjustment to the ALF environment (Armer, 1993; Parr, Green, & Behncke, 1989; Yee et al., 1999). Residential housing models were beneficial if found to fit or match the older adult's preference (Mor, Sherwood, & Gutkin, 1986).

Availability of services impacted the length of residency in an ALF. Those ALFs that provided additional services allowed for residents to age in place and avoided nursing home placement (Bowers, 1989; Lawton, Moss, & Grimes, 1985; Thompson, 1994). Of note, optimal outcomes are closely linked with the resident's financial ability to buy more services as the need arises. Study findings were inconsistent, however, on whether ALFs could improve or sustain physical and ADL functioning.

Lack of federal oversight and varying state regulations regarding the physical environment, service provision, and staff to resident ratio in assisted living facilities lead to inconsistent standards and quality of care. Indeed, the few studies available demonstrate that services vary among ALFs. The lack of standardized services is especially worrisome given the evidence that a significant proportion of ALF residents demonstrate similar physical, psychosocial, and cognitive needs as nursing home residents. The dearth of studies in this area, evidence of health care providers' lack of knowledge and confusion regarding ALFs' purpose and scope of services, the numerous terms used to describe various alternative living arrangements, and lack of regulatory oversight necessitate examining a number of questions. Who would benefit best from assisted living environments? At what point would the older adult be better served in a more protective but less homelike environment, such as a nursing home setting, taking into account autonomy, privacy, cost, and safety? What services should be provided at a minimum by all assisted living facilities? What are the features of various alternative housing arrangements that can differentiate the levels of care, for example residential home versus assisted living facility?

Findings from studying these questions will assist healthcare providers and policymakers in determining strategies to best suit the needs of an increasingly aging population.

Mary Hujer
Arlene Mann
Lorraine C. Mion

See also:
> **ACTIVITIES OF DAILY LIVING**
> **CAREGIVER**
> **FUNCTIONAL HEALTH**
> **MOBILITY**
> **QUALITY OF LIFE**

CAREGIVER

The term *caregiver* is defined as the individual who assists ill persons, helps with a patient's physical care, typically lives with the patient, and does not receive monetary compensation for the help. A more descriptive definition of a caregiver is a person who not only performs common caregiver responsibilities of providing physical, social, spiritual, nursing, and technical care but also advocates for the ill person within health care systems and society as a whole.

The caregiver role is often expected and prepared for in relationship to elders, but rarely is there preparation for caregiving to one's child (ventilator-dependent children) or one's spouse (technological dependency on lifelong hemodialysis or total parenteral nutrition). The caregiver's relationship with the patient, the caregiver's age and developmental stage, the patient's illness severity, the suddenness and amount of the change in the patient's need for caregiving have been predictive of caregiver burnout in various illness populations such as cancer care with home chemotherapy, cardiac rehabilitation, muscle deterioration, and disease victims (Biegel, Sales, & Schulz, 1991).

Defining the role and tasks taken on by a caregiver gives a much better description of the daily lives and potential problems these individuals experience. The typical role of the caregiver includes direct patient care, familial and societal responsibilities, and financial management of the home and medical care. Complex decisions must be made about finances, as well as deciding daily about the patient's status. Direct patient care is much more than physical care. It also necessitates learning large amounts of information about illness, symptoms, medications, and technological treatments and about how to relate to health care professionals (Smith, 1995). Caregivers also must be prepared for and able to respond to emergencies. Familial or household responsibilities include continuing the caregiver's life tasks, whether as breadwinner, housekeeper, or both. Caregivers also have many indirect activities related to direct care, such as establishing a care schedule, maintaining the inventory of supplies, and negotiating with third-party payers.

The indirect familial caregiver tasks include designating others to assist with patient care and other familial tasks, communication and exchanging information, and maintaining decision making among appropriate persons. Societal expectations of caregivers are assuming financial costs, planning for long-term care, and advocating for the patient's best interest. Society also expects caregivers to be knowledgeable about health services and reimbursement mechanisms (i.e., being their own case managers) to ensure effective yet efficient care. Caregivers also have numerous expectations for themselves and from others around them to perform various psychosocial tasks such as coping with changes in role, grieving the loss of health and personality of their loved one, releasing tension, resolving uncertainty or guilt, and providing positive regard for those with whom they interact.

Because the caregiver definition is laden with tasks and expectations, it is no wonder that the major area of research has been caregiver burden, measured as both subjective and objective strain. The majority of burden studies have been descriptive and correlational and have resulted in identification of multiple factors associated with caregiver burden. Major factors recognized as being significant for burden are the characteristics of the care needed by the patient, which are often measured as illness demands. Numerous demographic, life developmental stage, and social support variables have been studied in relation to caregiver burden (Braithwaite, 1992). Findings vary from study to study, but individual variables, such as gender, psychosocial adjustment, other life stressors, and the meaning of the care-giving experience to the individual, are influential yet not universally pre-dictive of caregiver burden (Biegel, Sales, & Schulz, 1991).

Historically, research on the topic of caregivers has come from the literature on aging in which burden and supportive interventions have been studied. Interventions tested include teaching mastery of caregiving tasks, social interventions such as support groups or telephone contacts, and direct clinical services such as counseling and respite care. Outcomes of many of these intervention studies indicated that, in the short term, the interventions may reduce caregiver stress in a limited way, but the burden returns when the interventions stop. Research with midlife caregivers re-veals the need for interventions on resource management (Smith, 1994b) and motivation to help (Smith, 1994a). Further research is needed to test more interventions and match the timing of the intervention with the developmental life stage of the caregiver.

Research should continue on the culturally related aspects of caregiving strategies used in various ethnic groups (Picot, 1995). Another contempo-rary focus in caregiving research should be the caregiving family, as research has clearly indicated that multiple members of families are involved in providing direct and indirect care both to the patient and in support of the primary caregiver (Smith, 1996). In addition to the caregiving family, the caregiving neighborhood or parish should be a focus of study. In some countries giving care is a way of life that extends to friends, neighbors, and society. In the Netherlands the term *mantlezorh* is used to define caregiving. This term is translated as the "care cloak," protecting not only the patient but also the caregiver. In this country, Share the Care, a program designed for the care of people with cancer, is an example of *mantlezork* (Capossela & Warnock, 1995).

Carol E. Smith

See also:
CARING
CERTIFIED NURSING ASSISTANTS
FAMILY CAREGIVING TO FRAIL ELDERS
FOSTER CARE
RESPITE CARE

CARING

There has been heightened interest in the concept of caring over the past 20 years. Many noted nurse theorists/philosophers and authors have written about the central role caring plays in our nursing ethic. Philosophy, theory, research, and practice models have emerged. Definitions of caring generally comprise five major conceptualizations (Watson, in press): caring as (a) a human trait, (b) a moral imperative, (c) an affect, (d) an interpersonal interaction, and (e) a clinical intervention. Research and theories of caring have come from many other fields, including feminist studies, sociology, education, philosophy, religious studies, ministry, ethics, arts, and humanities. Larson and Ferketich (1993) state, "Caring is defined as intentional actions that convey physical care and emotional concern and promote a sense of safeness and security in another" (p. 690). Swanson (in press) further defines caring as "a nurturing way of relating to a valued other toward whom one feels a personal sense of commitment and responsibility."

Several noted authors have conducted extensive reviews of the literature and specifically the research literature addressing caring (Sherwood, 1997; Swanson, in press; Watson, in press). Most of the authors in this field concur that the state of the science at this time is based on a very respectable amount of single, independent studies that identify and describe. The vast majority of the literature is qualitative in nature, describing caring as a concept, behavior, attitude, environment, or process. However, some focused attention has been given to instrument development and testing to measure this multidimensional phenomena (Center for Human Caring, 1997), with most attempting to describe caring behaviors, attitudes, or skills of nurses or student nurses.

Sherwood (1997) conducted a meta-analysis of 16 qualitative caring research studies in nursing. She described four patterns in the description of nurses' caring from the patient's perspective: interaction, knowledge, intentional response, and therapeutic outcomes. Those patterns, with explanatory themes, defined caring within the content, context, process, and outcomes related to therapeutic or healing outcomes. Two types of caring knowledge content and skills were found: person and technical-physical. Sherwood recommends that this review provides the structure to define therapeutics of caring operationally, providing a foundation and direction for future research.

Swanson (in press) conducted a literary meta-analysis of published nursing research on the concept of caring and to propose a framework. This quantitative analysis encompasses the review of over 130 caring research articles on empirical outcomes from 1980 to 1996. Her findings were congruent with Sherwood's data. The data collection was from a variety of sources: patient charts, observations of practice, and surveys or interviews of patients, families, nurses, students, teachers, and other health care professionals. The relationships investigated included nurse-colleagues, nurse-patient/family, student-teacher, student-student, student-patients, health care provider–patient/family, and family caregiver–family member. Research findings were categorized into five hierarchical levels: capacity, commitment/concern, conditions, caring actions, and consequences. Level I comprises characteristics of persons with the *capacity* for caring, whether inherent or environmentally enhanced or diminished. Level II, *concerns/ commitment,* focuses on beliefs and values that undergird caring actions. Level III describes *conditions:* patient-, nurse-, and organization-related circumstances that enhance or diminish the likelihood that caring will occur. Level IV describes *caring actions,* behaviors, or therapeutics. Level V focuses on *consequences of caring,* those intentional and unintentional outcomes of caring for provider and/or recipients of care.

The review of full texts, book chapters, and published theoretical and research articles over the past 16 years provides an inclusive repository of substantive knowledge developed toward the ongoing investigation of caring. Several criticisms have been levied about the state of the research to date. Some authors have raised the questions concerning the fact that, given the changes in health care today, with the relocation of patients to homes and community settings, a vast majority of the studies of nurses, patients, and students has taken place in acute care settings, with acutely ill clients. Future research should be conducted on community-based aspects of care and on recipients of care who are dealing with chronic or end-of-life issues. It is hypothesized that the responses and outcome findings will be vastly different in these populations. Questions about instrument development to date also have been raised. How can there be ontological congruence within instruments developed to measure a construct like caring with strategies such as forced choice, which violate basic tenets of a caring philosophy? Other authors express concern that our research is too individual, small, isolated, and focused and that it is time to move it forward.

The work of Sherwood (1997), Swanson (in press), and Watson (in press) all provide guidance for future directions for research. The assessment understanding of caring through a merging of qualitative and quantitative, data-based nursing studies will play a major role in specifying the processes and interventions resulting in critical patient care outcomes. This work is consistent with public demands for health care reforms and can provide a foundation and direction for practitioners in the 21st century. Given the state of knowledge to date, it is time to move toward more sound empirical nursing science studies that can ground our practice and demonstrate measurably improved outcomes.

Swanson (in press) suggests that investigations be directed toward areas such as (a) development of measures that quantify caring capacity; (b) examination of the effects of nurturing and experience on caring capacity; (c) development of measures to quantify conditions that may be competing variables when investigating links between caring actions and their outcomes; (d) moving investigations from the individual as unit of analysis to the study of aggregates; (e) development of clinical trials for the refinement of protocols for caring-based therapeutics toward tested effectiveness in promoting healthy outcomes; and further (f) caring as a measurable commodity in the promotion of health and well-being. Strategies of investigation that aim at new conceptualizations and models that explain, predict, and prescribe may lead to instrument development that will further our knowledge of effective caring and healing therapeutic interventions toward a mid-range, evidenced-based model of caring praxis.

SALLY PHILLIPS

See also:
   ACUTE CARE
   CAREGIVER

CERTIFICATION IN GERONTOLOGICAL NURSING

The American Nurses Credentialing Center (ANCC) randomly surveyed 1,040 Americans who expressed concern about quality healthcare. They found that 87% of those surveyed would feel more confident if nurses were board-certified specialists (ANCC, 1999).

Currently ANCC is the only certifying body specific to gerontological nursing. ANCC has been certifying nurses since 1973. Originally established by the American Nurses Association (ANA), the ANCC is now a separate corporation offering certification in 30 different specialty areas. The ANA Congress of Nursing Practice Standards guides the credentialing process. In 1991 the American Board of Nursing Specialties (ABNS), a national peer review program, was formed to ensure uniform standards for specialty nursing certifications. Both the ANCC and ABNS advocate for consumer protection by committing certified nurses to professional standards set by national nursing leaders.

Why is certification important? Licensure is a legal process that assures minimal competencies to those who practice nursing. Certification, a professional process, builds on that base toward excellence. Nurses who have met eligibility requirements, which are briefly discussed below, may take certification exams. It is through this certification process that nurses seek excellence in practice. The exam is not the end of the process, because nurses must maintain certification status by meeting continuing education requirements. Achieving excellence is a lifelong process.

Nurses who hold a baccalaureate (or higher degree) in nursing may be eligible for certification. The baccalaureate degree requirement began in 1998 as an effort to promote higher standards and uniformity. Candidates for the geriatric certification exam must have a minimum of 4,000 hours of gerontological nursing practice (2,000 hours must have been within the past two years). Eligibility requirements also include 30 hours of geriatric-focused continuing education. Currently there are over 21,000 certified gerontological nurses (ANCC, October 3, 1998). As of 1997 the majority of these nurses were employed in long-term care, hospitals, and home health.

Candidates seeking certification as Clinical Specialists in Gerontological Nursing must be licensed RNs with a master's or higher degree in nursing, with gerontological specialization. In addition, nurses must have practiced for one year following master's degree completion. There also must be recent patient care experience. These specialized nurses are considered expert in gerontological nursing, as is evidenced by their extensive knowledge of aging issues. Areas where specialists are employed include, but are not limited to, case management, education, consultation, research, and administration. Currently there are approximately 1,000 certified gerontological specialists (ANCC, Oct. 3, 1998).

Gerontological Nurse Practitioner (GNP)

The American Association of Colleges of Nursing encourages certification to aid in the regulation of advanced practice nurses (APN'S). Presently, APN practice requirements vary by state. For example, some states allow GNPs to practice without certification, while others require certification for practice. Certification is often a requirement in receiving reimbursement by third party insurers. GNP candidates must be licensed RNs possessing a master's or higher degree in nursing, with formalized education in preparation as a geriatric nurse practitioner. Approximately 3,000 GNPs are certified (ANCC, Oct. 3, 1998).

Continuing Nursing Education (CNE) is vital to achieving and maintaining certification status; criteria are available from ANCC. It is by CNE that high-level care can be achieved. ANA provides a position statement, providing guidelines for CNE, so nurses are assured quality educational programs. "The purpose of CNE is to build upon the educational and experiential bases of the professional nurse for the enhancement of practice, education, administration, research or theory development to the end of improving the health of the public" (ANA, 1997).

ANCC (Credenitaling News, Spring 1998a) conducted an informal survey examining the financial benefits of certification. Self-selected respondents (N = 152) reported monetary reward for obtaining certification status

(57%) ranging from the reimbursement of certification expenses to salary increases, with increases between $500 and $3,000 per year. In addition to providing financial information, responses included "personal satisfaction, gratification, pride, self-esteem, enhanced patient care, career development, peer recognition, professional credibility."

Certification research is in its early stages. ANCC has developed an Institute for Research, Education, and Consultation (IREC) to explore unanswered questions about nursing credentials. IREC is in the process of evaluating all credentialing agencies to have a better understanding of the certified nurse workforce. An initiative of IREC, the Nursing Credentialing Research Coalition (NCRC) is to "develop common demographic data sets for certified nurses; investigate whether practice outcomes vary between certified and noncertified nurses; examine the costs and benefits of nursing certification; and conduct market research designed to be of use to individual nurses" (ANCC, 1998a). The NCRC developed a demographic form to be utilized with certification applications; formed focus groups to evaluate various aspects of the certification process; and created the "Credentialing Organizations Survey Instrument" to aid in describing the certified nurse workforce in the United State (Cary, 1998). In addition, ANCC/IREC will be piloting a credentialing journal devoted to credentialing issues in nursing and other healthcare professions.

The certification process allows nurses to display professionalism. A volatile healthcare market and nursing's evolving, comprehensive credentialing process will help validate nursing's place in healthcare delivery.

ANNEMARIE DOWLING-CASTRONOVO

See also:
GERIATRICS
GERONTOLOGICAL CARE
GERONTOLOGICAL NURSING—ADVANCED PRACTICE

CERTIFIED NURSE ASSISTANTS

Unlicensed Assistive Personnel (UAP) who work in nursing homes are known as Certified Nurse Assistants or Aides (CNAs). The American Nurses Association defines a UAP/CNA as an unlicensed individual who is trained to function in an assistive role to the licensed nurse in the provision of direct and indirect care that is delegated and supervised by a registered nurse (ANA, 1992). Direct patient care activities are those related to Activities of Daily Living (ADLs) but may also include the collection of specimens and documentation. Indirect care activities are those related to environmental safety and cleanliness, patient transport, and maintenance of supplies. CNAs constitute 60%–70% of the nursing staff of long-term care (LTC) facilities, and provide as much as 70% of the direct care that is provided to nursing home residents. The CNA reports to the licensed nurse in charge of her residents. On average, in any given 24-hour period, residents in nursing homes receive 122 minutes of CNA time (Harrington, Carillo, Thollaug, & Summers, 1996). The following review focuses on recent research on the effectiveness of CNA educational programs, CNA practice models, CNA work satisfaction, resident care outcomes, and CNA's management of aggressive behavior. We conclude with suggestions for future research.

Mandatory education and training for nursing home CNAs was established by the Nursing Home Reform Act (Nursing Home Reform Law, 1987). The basic curriculum outlined by the federal government and the required training hours may be expanded by each individual state. Major topics within the curriculum include personal care of the elderly (e.g., bathing, feeding, dressing), communication and culture, age-related changes, resident rights, transferring residents, and death and dying. Each CNA must pass both written and performance-based competency exams in order to be certified. CNAs must be recertified every two years by providing evidence of at least 8 hours of continuing education annually, as well as demonstration of employment as a CNA for a minimum number of hours. Burns (1995) found that the OBRA-required curriculum is sufficient for the skills needed for standard resident care but that additional hours are needed for CNA-delivered care in subacute special-care units.

CNAs are expected to be able to read and follow their residents' care plans. Hence the CNA must have at least an eighth-grade level of reading proficiency. A study of the relationship between a CNA's literacy skills and job performance showed that CNA literacy was at a fifth grade level (Benjamin, 1995). The study further revealed that CNAs who spoke English as a second language scored lower on their estimated job performance.

Educational programs that draw on the lived experiences of CNAs may be more effective than standard inservice programs. In one study, a half-day training program using role-playing and material on normal aging to sensitize CNAs to the experience of being old elicited a significant improvement in CNAs' attitudes toward the elderly (Thomson & Burke, 1998). In another study, training materials developed from CNAs' workplace stories of abuse by residents and their families increased CNA job satisfaction (Braun, Suzuki, Cusick, & Howard-Carhart, 1997). R. M. Phillips and Baldwin (1997) describe a training program for CNAs that provides psychosocial care and facilitates the management of problem behaviors. The program improved CNAs' attitude and self-esteem, increased their motivation, and reduced lateness.

Workshops and research on the cultural differences between CNAs and residents is needed. In a study by Robinson (1994), CNAs from three black cultural groups (Afro-Americans, Haitians, and English-speaking Caribbeans) all had positive attitudes toward the elderly. However, the English-speaking Caribbean group expressed the most positive attitudes. All the CNAs expressed some negative attitudes toward families regarding their not taking care of their elderly relatives at home.

Permanent CNA assignments have largely replaced the team model for care delivery. Consequently, it is not uncommon for residents to have a new CNA assigned to provide their care every 2 weeks. Usually, each CNA on the day shift is assigned 6 to 8 residents, any or all of whom may be partially to totally dependent. The ratio on the evening shift is 1:12; and on the night shift, 1:15 or 1:20. Walker, Porter, Gruman, and Michalski (1999) found that, despite significant differences between nurses and CNAs about the feasibility of implementing individualized plans of care, both parties agreed that the barriers to individualizing care were inadequate staffing, poor staff attitudes, and poor communication within the team. The authors suggested that staffing numbers should consider the type of resident referred to in the ratio.

A "primary care" nursing-assistant model that was tested both in a small rural and a large urban nursing home revealed that having a permanent CNA caregiver, a team approach, and systematic communication all significantly improved resident behavior, affect, and social interaction (Teresi et al., 1993). The "empowered aide model," TEAM, was specifically developed for nursing home CNAs, and goes beyond the traditional concept of a team. It has four components, each of which requires administrative, structural, and operational support: (a) empowerment—the ability to make job-related decisions with the resident and independently; (b) organization—the resident-CNA assignment should be thoughtful, consistent with characteristics of resident and caregiver, and continuous; (c) education—for managing stress and dealing with difficult behaviors; and (d) teamwork—enhanced between-shift CNA communication, unit-based meetings, and the sharing results of continuing quality-improvement studies (McAiney, 1998).

A practice model should enhance resident autonomy and dignity. Kane et al. (1997) reported that residents attached importance to choice and control over their own bedtime and rising time, food, roommates, care routines, use of money and the telephone, getting in touch with their physician, and trips. CNAs placed a lower emphasis on telephone use and control of personal money and a higher emphasis on control and choice over activities. Interestingly, CNAs within this study ranked visitors as highly important, whereas residents ranked them last. Perhaps this reflects the "fact" that nursing-home staff are "family" to the residents. Hence, the traditional visitor is not as highly valued by the residents. Of 134 CNAs, 87% felt that they knew a given resident's plan of care and physical needs, but only 50% were aware of the resident's personal tastes. Fewer CNAs were knowledgeable about the resident's family situation, former occupation, or interests. Overall, residents were dissatisfied with their degree of control and choice, and CNAs were not optimistic that residents could achieve the degree of choice and control they desired.

Instability within the workforce affects the budget and more importantly, resident outcomes. Factors associated with job satisfaction are the opportunity for: (a) growth and development, (b) job security, (c) socialization, and (d) challenge (Atchison, 1998). Causes of turnover include: inadequate preparation for CNA roles and responsibility, management that is insensitive to the stress of the CNA job, and a failure to create practice models that are responsive to resident-care needs.

CNA wages and benefits continue to influence job satisfaction and turnover. Ramirez, Teresi, Holmes, and Fairchild (1998) found that frequent changes of assignments, insufficient team meetings, having many bowel-incontinent and heavy-care residents, and racial bias (a stressor) were significantly related to job dissatisfaction and burnout. Caudill (1989) observed that CNA involvement in care planning and evaluation—hallmarks of a team care model—significantly reduced turnover. Monahan and McCarthy (1992) found, in their study of seven rural nursing homes, that attachment to others, teamwork, good management, and a sense of humor were important retention factors. Major points of dissatisfaction within this study included problems with supplies, inappropriate rules and regulations, supervisors who didn't listen to their problems, and the perceived lack of time to give quality care. Additional points of dissatisfaction might be found in studies conducted in high-cost and culturally diverse urban settings.

A small sample of CNAs (n = 30) stated that quality of care means giving care you would want for yourself. According to the findings of this study, quality of care is achieved by providing personalized care and doing extra things for the resident. Quality care includes keeping the person dry, clean, and meeting their physical needs. Other components of quality care are giving residents love, kindness, and gentleness (Finnick, Reis, & Drobits, 1990). The CNAs in this study felt that quality care requires a good attitude, sufficient staff and supplies, and adequate training. In their view, toileting assistance and interaction (e.g., orienting and emotional support) were important markers of quality care. However, the researchers saw scant evidence of these two activities.

Ryan (1997) found that CNAs experienced anxiety when feeding residents with swallowing disorders. Overall, CNAs preferred spoon-feeding over artificial feeding, and felt that it was easier to care for a resident with a gastric feeding tube rather than a nasogastric tube. The majority of CNAs within this study, most of whom were Southern Baptists, felt that it was legally and ethically acceptable to withhold nutrition. Furthermore, they perceived no difference between stopping artificial feeding and never starting it. Interestingly, 35% of the CNAs did not know if the interdisciplinary team was aware of a resident's advance directives with regard to artificial nutrition.

Schell and Kayser-Jones (1999) found that inadequate staffing led to hurried, "mechanistic" care at mealtimes. The authors' recommendations included role-taking—seeing the world from the resident's perspective, addressing the resident, attending to the social value of mealtime, and "sharing the experience" by eating with the resident, as a means of eliciting compassionate care.

Learned helplessness in nursing-home residents is only a partially understood phenomenon in nursing homes. The role of caregivers' actions in allowing and encouraging this behavior is of great concern. An educational intervention to change CNAs' behavior demonstrated that the experimental group was less supportive of residents' unnecessary independence than was the control group (Bandriet, 1993). Barriers to maximizing resident independence included limited time, insufficient communication, inadequate administrative support, not being involved in resident care decisions, fear of weight loss and dehydration, and rigid routines.

Two studies of CNAs and end-of-life care are worth noting because of their relevance to management acts, education, and outcomes. Robbins, Lloyd, Carpenter, and Bender (1992) found that the ethnicity of supervisors influenced their perceptions of death anxiety among CNAs. Miskella and Avis (1998) reported that CNAs felt unprepared, unsupervised, and isolated in their role in death and dying care. The authors suggested that the values and perceptions of these staff may influence the quality of their end-of-life caregiving.

Only recently has research focused on verbally and physically aggressive resident behaviors, in an attempt to better manage these problems within the LTC environment. Goodridge, Johnston, and Thomson (1996) found a statistically significant relationship between staff conflict with residents, and residents' aggressive behavior. Less than 0.3% of residents' aggressive behaviors (commonly occurring during residents' personal care or wanting to go outside the nursing home), are reported or recorded by CNAs. The nursing assistants in this study expected to be physically assaulted 9.3 times per month on average, and verbally assaulted 11.3 times per month. CNAs react with anger, sadness, frustration, and indifference but simultaneously need to cope with feelings of responsibility and helplessness (Gates, Fitzwater, & Meyer, 1999).

An observation of CNAs providing care to residents with dementia revealed that some CNAs intuitively provided care that reduced residents' agitation or aggression (Anderson, Wendler, & Congdon, 1998). These CNAs had a structure or "foundational pattern" of respect for adults and positive family and personal values. The combination of this pattern and the home's active support of teamwork and adequate orientation to the resident resulted in effective care for residents with dementia. An educational program on the management (and reporting) of assaultive behaviors, combined with administrative support, may achieve positive outcomes for residents as well as staff (Cohn, Horgas, & Marsiske, 1990; Wilkinson, 1999).

A study of the relationship between aggressive behavior revealed that RNs selected fewer resident behaviors requiring physical intervention than did CNAs (Haber, Fagan-Pryor, & Allen, 1997). Both CNAs and RNs opted for therapeutic communication for behaviors that included scowling, appearing tense, irritability, and challenging and/or complaining behavior. Interestingly, CNAs and RNs agreed equally on the use of verbal and chemical intervention as a means of limiting use of physical restraints.

Despite the high ratio of CNAs to professional nursing staff, little nursing research is available to provide information about these highly utilized LTC employees. Further research is needed on how to effectively educate CNAs to provide the best resident care possible. Few practice models are available to provide a framework for the role of a CNA within an interdisciplinary team. Further research is needed on developing effective models to improve resident care. Given the heavy workload, recruitment and retention of CNAs is among the major problems facing LTC management. In some areas of the country turnover is as high as 130% annually. In addition, the work satisfaction of CNAs is likely to be closely linked to resident outcomes. Yet research is sparse in these areas. Future research may provide information on both variables, as well as on the relationship between them.

ETHEL MITTY

See also:
AGGRESSIVE BEHAVIOR
ALZHEIMER'S DISEASE
ALZHEIMER'S DISEASE—SPECIAL CARE UNITS IN LONG-TERM CARE
LONG-TERM CARE DEMENTIA

CONTINUING CARE RETIREMENT COMMUNITIES

A continuing care retirement community (CCRC) is a type of facility that provides housing, meals, and other services, including nursing home care, for older adults in exchange for a one-time capital investment or entrance fee and a monthly service fee. Most CCRCs are sponsored by religious or other nonprofit organizations, but for-profit organizations have entered into the retirement business as well. The CCRC is usually constructed as a village or community, and the individual remains within this community for the remainder of his or her life. All CCRCs have a written contract that residents must sign. The terms of the contract vary and have been separated into three categories by the American Association of Homes for the Aged: Type A homes are "all-inclusive" as they offer guaranteed nursing care in the nursing facility at no increase in the residents' monthly fee; Type B CCRCs do not guarantee unlimited nursing home care, but have a contractual agreement to provide a specific number of days per year, or lifetime, of the resident in the nursing facility; Type C CCRCs are based on a typical fee-for-service approach. Financial stability, particularly of Type A and Type B CCRCs, depends on high occupancy rates in the independent-living apartments, and on maintaining the residents' optimal health and function, this requiring fewer healthcare services.

The number of CCRCs has increased dramatically (50%) during the 1980s and has continued to grow in the 1990s. CCRCs are located throughout the United States, although five states (Pennsylvania, California, Florida, Illinois, and Ohio) are home to more than one-third of the nation's CCRCs. Despite the growth of CCRCs, they now account for a smaller percentage of senior housing overall, due to the dramatic increase in assisted living facilities.

Generally, older adults who live in CCRCs are those who were never married, or married without children, are well educated, and are "health-conscious" (Krauskopf, Brown, Tokarz, & Bogutz, 1993; Petit, 1994; Resnick, 1989; Resnick, 1998b). Initially, CCRCs were for affluent older adults. However, CCRCs are becoming more affordable and are attracting those with more moderate incomes (Kitchen & Rouche, 1990). The decision to move into a CCRC requires a good deal of planning and adjustment for older adults, especially if they are relocating to another city or state, and/or moving from a large home to a smaller apartment.

CCRC residents' overall use of Medicare-covered medical services is no different from that of older adults who live in traditional community settings, with the exception of lower expenditures for hospital care (Ruchlin, Morris, & Morris, 1993). The types of healthcare services provided vary based on the facility. Most facilities have a nurse responsible for those in independent living to help with routine care activities, such as dressing changes, administration of injectable medications, and health screenings. It is these nurses who are the first to respond to emergencies, and often the first to identify changes in the older resident. Depending on the CCRC, there may also be a geriatric nurse practitioner available for daytime management of acute and chronic problems, and a cadre of primary and specialty physicians. The availability of healthcare is seen as a major advantage to living in a CCRC, and the focus on health promotion and disease prevention is important to residents. The residents' focus on health and maintenance of health, supported by managers within these systems (Hurley, 1991; Moore, 1998), makes the CCRC an ideal environment for geriatric nursing research.

The initial research in CCRCs focused on the residents' adjustment to the community, and the impact this had on the residents. Resnick (1989), using a qualitative approach, described the challenges of adjustment to a CCRC and identified groups of individuals who were particularly at risk for relocation stress: those who had experienced a recent loss; those with a decline in mental status; and the young-old (60–70) age group. Anticipating problems and letting residents know that they might have certain feelings helped residents in the adjustment process. The study also identified the need for frequent follow-up in the first 6 months to a year following move-in, as many residents did not begin to grieve over their losses until they fully completed the work of the move. Petit (1994) implemented the findings of this work as she developed the role of the wellness nurse in a CCRC.

Most of the nursing research done in CCRCs has been on the health practices and health promotion of residents (Adams, 1996; Crowley, 1996; Resnick, 1998b; Resnick, Palmer, Jenkins, & Spellbring, in press; Resnick, manuscript submitted.). The research generally consists of descriptive surveys in which residents are asked about specific health behaviors, such as getting vaccinations, monitoring cholesterol and dietary fat intake, exercise activity, alcohol and nicotine use, and participation in health screenings— including mammograms, Pap tests, stools for occult blood, or prostate examinations. The majority of residents in the CCRCs studied got yearly flu vaccines, and a pneumonia vaccine, and approximately 61% had received an up-to-date tetanus booster. A smaller percentage, approximately 30%, monitored their diets. About 50% of those living in CCRCs drink alcohol regularly, only 11% use nicotine, and under 50% exercise regularly.

With regard to cancer screening, about 40%–50% of the residents get yearly mamograms, 31%–37% get pap tests, 65%–80% get prostate examinations, approximately 60% have stools checked for blood yearly, and a little over 50% regularly monitor their skin for abnormal growths. Overall, there is better participation in health-promoting activities on the part of older adults living in CCRCs when compared to older adults in the community at large (Blustein & Weiss, 1998; Smith, Zhou, Weinberger, Smith, & McDonald, 1999). However, the findings suggest that even in this population continued education is needed to encourage personal decision making related to health-promoting activities. The findings can also be used to develop interventions to improve specific health behaviors.

In addition to a description of the health-promoting behaviors of these individuals, consideration has been given to factors that influence residents' willingness to engage in these activities. Combined qualitative and quantitative approaches were used to explore this question (Resnick, 1998b; Resnick et al., in press; Resnick, manuscripts submitted). Common themes were identified by the open-ended interviews and indicated that the most common reasons for not engaging in specific health activities were: (1) never being told to by a primary healthcare provider; (2) not wanting to do anything even if the tests were abnormal; (3) feeling they were too old; and (4) a desire to contract the known illness so as to hasten death.

Exploratory regression analyses (Resnick, 1998b) and path analyses using structural equation modeling (Resnick et al., in press; Resnick, manuscript submitted) were done to test predictors of health-promoting activities in general, with special attention given to factors that predicted exercise behavior. Age was the only variable that was significantly related to these behaviors and accounted for 7% of the variance. With increased age, the residents participated in fewer health-promoting or health-preventive behaviors. Age, gender, physical and mental health, self-efficacy expectations, and outcome expectations directly and/or indirectly influenced exercise behavior in the residents. The influence of these variables on exercise behavior was supported in a qualitative study (Resnick & Spellbring, in press) that focused on factors that helped older adults in a CCRC adhere to a regular walking program, and on factors that decreased their willingness to adhere to one.

Crowley (1996) also considered the health behaviors of older adults in a CCRC, and the outcomes of a wellness program that encouraged regular exercise. A total of 21% of the 225 residents exercised, and case reports identified positive outcomes, such as weight loss and improved recovery following a fracture.

Falls, a common problem for the older adult in any setting, are another area that has been studied in CCRCs. Resnick (in press) explored the incidence and predictors of falls in a CCRC, and stressed the importance of considering falls within each specific community because environmental risks and activity patterns may be very different. In the community studied, falls generally occurred between noon and midnight, within the residents' apartments, and when walking (63%) or transferring (19%). Only sixteen (10%) of the falls resulted in a fracture. The number of falls was the only variable associated with having an injurious fall. Individuals who had atrial fibrillation or neurological problems, or were not married, or did not adhere to a regular exercise program were more likely to have multiple falls. Crowley (1996) also considered the number of falls within a CCRC, and noted that over a 5-year period there were 427 falls involving 139 residents, but only 21 of the falls involved residents who exercised regularly.

Some research (Resnick, 1998a, 1999) has considered the functional performance of residents who live in the long-term-care areas, or "health centers," within the CCRC. Resnick (1998a, 1999), using a combined qualitative and quantitative approach, explored what increased or decreased the residents' willingness to participate in, and actual performance of, activities of daily of living, such as bathing, dressing, and ambulating. Common themes identified as influencing performance of functional activities included personality (i.e., determination); belief in their individual ability; the unpleasant sensations associated with the activity; goals; and fears, such as the fear of falling. Quantitative findings indicated that motivation (self-efficacy expectations, outcome expectations, and the personality component of motivation) and physical condition (standing balance and lower-extremity contractures) were the most important predictors of functional performance in these individuals.

Russell (1996) considered the care-seeking behavior of older adults living in a CCRC. This was a qualitative study using ethnographic field research that incorporated semistructured interviews, participant observation, and focus-group interviews. The care-seeking process was described as sequential phases and stages that evolved over time.

CCRCs continue to be a viable living environment for older adults. For these facilities to keep costs down and remain lucrative, it is imperative that there be a focus on maintaining health and function. Most of the nursing research has been qualitative and/or descriptive in nature, and has focused on health promotion. Continued research needs to build on these preliminary findings and begin to develop and test interventions that may help older adults in CCRCs maintain their health and function. For example, one current investigation involves exploring the outcomes of a restorative care program for residents in the health center of a CCRC. Many CCRCs have "wellness programs" that are nursing-driven. The outcomes of these programs need to be considered from both a health perspective and a fiscal perspective. Other important areas of research within CCRCs that nursing has not yet considered include relocation to different levels of care, healthcare utilization patterns, and the impact this has on nursing care services and end-of-life care.

Barbara Resnick

See also:
ACTIVITIES OF DAILY LIVING

ASSISTED LIVING
BREAST CANCER SCREENING
EXERCISE
FALLS
FUNCTIONAL HEALTH
HEALTH CARE FINANCING ADMINISTRATION

DEMENTIA: LONG-TERM CARE

Approximately 4.8 million Americans suffer from dementia. This number is expected to almost triple by 2050 (Alzheimer's Association, 1997). Costs to society related to dementia exceed $111 billion annually, but do not reflect the toll this disease takes on humanity. People with dementia (PWD) experience severe cognitive changes and often display problematic behaviors (70%–90% of PWD). These characteristics can overwhelm home caregivers, and force them to place PWD in nursing homes (Post & Whitehouse, 1995) whose environments are often overresponsive and overprotective and do not consider the PWD's preserved strengths and abilities (Baltes & Horgas, 1997). However, federal legislation has sought to increase the autonomy of PWD by mandating a reduction in chemical and physical restraints in nursing homes (OBRA 1987) and by developing programs to prevent or delay institutionalization (Social HMO Consortium, 1998). Recently, the National Institutes of Health received $50 million in federal funds to launch an Alzheimer's-disease-prevention initiative, which includes testing new methods to improve quality of life ("an individual's subjective experience and evaluation of their life circumstances" [Brod, Stewart, & Sands, 1999]), prevent excess disability (functional impairment greater than actual impairments warrant [Brody, 1971; Sabat, 1998]), and develop affordable systems of care (Alzheimer's Association, 1999). Improving the psychological well-being of PWD, especially those in advanced stages of disease, will require aggressive medical interventions and/or palliative treatment and hospice care. The palliative care approach provides more appropriate care, and saves healthcare resources (Volicer, 1997). The Chronic Care Consortium has developed a care model that emphasizes disability prevention, acknowledges the heterogeneity of PWD and their caregivers, and builds on their strengths and abilities to prevent, delay, or minimize disability and lessen caregivers' health risks (National Chronic Care Consortium, 1999). Kane, Kane, and Ladd (1998) assert that long-term care programs must preserve the dignity and autonomy of PWD and allow them to live as meaningfully as possible.

In trying to promote autonomy, researchers have discovered that PWD can improve or maintain their functional performance (Beck, Heacock,

Rapp, & Mercer, 1993; Beck et al., 1997) with interventions that engage their procedural memory and priming responses (Knopman, 1991), important components of Activities of Daily Living (ADLs) (i.e., eating, bathing), which seem relatively resistant to dementia (Desgranges, Eustache, Rioux, De La Sayette, & Lechevalier, 1996). Grafman et al. (1990) showed that PWD could perform ADLs when they had the physical capability and understood the task. Interventions tested on various ADLs have shown the effectiveness of guidance as an alternative to total care (Beck et al., 1993; Beck et al., 1997; Coyne & Hoskins, 1997; Nolen & Garrard, 1988; Reichenbach & Kirchman, 1991; Rosswurm, 1989). Strategies include reducing unrelated cognitive demands (Beck et al., 1993; Grafman et al., 1990), verbal prompts (Coyne & Hoskins, 1997; Grafman et al., 1990; McEvoy & Patterson, 1986; Osborn & Marshall, 1993; Zanetti et al., 1997), directions to correct mistakes (Bonder, 1993; McEvoy & Patterson, 1986), and positive reinforcement (Coyne & Hoskins, 1997). Further, breaking the task down into simple steps (Beck et al., 1993; Grafman et al., 1990) and modeling the behavior (McEvoy & Patterson, 1986) have fostered functional improvements. Levels-of-assistance strategies allow caregivers to use the least amount of assistance necessary to complete the task, and support the PWD's autonomy (Beck et al., 1997; Tappen, 1994). Also, low light (Ford, Fox, Fitch, & Donovan, 1987) and music (Ragneskog, Kihlgren, Karlsson, & Norberg, 1996) have increased food consumption. Scheduled toileting, habit training, and prompted voiding have helped in toileting (Ouslander & Schnelle, 1993; Simmons & Schnelle, 1999).

Problematic behaviors, such as agitation, aggression, and wandering have a negative impact on PWD and others including caregivers. Since 1992, many studies have tested interventions to curb problematic behaviors in PWD. Treatments fall into three categories: sensory stimulation, psychosocial strategies, and care-environment alterations. The studies with interventions that significantly reduced problematic behaviors follow.

Among sensory treatments, researchers have most often employed music (Casby & Holm, 1994; Clark, M. E., Lipe, & Bilbrey, 1998; Gerdner, in press; Gerdner & Swanson, 1993; Goddaer & Abraham, 1994; Tabloski, McKinnon-Howe, & Remington, 1995; Thomas, Heitman, & Alexander, 1997), followed by non-music auditory stimulation (Burgio, Scilley, Hardin, Hsu, & Yancey, 1996; Camberg et al., 1999; Woods & Ashley, 1995), bright light (Lovell, Ancoli-Israel, & Gevirtz, 1995; Mishima et al., 1994), exercise (Holmberg, 1997; Namazi, Gwinnup, & Zadorozny 1994), touch/massage (Snyder, Egan, & Burns, 1995; Woods, Craven, & Whitney, 1993), and increased visual contrast (Koss & Gilmore, 1998) and cues (Bourgeois, Burgio, Schulz, Beach, & Palmer, 1997). Psychosocial treatments have included matching language complexity to comprehension level (Hart &

Wells, 1997), video respite (Lund, Hill, Caserta, & Wright, 1995), a sensory-integration group (Robichaud, Hebert, & Desrosiers, 1994), and a wellness group (Lantz, Buchalter, & McBee, 1997).

Care-environment alterations often combine approaches such as specialized training for nursing staff, specialized activities, decreased resident-to-staff ratios, reduced psychotropic medications, and reinforcement of staff by means of feedback and education (Matteson, Linton, Cleary, Barnes, & Lichtenstein, 1997; Matthews, Farrell, & Blackmore, 1996; Rovner, Steele, Shmuely, & Folstein, 1996). Other alterations included background nature sounds and scenes (Whall et al., 1997), and a combination of psychosocial and physical environment changes (Hoeffer, Rader, McKenzie, Lavelle, & Stewart, 1997).

Since no effective treatment exists to prevent or reverse Alzheimer's disease, caregivers focus on the improvement and maintenance of quality of life (Volicer & Bloom-Charette, 1999). Interest in studying the quality of life for PWD is growing. Volicer and Bloom-Charette (1999) have identified three main areas that determine quality of life: meaningful activities, medical issues, and psychiatric symptoms. Quality of life is a difficult concept to measure in persons in the advanced stages of Alzheimer's disease because cognitive impairment impedes their ability to discuss their feelings (Volicer & Bloom-Charette, 1999).

New tools to measure this quality of life include: Dementia Quality-of-Life Instrument (DQoL) (Brod, Stewart, Sands, & Walton, 1999), Quality of Well-Being (QWB) (Kerner, Patterson, Grant, & Kaplan, 1998), and Quality of Life in Alzheimer's Disease (Lawton, 1994; Lawton, Haitsma, & Klapper, 1996).

Approximately two-thirds of PWD live at home (Alzheimer's Association, 1996). Living with and caring for a PWD is associated with impaired mental and physical health, social isolation, and family conflict (Collins, Stommel, Wang, & Given, 1994; Davis, 1997; Dempsey & Baago, 1998; Donaldson, Tarrier, & Bruns, 1998; Gallagher-Thompson & Powers, 1997; Kiecolt-Glaser, Dyer, & Shuttleworth, 1988; Schulz, O'Brien, Bookwala, & Fleissner, 1995; Pearson et al., 1993).

Interventions to alleviate caregiver stress and depression include in-home psychoeducational programs (Buckwalter et al., 1999; Buckwalter et al., in press; Mittelman et al., 1995) and the use of adult day care (Zarit, Stephens, Townsend, & Green, 1998). Further, a comprehensive caregiver support-and-counseling program lengthened the time that spousal caregivers were able to care for patients at home, particularly during the early-to-middle stages of the disease (Mittleman, Ferris, Shulman, Steinberg, & Levin, 1996). Another promising intervention is the provision of information and emotional support for family caregivers via a telecommunication system (Wright, Bennett, & Gramling, 1998).

Assisted living is another option for persons in the early stages of PWD who are no long able to function independently in their own homes. Separate living conditions are provided for each individual, with the provision of services being tailored to the individual needs of the person. This helps to promote as much independence as possible (Forbes, C. S., 1997; Grant & Sommers, 1998).

Due to the stress and demands of caregiving over time a large percentage of PWD eventually require placement in long-term care facilities. Approximately 70% of persons residing in long-term care facilities have dementia (Chandler & Chandler, 1988; Rovner, 1990). As a result, Special Care Units (SCUs) were established to tailor care to the unique needs (i.e., functional impairment, problematic behaviors) of PWD. Ideally these include a safe physical environment that supports and maximizes the functional abilities of PWD, and a trained interdisciplinary staff to develop and implement a plan of care based on the individual needs of the PWD (Alzheimer's Association, 1992).

In 1995, 10.4% of all Medicare- or Medicaid-certified nursing facilities were estimated to have SCUs (Phillips et al., 1999). The establishment of SCUs is increasing, despite conflicting research findings on their efficacy. Sloane and colleagues (1991) identified a statistically significant reduction in the use of physical restraints (but not chemical restraints) in persons residing in a SCU compared to those residing on an integrated unit. Similarly, Swanson and colleagues (1993) reported a significant reduction in catastrophic reactions and other problematic behaviors in patients residing on a SCU compared to an integrated unit. Studies have not shown that SCUs result in an improvement in the functional status of PWD (Phillips et al., 1997; Swanson, Maas, & Buckwalter, 1994).

The transfer of a PWD from home to a long-term care facility is a difficult transition for many family members who have been the primary caregivers for an extended period of time. Maas and Swanson (1991) developed the Family Involvement in Care (FIC) protocol as a means of easing this transition, promoting a cooperative relationship between family and staff, and enhancing the quality of care for PWD.

There is a need to further investigate the various types of living environments available for PWD, and the outcomes associated with these alternative residences. Also, there is a need to study the wide range of community services for PWD and their family members (i.e, respite, adult day-care, support groups) with a focus on the content and quality of the services provided. Other issues include geographic location with regard to access and utilization, cost-effectiveness, and acceptability on the part of the client and their family (Montgomery, 1996). Much research is also needed to address the racial, ethnic, and cultural issues related to the care of a PWD.

Linda A. Gerdner
Valorie M. Shue
Cornelia K. Beck

See also:
    AGGRESSIVE BEHAVIOR
    ALZHEIMER'S DISEASE
    ALZHEIMER'S DISEASE: SPECIAL CARE UNITS
    CERTIFIED NURSE ASSISTANTS
    COGNITIVE DISORDERS
    COGNITIVE IMPAIRMENT
    WANDERING
    COGNITIVE INTERVENTIONS

END-OF-LIFE CHOICES: DECISION MAKING

The American Nurses Association (1992) has issued four position statements on nursing's role in end-of-life decisions. These statements concerned the Patient Self-Determination Act (PSDA), comfort and pain relief for dying patients, nurses' involvement in decisions to forgo artificial nutrition and hydration, and do-not-resuscitate (DNR) orders. The Patient Self-Determination Act statement addressed the nurse's responsibility to facilitate informed decision making. The statement on forgoing artificial nutrition and hydration spoke to the ability of "competent adults" to evaluate and express their values and their right to have those preferences respected; this included the individual's preferences as expressed in an advance directive. Individuals who have "never been competent" included mentally disabled and mentally ill individuals. The DNR statement indicated that nurses' concerns with DNR orders included lack of documentation regarding how a DNR decision was made. It addressed the rights of competent as well as incompetent patients (through their surrogates). However, none of these statements addressed the nurse's role, responsibility, and participation in determining a patient's capacity to make these decisions nor in assessing the patient's understanding of the decisions made. All four statements fail to distinguish between legal competency and clinical capacity.

Nursing research on nurses' actions with regard to assessment of decisional capacity and decision making about end-of-life choices is sparse. In a review of 182 charts, Palmateer and McCartney (1985) found that nurses used the term *disoriented* to describe mental status and rarely provided a behavioral description of "confusion." Their survey of nurses revealed that less than half of nurses interviewed knew about the early changes indicative of dementia. Brady (1987) reported that nurses documented that patients were confused when they exhibited disruptive or resistive behavior. Using a small convenience sample ($N = 70$) composed of undergraduate and graduate nursing students from a university-based school of nursing, psychiatric mental health nurses, and home health nurses, Weisensee and colleagues (Weisensee, Kjervik, & Anderson, 1994) found that nurses inadequately document nursing home residents' memory deficits or ability to follow simple directions and used short-term memory loss as a sign of incompetence. They report that a national survey of schools of nursing found that most nursing students receive some age-related content but that faculty preparedness in this area is extremely variable (Solon, Kilpatrick, & Hill, 1988).

Williams and Engle (1995) found that health care professionals, overall, predominantly used orientation and verbal function as indices of competence. In their interview survey, it appeared that nurses did not use decision-making ability or comprehension of a decision's consequences as criteria in their assessment. They suggest that nurses may be using the terms *alert* and *oriented* interchangeably. In general, these studies were limited by their small sample size and by the fact that standard definitions for key terms, such as *decisional capacity, confusion,* and *disorientation* were not established a priori.

There are several fruitful areas for nursing research. Consistent with nursing's role in encouraging and assisting patients to make decisions about end-of-life choices, it is vitally important to learn how nurses differentiate between competence and decision-specific capacity: what cues and patterns they look for and how this affects their conclusions, actions, and plans of care. *Competence,* a legal term, is presumed unless there is evidence that, overall, an individual is unable to manage personal or financial affairs, or both. *Capacity,* a clinical term, is based on the observation or test of specific abilities: (a) to make a choice, (b) to understand the situation and its implications, (c) to manipulate information rationally, and (d) to appreciate the nature of the situation (i.e., its consequences pursuant to giving or withholding consent).

A universal view of capacity as either fully present or absent is not supported medically or legally. For medical decision making, the specific competence needed to appreciate the nature, consequences, and alternatives of treatment options is known as decision-specific capacity. An individual may be capable of making some decisions but not others. Most older people retain sufficient cognitive capability to make some, but not necessarily all, decisions. Research has shown that physicians and psychiatrists know the legal standard for competence but apply it incorrectly, thereby undermining patient autonomy (Markson, Kern, Annas, & Glantz, 1994). Nothing is known about how well nurses approximate patients' mental status and decisional capacity in comparison to their professional colleagues.

Another area of research is nurses' understanding of the purposes of mental status assessment tests. Often used as a surrogate for decision-making capacity, tests such as the Mini-Mental Status Examination (MMSE) or Short Portable Mental Status Questionnaire (SPMSQ) were not designed or validated as tests of legal competence or decisional capacity (see Mezey, Stokes, & Rauckenhurst, 1995). Low scores do not automatically imply a complete absence of decisional capacity, nor do high scores confirm its presence. As found by others, Mezey, Teresi, Mitty, Ramsey, and Goldstein (1997) demonstrated that nursing home residents with mild Alzheimer's disease/dementia retain the ability to make a treatment choice. Even some residents with extremely low MMSE scores had sufficient decisional capacity to execute a health care proxy. These are residents who are frequently denied the exercise of their right to make this kind of health care decision on the basis of mental status assessment scores. Understanding, a key aspect of capacity, can be affected by language skills and nuance, sensory deficits, illness, depression, anxiety, medication, and education. Nursing research in this area might compare patients' ability to follow simple directions for self-care with their scores on standardized mental status assessment tests.

Capacity determination should rely on a composite picture of clinical data, not the least of which should be observations of an individual's functional ability. Such observations in a clinical or domiciliary setting would include a person's orientation, behavior, memory, ability to follow simple directions, ability to communicate and state wishes, and compliance with care regimens. Appropriate assessment of an individual's ability to make end-of-life choices should prevent two types of errors: (1) preventing competent individuals from making their own decisions and (2) failing to protect incompetent individuals from the harmful effects of a poor decision. An individual with limited verbal and social skills might be incorrectly assessed as incapacitated, whereas an individual with appropriate and acceptable verbal and social skills might be assessed as capable of reaching a health care decision when they are, in fact, incapable of doing so.

Research on the validity and reliability of nursing observations might remove barriers to patients' exercise of their right to make end-of-life decisions and prevent these kinds of errors. Physicians as well as the courts rely on nursing data, and thus it is urgent to investigate nurses' operative definitions of key mental status and cognitive, affective, and behavioral descriptors within and across settings and by level of professional education. Such research also could include faculty knowledge and understanding.

Basic descriptive research is needed on nurses' understanding of end-of-life decision making, for example: What is their knowledge about how advance directives (i.e., living will and durable power of attorney for health care) facilitate autonomous decision making? What is their understanding of the differences between withholding, withdrawing, and forgoing treatments or interventions? How do nurses assess whether or not a patient understands the particular decision(s) to be made or that have been made? Nurses are instrumental in helping proxy decision makers learn more about what individuals want and do not want at the end of their lives and understand the treatment options. Yet nothing is known about nurses' roles in proxy decisions nor about how nurses interpret, document, and communicate a patient's verbal instructions. Finally, additional research is needed about nurses' experiences with and communication of the patient's interest in assistance with dying.

ETHEL L. MITTY
MATHY D. MEZEY

See also:
  ADVANCE DIRECTIVES
  AGEISM
  CHRONIC ILLNESS
  QUALITY OF LIFE
  TERMINAL ILLNESS

FALLS

A fall is an unintentional slip, trip, or drop from an upright position, resulting in the person landing on the floor. A near fall occurs when an environmental object or person prevents the person falling from landing on the floor. A fall may be associated with a fear of future falls; and subsequently, persons may restrict their activities or seek assistance, making them more dependent and less active. Injury, disability, and death are serious sequelae of falls, making this a critical issue to the person, the nurse, and society.

Risk Factors

Although the etiologies for a fall and near fall may be similar, persons at risk for each type may be different. Research has focused primarily on falls. Being female and over 65 years of age have been found to be risk factors for falls in all settings (community, long-term care facility, and hospital). However, these factors have very low sensitivity for identifying those at greatest risk. Thus, the number of risk factors has been used as an indicator of the degree of risk.

Most research on falls has not been guided by theory. However, the ecological model of functional health (Hogue, 1984) describes the interaction among environment, personal competence, and cognitive appraisal as contributing to falls. This model provides direction for identifying sets of factors that predict the probability of falls. Environmental risk factors include poor lighting, low contrast among important elements of the environment (e.g., poor contrast between edge of step and next step or between floor and wall), clutter and loose objects on the floor (e.g., children and rugs). Although not commonly categorized as environmental factors, other risk factors are medications, treatments for disease, and policies of health care facilities (e.g., use of restraints or ensuring exercise). These environmental factors may increase the risk of falls, but the personal competence determines whether an individual can recover from an unexpected disruption in posture.

The physical competencies associated with falls include poor balance, poor muscle strength, postural hypotension, impaired gait, and sensory losses (e.g., poor vision, impaired proprioception, and altered vibratory and vestibular information). Psychological competencies include cognitive impairment and depression. Cognitive appraisal, as an evaluative judgment of the environment and personal competencies, contributes to falls in this model but was rarely considered in past research on falls. However, cognitive appraisal is required for persons to determine their ability to move about safely and to identify hazards in the environment; it is integral to decisions about how and when to participate in activities. The accuracy of such judgments will affect whether activities are appropriately limited or adaptations are made in performing them.

Prevention and Intervention Programs

Most fall prevention programs in hospitals and nursing homes use risk factors to identify those persons at highest risk for a fall. Nearly all fall prevention programs include age, gender, and number of medications to identify those at risk. The most frequent interventions used in these programs focus on removing hazards from the environment, instructing the person to ask for help when ambulating or transferring, and ensuring that the person can easily call for help. In some nursing homes, motion monitors are placed on a wrist or ankle that send sound signals to alert the nursing staff when the person moves. However, these programs do not address the physical and psychological factors that place a person at risk for a fall.

Removing environmental hazards in the home has had limited success in reducing the rate of falls. In the community, investigators have assessed these hazards and developed individualized interventions to remove or minimize them. Investigators noted that many elderly adults were willing to make only a few changes and were more interested in interventions directed at physical risk factors. Moreover, Northridge, Nevitt, Kelsey, and Link (1995) demonstrated only a weak association between home hazards and falls, and the vigorous elderly adult was more likely to fall when more hazards were present than was the frail elderly adult.

Research of interventions targeted to specific physical risk factors is emerging. In a meta-analysis of exercise interventions in the program Frailty and Injuries: Cooperative Studies of Intervention Techniques (FICSIT), exercise reduced the rate of falls in elderly adults in nursing homes and in the community (Province et al., 1995). These results may be attributed to exercise-related increases in muscle strength and balance and improvements in gait.

Although exercise is a promising intervention to reduce falls, multidimensional interventions targeted to physical, psychological, and environmental factors associated with falls may be more effective. For example, Tinetti and associates (1994) demonstrated the effectiveness of an intervention that included assessment of risk factors for falls in elderly adults living in the community, and then they implemented an individualized treatment program targeted at each risk factor. This multidimensional program reduced the rate of falls and can be used as a model to develop similar interventions for evaluation in other settings.

Although research on falls started in the 1950s, more is needed to develop risk assessments that have adequate sensitivity and specificity and to develop more effective interventions targeted either to the specific populations at greatest risk for falls or to specific risk factors. This knowledge will provide direction for nursing assessment and intervention.

BEVERLY L. ROBERTS

See also:
ACTIVITIES OF DAILY LIVING

FUNCTIONAL HEALTH
GERONTOLOGIC CARE
MOBILITY
NEUROBEHAVIORAL DISTURBANCES OF THE OLDER ADULT:
  DELERIUM AND DEMENTIA
PHYSICAL RESTRAINTS FOR THE ELDERLY

FAMILY CAREGIVING TO FRAIL ELDERS

Family caregiving to frail elders is defined as the processes by which family members provide care, support, and assistance to elders who require help because of illness, memory problems, or frailty. For many years the family has provided the majority of long-term care to frail elders in community settings. Indeed, the health care system could not meet the needs of frail elders without the care provided by informal caregivers. In the past decade, changes in health and social policies have meant that the family is increasingly expected to assume a role in the acute care of elders in the home.

Because of their expertise in care processes, nurses are in a position to assist families in developing the knowledge and skill needed to provide care to frail older family members. Assisting families in this way has traditionally been the responsibility of home health nurses, but the increasing use of outpatient strategies to manage complex health problems in combination with early hospital discharge and use of skilled nursing facilities for acute care means that nurses in many settings have the potential to influence family caregiving.

Research on family caregiving to frail elders in the United States began in the late 1970s with the publication of a cross-national survey that debunked the myth that the American family abandons its elders to nursing home care (Shanas, 1979). Since that time, data from multiple national studies indicate that families provide over 80% of the personal and medically related care given to community-residing elders and that most caregivers are women, spouses, or adult children, retired and in poorer health than would be expected based on their age and gender. Primary caregivers often spend more effort in caregiving activities than a full-time job requires.

The first wave of research on caregiving focused on describing its negative effects on the caregiver, known variously as burden, strain, and stress. This work provided unequivocal evidence that caregiving for elders is difficult for the caregiver. It also led to an understanding of some of the factors that predict the negative responses to caregiving. Being female rather than male and being the spouse of the care receiver rather than a nonspouse are linked to higher levels of strain. High elder dependency is associated with higher levels of strain. Caregivers who provide more care report more strain. Higher levels of such variables as affection, reciprocity, mutuality—all related to the quality of the relationship between the caregiver and care receiver—are associated with lower levels of strain. Likewise, higher levels of feelings of preparedness for caregiving are associated with lower levels of strain.

Less is known about positive responses to caregiving. Some studies indicate that caregivers experience satisfaction with and personal meaning from the caregiver role. Such rewards of caregiving are associated with lower levels of strain.

The quality of care provided by families needs further exploration. To date, most of the work in this area has focused on the recognition of poor-quality care and abuse—two important areas for nursing. Nursing interventions, however, are often focused on improving the quality of care provided by families; thus, we need a better understanding of good-quality family care.

The phenomenon of caregiving to persons with dementia has been explored more fully than caregiving to other special populations. Families find the secondary symptoms of dementia (e.g., wandering, agitation) particularly difficult. Increasingly, researchers are investigating caregiving in other special populations (e.g., cancer, Parkinson's disease). Recent studies have compared caregiving processes by race and ethnicity. This is an extremely complex area of research. For example, there is some evidence that caregiving processes are similar between Black and White families; measures used in these studies were developed in the dominant White culture and may not be appropriate for other groups. Concepts such as filial piety have been identified in studies of family care in Asian cultures. Evidence supports the existence of both similarities and differences in caregiving by culture and national origin.

Two excellent summaries of early caregiving research can be found in Horowitz (1985) and Givens and Givens (1991). The interested reader is referred to these sources for thoughtful analyses of the research on family caregiving in relation to nursing research and practice.

Although numerous theoretical perspectives have been brought to bear on family caregiving, two have had a major influence on knowledge development in nursing: theories of stress and coping and interactionist theories. Researchers who focus on family caregiving to elders with dementia and on the caregiver have tended to approach this area from the intraindividual perspective of stress and coping theory, whereas researchers interested in explicating caregiving processes and on improving care to the frail elder through work with the family have used the interpersonal interactionist perspective. Theoretical perspectives have influenced instrument development in caregiving. Measures of such concepts as caregiver stress and burden are used by researchers focused on stress and coping. Measures of such concepts as role strain and rewards are used by researchers focused on interactional caregiving processes.

Finally, more attention is now being given to interventions with caregivers or caregiving families; see Gallagher, Lovett, and Zeiss (1989), Collins, Givens, and Givens (1994), and Archbold and Stewart (1996) for a review of caregiving interventions. Nurses have been active in developing, administering, and evaluating psychoeducational interventions, expanded in-home care, transitional care models, and cognitive stimulation. Nurses are an important component of health services interventions for frail elders and their families (e.g., the channeling demonstrations, the social health maintenance organization). One conclusion from reviewing this work is that nurses have a key role in preparing and supporting families in caregiving activities and in identifying high-risk caregiving situations. Because of the increasing reliance on the family for care of frail elders, it is possible that too great a burden has been placed on the smallest social unit in society. It is critical that we turn our attention to understanding the costs to families of such changes in policy.

PATRICIA G. ARCHBOLD
BARBARA J. STEWART

See also:
ACTIVITIES OF DAILY LIVING
CAREGIVER
FOSTER CARE
FUNCTIONAL HEALTH
RESPITE CARE

GERIATRICS

Geriatrics evolved from the Greek word *geras,* "old age," and it refers to the branch of medicine that covers the diagnosis and treatment of the diseases and syndromes that occur in old age. A board-certified medical practitioner of geriatric medicine is called a geriatrician. In the lay press the term has sometimes been overgeneralized to include comprehensive health care and preventive services for older adults, but this obfuscates the precise original meaning of the term.

In the specialty of nursing devoted to care of the aged, there has been considerable overlapping of words and definitions, linguistic confusion, and philosophical controversy. These problems led to attempts to clarify and specify terminology and make the terms fit the consensual philosophy and goals of practitioners within the specialty. The debate about proper terminology will continue into the next century and may become even more heated as the absolute numbers and subsequent health care needs of older adults escalate through at least 2030.

A specialty referred to as geriatric nursing was first suggested in an anonymous 1925 editorial, "Care of the Aged," in the *American Journal of Nursing*, and the first nursing textbook on the topic was published in 1950 (Burnside, 1988). However, the actual birth of the specialty occurred in 1962, when the American Nurses Association (ANA) formed the Conference Group on Geriatric Nursing Practice. In 1966 the ANA officially created the Division of Geriatric Nursing, and in 1976 the name was changed to the Division of Gerontological Nursing (ANA, 1982). The ANA published the first set of *Standards of Practice for Geriatric Nursing* in The *Journal of Gerontological Nursing* began operation in 1975, and *Geriatric Nursing* was first published in 1979. The titles of these two journals and the ANA division's name change reflect the ongoing debate about proper terminology for this nursing specialty.

Many people rejected the term *geriatrics* because it did not properly reflect nursing's interest in the entire continuum of health and disease, including health promotion, disease prevention, care of acute illness, and long-term care. Others rejected it on narrower terms, saying that it did not convey inclusion of the art of nursing.

Although the ANA division's name change to the Division of Gerontological Nursing pleased some nurses, others said it introduced a new error in terminology. The main criticism about this new label was that gerontology refers to the study of or science work about the aging processes and the biological, psychological, sociological, and economic experiences of normal aging (Lueckenotte, 1996). Using an "ology" term did not logically lend itself to the name of a clinical specialty in a practice field. This problem led some leaders in the field to lobby for the term *gerontic nursing* to identify the specialty. Gerontic nursing as defined by Gunter and Estes (1979) is more philosophically palatable than geriatric nursing and more linguistically correct than gerontological nursing. Gerontic nursing was defined as a nursing specialty that includes the art and practice of nurturing, caring, and comforting older adults. Supporters of this term maintained that it included both the science and the art of nursing.

A review of the titles of the most popular clinical textbooks in the field today showed that the field of medicine clearly uses the term *geriatric medicine* in the titles of its textbooks, but nursing is more ambivalent. Nursing textbook titles include such terms as gerontological nursing, clinical gerontological nursing, gerontologic nursing, gerontic nursing, and geriatric nursing; however, the latter two are in the minority. Lueckenotte, in her 1996 textbook, goes so far as to say that geriatrics is a branch of medicine, that it has limited application to nursing because of its disease orientation, and that it generally is not used to describe nursing care of older adults. Gerontic nursing never became commonly accepted, and it now seems very dated in its conceptualization. As Gunter and Estes (1979) defined the term, it would not include health promotion, risk reduction, or disease prevention (primary and secondary prevention). So in today's reality it would not be inclusive enough to meet the health care goals and client needs of the 21st century.

An ideal term for this nursing specialty would cover the full range of knowledge needed and services to be provided in this practice field that has age of client as its sole parameter. The specialty is practiced at all levels of the health continuum, with persons who are aged 60+ to 115+, in any and all types of settings where older adults are to be found, and for periods of time that stretch from minutes to decades. Finding a fitting replacement for the term *geriatrics* or *geriatric nursing* has already challenged some of the best minds in the profession for over 30 years. The search for an ideal term is not likely to end soon.

JOANNE SABOL STEVENSON

See also:
DEPRESSION AMONG OLDER ADULTS
ELDER ABUSE
FAMILY CAREGIVING TO FRAIL ELDERS
GERONTOLGOICAL CARE
GERONTOLOGICAL NURSING—ADVANCED PRACTICE

GERONTOLOGICAL CARE

Gerontology emerged as a field of inquiry in the 20th century, but there is little agreement as to what gerontology is. According to the National Institute on Aging (NIA), scientists study aging from the broadest biological, medical, behavioral, and social perspectives in order to understand its fundamental processes and mechanisms (Achenbaum, 1995). This breadth of scope is both an asset and a liability because there is no single disciplinary perspective, few models and support for interdisciplinary work, and no common core of disciplinary knowledge to unify the field. Thus, the theory and practice of gerontology is often fragmented among multiple disciplines, each with its own traditions, theories, methods, and body of knowledge (Estes, Binney, & Culbertson, 1992).

The terms *gerontological/geriatric* nursing are often used interchangeably. In this section the former term is used, as it encompasses the study of aging, geriatrics (the medical treatment of old age and its disease), geriatric nursing, and research. Gerontological nursing practice standards were first published in 1967, and since then several reviews have assessed the state of gerontological nursing and research, including those by Adams, Basson, Brimmer, Gunter and Miller, Kayser-Jones, Rempusheski, Robinson, and Wolanin. These reviews and others in the *Annual Review of Nursing Research* and *Advances in Gerontological Nursing* indicated a steady increase in gerontological nursing research over the past 30 years. They also argued for more systematic investigations of interventions targeted to both older adults and the health care system that serves them.

Importance of Gerontological Nursing Research

Tripp-Reimer (1994) noted that interacting societal and professional factors create a current imperative for gerontological nursing research. The continuing growth of older adults (currently 13% of the U.S. population and estimated at 22.9% by 2050), the heterogeneous characteristics of the aging population, economic incentives to develop cost-effective interventions (elders account for 40% of health care expenditures), and national health objectives press for more gerontological research, especially on the effectiveness of interventions to address these diverse issues.

Early research was largely atheoretical, hindering development of a knowledge base. According to Murphy and Fenton (1991), only 59% of the 142 studies they reviewed evidenced an explicit theory-research link. Recently, nurses have used a number of conceptual models and theoretical frameworks to guide research. These include reactance (Meddaugh), behavioral theories (Whall & Boehm), basic need model (Nelson; Rossby, Beck, & Heacock), person-environment fit and interaction (Kayser-Jones; Maas and colleagues; Wyman), and stress and coping models (Archbold and associates; Hall & Buckwalter). Glick and Tripp-Reimer (1996) recently published an integrative model depicting the scope of gerontological nursing encompassing three spheres (elder, environment, and nursing) and designed to assist nurses to provide comprehensive and contextually relevant care.

Current reviews of research concentrate on single topics such as hypertension, caregiving, incontinence, confusion, sleeplessness, or dyspnea (Tripp-Reimer, 1994). Although most research has been descriptive, more nurses are using the existing knowledge base to identify and test interventions. The generalizability of gerontological research findings has been limited by methodological and measurement difficulties (i.e., inadequate sample sizes and sampling plans, lack of rigorous designs, insufficiently operationalized interventions, and inappropriate, ill-defined, insensitive, incorrectly timed or invalid outcome measures), but nurses have begun to address these methodological issues. It is important to note that there are recently issued clinical practice guidelines addressing common gerontological care issues such as pressure ulcers, cataracts, dementia, and incontinence.

Gerontological Nurse Researchers

Any compilation of this nature risks the omission of key topics, individuals, and studies. With this limitation in mind, selected nurse researchers and their areas of investigation are briefly highlighted. By no means exhaustive, these exemplars include caregiving, abuse, incontinence, confusion, and pressure ulcers—areas in which gerontological nursing research has made a significant difference in elder care.

Caregiving. Providing care for someone with a chronic illness can result in negative emotional, physical, financial, and social sequelae. The work of numerous gerontological nurse researchers (e.g., Given, Collins, Archbold, Wykle, Wright, Stewart, Hall, Farran, Davis, and others) in the areas of theory testing, interventions, outcomes, and advances in measurement has made a substantial contribution to our understanding of the caregiving experience and its multifaceted impact, particularly on family caregivers. In institutional settings, Chiverton, Burgener, Maas and associates, and Beck and colleagues have focused attention on the role of both professional and assistive personnel and its effect on care-recipient and family outcomes.

A related dimension of research in which nurses have played a key role is the etiology, identification, and intervention of elder mistreatment. The work of Fulmer, Phillips, and Rempusheski is notable in this area.

Urinary incontinence. Another common and costly gerontological condition is urinary incontinence. Nurse researchers such as McCormick, Wells, McDowell, Dougherty, Colling, and Wyman have increased our understanding and treatment of this condition in both community-dwelling and institutionalized elders. Their investigations to prevent, reverse, or reduce the negative physiological, psychological, and social effects of incontinence have ranged from the development of procedures testing pelvic floor muscle strength to nursing home staff interventions such as prompted voiding.

Acute and chronic confusion. Acute confusion can be caused by a variety of physiological, psychological, and environmental factors and is associated with high morbidity and mortality in older adults. Wolanin and Philips authored a seminal text on confusion, paving the way for others to study this pervasive condition in various patient populations. Champagne, Foreman, Neelon, Vermeersch, and M. Williams have elucidated the incidence and risk factors associated with acute confusion and developed methods to effectively capture this elusive phenomenon.

Most care needs of chronically confused elders, such as those with Alzheimer's disease, are met through nursing management strategies. Important advances have been made by Abraham, the Quayhagens, and Beck in the area of cognitive remediation; by Maas and colleagues, Mathew, and Hall in evaluating environmental designs; by Ryden, Snyder, Rader and associates, Beck, Burgener, Whall and colleagues, and Baldwin in diminishing disruptive behaviors; and by Beck and others in dressing behaviors. Gerontological nurse researchers have evaluated selected interventions to enhance sensory stimulation, such as music (Gerdner, Swanson, Abraham), exercise (Meddaugh), dolls and stuffed animals (Bailey), and animals (Baun, Kongable), and biobehavioral interventions for sundowning (Evans), wandering (Algase), and improved food consumption (Mion, Kayser-Jones), to name but a few.

Pressure ulcers. Nurse researchers also have made significant contributions to the etiology and treatment of pressure ulcers, a pervasive gerontological problem. Norton, Gosnell, Braden, and Bergstrom have been instrumental in developing risk assessment tools. Frantz evaluated prevention and treatment of pressure ulcers in a variety of settings, using transcutaneous electrical stimulation techniques, and developed measures to capture wound healing in elders.

Conclusion

As noted by Williams (1988), "research and care require each other; they interact with each other; they benefit from each other . . . this applies to all aspects of care for older people, personal care, preventive and therapeutic health services, social services, and the organization and financing of care" (p. 579). The scope of gerontology, a relatively new multidisciplinary field, is very broad. Nurses have made substantial contributions to research in the psychological, environmental, physiological, and sociological care of older adults, as supported by reviews of theory-research linkages (Murphy & Fenton, 1991), the usefulness of gerontological research for practice, and meta-analyses of gerontological research and theory. Nonetheless, Achenbaum (1995) cautions: "Gerontology will continue to open new frontiers of knowledge as long as highly trained scholars are willing to cross the boundaries of their own scientific training and appreciate the rewards of broadening their fields of vision" (p. 268).

KATHLEEN C. BUCKWALTER
SUSAN GARDNER

See also:
   CAREGIVER
   COGNITIVE DISORDERS
   GERIATRICS
   GERONTOLOGICAL NURSING: ADVANCED PRACTICE
   PRESSURE ULCERS
   URINARY INCONTINENCE

GERONTOLOGICAL NURSING—ADVANCED PRACTICE

The proliferation of Advanced Practice Nurses (APNs) during the last three decades has been shown to improve the quality of patient care, increase patient and staff satisfaction, and be cost effective across various health care settings (Feldman, Ventura, & Crosby, 1987; Master et al., 1980; Miller, 1997; Naylor et al., 1999; Ramsay, McKenzie, & Fish, 1982; Sox, 1979; Spitzer et al., 1974).

Types of Geriatric Advanced Practice Nurses (GAPNs)

During the late 1960s to 1970s graduate nursing programs began developing specialties in gerontological nursing. GAPN is an umbrella term that refers to Geriatric Nurse Practitioners (GNP) or Gerontological Clinical Nurse Specialists (GCNS). Currently there are over 3000 certified GNPs and nearly 1000 certified GCNS (AACN, 1999). These APN subgroups presently require gerontological-focused graduate education. GCNS roles include educator, researcher, practitioner, manager, and consultant. In addition to the GCNS roles, GNPs have the ability to perform advanced health history taking and physical assessment, diagnosis, and to prescribe appropriate medical treatments—including pharmaceuticals. Scopes of practice for the GCNS and the GNP vary among states. Literature demonstrates more similarities between nurse practitioners (NPs) and clinical nurse specialists (CNS) than differences. Nursing leaders debate role integration (Fenton & Brykczynski, 1993; Soehren & Schumann, 1994).

Naylor, Munro, and Brooten (1991) explored measurable outcomes validating APN practice: mortality, morbidity, LOS, functional status, mental status, stress level, and patient satisfaction, burden of care, and cost of care. Feldman, Ventura, and Crosby (1987) critically reviewed 56 studies focused on NP effectiveness in areas ranging from pediatrics to long-term care facilities. Overall these studies demonstrated consumer acceptance and satisfaction with NPs; physician-comparable quality of care; increased productivity; cost savings; saved physician time; effective management of both preventive care and care of the chronically ill; and improved patient education. The literature has GAPNs in a favorable light.

GAPN—Long Term Care (LTC)

The role of the GAPN has impacted the quality of care in LTC populations as evidenced by decreased hospitalizations, reduced pharmaceutical usage, cost savings, and improved patient-family-staff satisfaction. GAPNs have played a vital role in reducing restraints in this population (Evans et al., 1997). Using a quasiexperimental design, Kane and colleagues (1989c) compared data of pre- and post-GNP time periods in 60 nursing homes (30-GNP; 30-control) dispersed throughout eight western states. The authors also examined various issues surrounding the role of a GNP as a nursing home employee. A 1-year retrospective data analysis for 1,077 LTC residents compared 414 residents followed by GNP/MD teams and 663 residents followed by MDs. Patients of the GNP/MD teams yielded a $72 per resident per month savings (Burl, Bonner, Rao, & Khan, 1998). GNPs once again proved to be cost-effective.

GNPs may succeed in management. Grzeczkowshi and Knapp (1988) evaluated a 120-bed nursing home after a GNP became the Director of Nursing. The findings demonstrated fewer medications, lower rates of urinary/respiratory tract infections, decreased utilization of indwelling urinary catheters, and less decubiti. It was hypothesized that GNPs' extensive geriatric education and ability to work well within interdisciplinary teams yield effective patient care.

GAPN—Acute Care

Given the advanced education in geriatric issues such as falls, restraint usage, delirium, polypharmacy, and normal versus abnormal physical changes, the GAPN plays a vital role in acute-care management of frail elders. Often GAPNs anticipate these conditions and provide early intervention. Models of care that have improved hospitalized care to the elderly include geriatric evaluation teams, Nurses Improving Care to the Hospitalized Elderly (NICHE), Geriatric Resource Nurse (GRN), Case Management (CM), Geriatric evaluation and management (GEM) units, and Acute Care of the Elderly (ACE) units. GAPNs have been integral members of these models of care (Paier & Strumph, 1999).

A retrospective analysis of geriatric nursing home patients admitted to an acute-care facility demonstrated a mean decrease of 2.78 ($p < 0.05$) days in length of stay (LOS) when care involved a GNP (Miller, 1997). Naylor et al. (1999) went further than evaluating "in-house" statistics. Their randomized clinical trial included 363 patients (186 control; 177 intervention) with follow-up data collection up to 24 weeks posthospital discharge. In the intervention group, GAPNs were responsible for Comprehensive Discharge Planning (CDP) and home follow-up protocol. A few outcome measures were hospital readmission, recurrence or exacerbation of the index hospitalization DRG, comorbidity, cumulative days of rehospitalization, functional status, depression, and patient satisfaction. The findings at 24 weeks demonstrated that GAPN patients experienced 270 days of hospitalization, as opposed to 760 days for patients in the control group. GAPN patients yielded a Medicare saving of almost $600,000. Other findings including functional status, depression scores, and patient satisfaction were similar in both study groups.

GAPN—Home Care

Case studies in home care describe the accessible, comprehensive, accountable, continual, and collaborative care delivered by GNPs (Burns-Tisdal & Goff, 1989). Alessi and colleagues (1997) studied 414 home clients (random: 215-intervention and 199-control). The intervention group had GNPs perform comprehensive geriatric assessments (CGAs) annually for 3 years along with quarterly follow-up visits. The authors examined the GNPs healthcare recommendations made to clients and proposed that repetitive reinforcement and the GNP-patient relationship contributed to achieving patient adherence to therapies. This warrants further investigation.

The Program of All-inclusive Care for the Elderly (PACE), a program developed in San Francisco known as On Lok in 1971, focuses on day health and social services to enable frail elderly to remain in the community. PACE's model requires GAPNs in the interdisciplinary team. PACE programs now exist in nine states (Eng, Pedulla, Eleazer, McCann, & Fox, 1997).

GAPN—Ambulatory Care

GNPs have provided effective ambulatory care. McDowell, Martin, Snustad, and Flynn (1986) performed a retrospective review of 800 patients and found that a GNP's care was comparative to two internal-medicine board-certified physicians with geriatric experience in university-based settings. Polypharmacy and functional status were the measurements used to compare GNP and MD care. Mahoney (1994) compared medication usage of NPs and MDs. Three geriatric vignettes designed by GNPs, geriatricians, and geriatric pharmacists were presented to 373 MDs and 118 NPs. Analysis of the MDs and NPs was discussed. NPs utilized fewer drugs. The NP sample was not specifically limited to GNPs; family and adult nurse practitioners (APN, FNP) were included in the sample. Geriatric experience and prescribing experience proved to be significant factors affecting the appropriate prescription. Mahoney proposed that gerontologic education for the APNs and FNPs would ensure proper pharmaceutical usage for the elderly.

Future Directions

Meta-analysis methods have allowed researchers to examine conflicts in the data and deduce clearer and more conclusive findings; this research further validates GAPN practice. Future research needs to be rigorous with attention to: (a) conceptual definitions including sensitivity of outcome measures, study of the process not the provider, relationship between the process and outcomes of care; (b) measurement of variables; and (c) methodology including more blinded randomized trials with attention to internal and external validity (Brown & Grimes, 1995).

ANNEMARIE DOWLING CASTRONOVO

See also:
    ACUTE CARE
    CERTIFICATION IN GERONTOLOGICAL NURSING
    GERONTOLOGICAL CARE

HEALTH CARE FINANCING ADMINISTRATION

The Health Care Financing Administration (HCFA) of the Department of Health and Human Services is the federal agency that administers the Medicare and Medicaid programs. It also regulates all U.S. laboratory testing (except research) through the Clinical Laboratory Improvement Amendments program (United States Health Care Financing Administration, 1997c). The HCFA's roles include purchasing health care services, conducting research on health care management, treatment, and financing; establishing reimbursement policies; and evaluating health care facility and services quality. The HCFA oversees about 17,400 nursing homes and 9,800 home health agency inspections each year (United States Health Care Financing Administration, 1997d). Title XVIII, Medicare, and Title XIX, Medicaid, of the Social Security Act were enacted in 1965. As of 1997 more than 74 million Americans receive health care through Medicare and Medicaid. Most of the care is provided through the fee-for-service delivery system, although many recipients receive care through managed care plans. The HCFA is important to nursing for health care service reimbursement, funding for nursing research, and monitoring for quality nursing and other health care.

Medicare is the nation's largest health insurance program, covering 38 million Americans. The HCFA expects to spend $210.9 billion for Medicare in 1997. Medicare provides insurance to people 65 years and older, the disabled (5 million), and those with permanent kidney failure (275,000). Medicare is hospital insurance (Part A) and medical insurance (Part B). Part A provides coverage of inpatient hospital services, skilled nursing facilities, home health services, and hospice care. Part B helps pay for the cost of a nurse practitioner, nurse midwifery, physician services, outpatient hospital services, medical equipment and supplies, and other health services and supplies. Part A is financed through a part of the Social Security payroll tax, although Medicare beneficiaries must pay deductibles ($760 in 1997) and coinsurance. General tax revenues fund about 75% of Part B expenditures, although beneficiaries must pay monthly premiums for coverage ($43.80 in 1997) as well as deductibles and coinsurance (United States Health Care Financing Administration, 1997a).

Medicaid is a program that provides medical assistance for certain individuals and families with low incomes and resources. The program is jointly funded by federal and state governments and varies from state to state and within states over time as to eligibility and covered benefits. States provide medical care to eligible needy persons within broad federal guidelines. Each state "1. establishes its own eligibility standards; 2. determines the type, amount, duration, and scope of services; 3. sets the rate of payment for services; and 4. administers its own program" (United States Health Care Financing Administration, 1997b).

Title XIX requires that states provide specified basic services to the categorically needy population in order to receive federal matching funds. These services are

> inpatient hospital services; outpatient hospital services; physician services; medical and surgical dental services; nursing facility (NF) services for individuals aged 21 or older; home health care for persons eligible for nursing facility services; family planning services and supplies; rural health clinic services and any other ambulatory services offered by a rural health clinic that are otherwise

covered under the State plan; laboratory and x-ray services; pediatric and family nurse practitioner services; federally-qualified health center services and any other ambulatory services offered by a federally-qualified health center that are otherwise covered under the State plan; nurse-midwife services (to the extent authorized under State law); and early and periodic screening, diagnosis, and treatment (EPSDT) services for individuals under age 21. (United States Health Care Financing Administration, 1997c)

If states choose to provide Medicaid to the medically needy, they must provide the following additional services:

prenatal care and delivery services for pregnant women; ambulatory services to individuals under age 18 and individuals entitled to institutional services; home health services to individuals entitled to nursing facility services; and if the State plan includes services either in institutions for mental diseases or in intermediate care facilities for the mentally retarded (ICF/MRs), it must offer either of the following to each of the medically needy groups: the services contained in 42 CFR sections 440.10 through 440.50 and 440.165 (to the extent that nurse-midwives are authorized to practice under State law or regulations); or the services contained in any seven of the sections in 42 CFR 440.10 through 440.165. (United States Health Care Financing Administration, 1997c)

States may also provide optional services and receive federal funding for those services. Such services include "clinic services; nursing facility services for the under age 21; intermediate care facility/mentally retarded services; optometrist services and eyeglasses; prescribed drugs; TB-related services for TB infected persons; prosthetic devices; and dental services" (United States Health Care Financing Administration, 1997c).

Each state's Medicaid plan must allow recipients freedom of choice among health care providers participating in Medicaid. The waivers 1915(b) and 1115(b) allow states to pay for Medicaid services through managed care organizations. In 1995 about 25% of Medicaid recipients were in managed care organizations. The portion of the Medicaid program that is paid for by the federal government is based on each state's average per capita income and ranges from 50% to 83%.

The HCFA is the federal agency that manages the Medicare and Medicaid programs. Medicare is the national health insurance program for the elderly, the disabled, and those with permanent kidney damage. Medicaid pays for health care for people with low incomes and is jointly funded by the federal government and states.

Christine T. Kovner

See also:
HEALTH MAINTENANCE ORGANIZATIONS

HEALTH MAINTENANCE ORGANIZATIONS

Historically, most physicians were paid on a fee-for-service basis. The physician received a payment for each patient encounter or other service from the patient receiving the care or from someone paying on behalf of the patient, such as an insurance company. Recently, health care has become "managed." Managed care systems integrate the financing and delivery of care and include financial incentives for people to use providers within the system. Health maintenance organizations (HMOs) are a type of managed care system.

Health maintenance organizations provide a defined set of health care services to persons for a predetermined periodic fixed prepayment unrelated to the actual services received and restrict their members to specific health care providers. In many cases the providers are paid a periodic payment unrelated to the services rendered. This payment method is called capitation. The providers receive a periodic fee whether or not they provide care. In HMOs there is a financial incentive to provide fewer health care services, and many people are concerned that the HMOs may not provide needed care. On the other hand, many traditional fee-for-service insurance plans have not reimbursed for preventive care. HMOs provide preventive care as part of the benefit package.

HMOs have a database on the health services the members receive. The database provides an opportunity for nurse researchers to study the health of people across settings. Many HMOs provide health promotion services, and studies could identify how these services are provided and the impact they have on people's health.

HMOs limit people's choice to a specific group of providers. Providers who are not part of these groups have few patients from HMOs. Nurses are anxious to become part of the group that is approved to provide care to HMO members.

HMOs provide a set of health care services for a fixed prepayment unrelated to the amount of health care services provided. This is beneficial to clients in need of extensive health care and clients involved in health promotion. Also, HMOs have given opportunities for nursing in the areas of research and health provider.

CHRISTINE T. KOVNER

See also:
  HCFA

HOMELESSNESS

Older homeless persons have been largely neglected in the nursing literature. Existing studies of homeless elders describe individual risk factors for homelessness among the aged but offer only a limited understanding of the magnitude of the problem. General health patterns of older homeless men and women, homeless elders' use of healthcare services, and real and perceived barriers to care all grant us further insight regarding homeless elders (Kutza & Keigher, 1991; Vance, 1994). There is also a dearth of healthcare policy and clinical-intervention research that addresses the unique and complex healthcare needs of this vulnerable—and often invisible—population of elders.

A key problem in studying the aging homeless is the lack of a clear definition of "older homeless" individuals. Some researchers—noting that homeless individuals look and behave 10–20 years older than they should, and that they have significant physical and psychological health problems— define the older homeless person as any homeless individual over the age of 50 (Cohen, 1999; Cohen & Sokolovsky, 1989; Crane, 1994; Gelberg, Linn, & Mayer-Oakes, 1990). Using age 50 as the criterion for identifying elderly homeless people, Burt (1996) widely estimates that there are between 60,000 and 400,000 older homeless in the United States today and predicts that these figures will double by 2030.

Several studies report that older homeless persons are mostly male Caucasians (Gelberg et al., 1990; Rossi, 1989), whereas younger homeless tend to be nonwhite men, women, and children (Hopper & Milburn, 1996). Although women outnumber men in the general population aged 50 and older, men outnumber women four to one among the aging homeless population (Bissonette & Hijjazi, 1994). A Chicago-based study found that older men were homeless roughly 50% longer than older women (Rossi, 1989). In New York City, older women tended to become homeless in their mid-fifties, while older men reported living on "skid row" since their mid-forties (Cohen, C. I., & Crane, 1996).

Given the predominance of older homeless males, it is not surprising that most studies of the physical and/or mental-health needs of homeless elders have focused on small convenience samples of homeless elderly men (Harris & Williams, 1991; Teresi, Holmes, & Cohen, 1988), or have lumped men and women together without addressing age- or gender-specific health concerns (Damrosch & Strasser, 1988; Lafluente & Lane, 1995; Reilly, 1994). For example, Lafluente and Lane's (1995) phenomenological study investigated social disaffiliation among 10 homeless men between the ages of 20 and 61. Montgomery's (1994) analysis of homeless women included 7 women of mixed race between the ages of 35 and 53. Ugarriza and Fallon (1994) suggest that studying homeless women in general may be difficult because women do not access public healthcare facilities as readily as homeless men. When they do seek health services, it is often for prenatal care or care for dependent children (Adkins & Fields, 1992). Therefore, older homeless women are less likely to make contact with the healthcare system and are often overlooked in clinical research.

Despite the abundance of research on homeless older men, numerous studies have established that older homeless persons suffer substantially more physical illnesses than do younger homeless adults and nonhomeless elders (Atkinson, Turner, & Tolson, 1998; Reilly, 1994). To date, one of the most comprehensive examinations of homeless persons' health used objective and self-reported measures of physical health. It was undertaken as part of a study of 521 homeless men in two Los Angeles beach communities (Gelberg et al., 1990). The results indicated that homeless men older than 50 suffered more chronic illness and had more functional disabilities than did younger individuals, and that the 50-and-over sample demonstrated patterns of illness that were similar to those of adults 65 and older in the general population (Gelberg et al., 1990). Because their illnesses often go untreated, illness among homeless adults leads to higher mortality rates than does illness among their nonhomeless peers (Hwang, Orav, O'Connell, Lebow, & Brennan, 1997).

Many of the health problems experienced by older homeless persons are exacerbated by substance addiction (Atkinson, Turner, & Tolson, 1998). DeMallie, North, and Smith (1997) also noted higher rates of lifetime histories of alcohol abuse or dependence among homeless individuals age 50 and older.

While alcohol misuse and prescription-drug dependence are more prevalent among older adults (Gurnack, 1996; Finlayson, 1998), the prevalence of heroin abuse, crack cocaine abuse, and the abuse of other substances is also rising among aging baby boomers (Gurnack & Schonfeld, 1998). The increase in the abuse of substances in the geriatric population creates new challenges for healthcare professionals, since most models of assessment, treatment, and intervention focus on older problem drinkers (Adams, Barry, & Fleming, 1996; Atkinson et al., 1998; Dupree & Schonfeld, 1998).

Heavy alcohol consumption among individuals over the age of 65 in the general population has been associated with decreased bone density, an increased risk of hip fracture from falls, and motor vehicle accidents (Felson, Kiel, Anderson, & Kamel, 1988). A large cross-sectional study by Adams, Yuan, Barboriak, and Rimm (1993) reported that alcohol-related hospitalizations among elderly U.S. residents in 1989 occurred at the same rate as for myocardial infarction, at a cost of 2.3 million dollars. Alcohol was implicated in the hospitalization of 54.7 per 1,000 men compared to 14.8 per 1,000 women. Given that older homeless men outnumber older homeless women in the United States, the connection between health and substance addictions is an important area for further nursing research.

There is also compelling evidence that homeless elders have higher overall rates of mental illness than the general older population (Crane, 1998; Harper & Lacey, 1993). Wallsten (1992) estimated that 10%–15% of homeless elders have a serious or chronic mental illness, including alcohol abuse, drug abuse and dependency, anxiety disorders, depression, and schizophrenia. Crane (1992) interviewed 50 homeless individuals over the age of 60 in central London and noted a profound link between mental-health problems and elder homelessness. Even so, few nursing studies address mental-health needs or assess the possibility of alcohol-related dementia among older homeless persons. There has also been limited research examining drug misuse among older persons and its long-term effects on physical, psychosocial, and spiritual health. Comprehensive population surveys that address widespread drug misuse often fail to identify older drug misusers, even though risk factors such as the presence of physical illness, chemical abuse, cognitive impairment and/or psychiatric disease, inadequate social support, and a history of victimization have all been linked to homelessness among the elderly (Cohen, C. I., 1999).

Given the rise in the number of homeless elders in American society, nurses need to conduct scientific research that soundly measures the complex parameters of elder homelessness. Outcome data must be gathered to provide an accurate description of homeless elders and their healthcare needs, as well as any root problems that may be contributing to prolonged homelessness. Only then can programs be designed to address the specific needs of older homeless persons, policy be developed to respond to this growing social problem, and adequate resources be allocated to implement both practice and policy.

BARBARA L. BRUSH

See also:
   ADULT FOSTER CARE
   ALCOHOLISM
   DEPRESSION AMONG OLDER ADULTS
   RESPITE CARE

HOSPICE

Definition

Hospice has been defined as a concept of care, a program of care, and a place for care. Hospice as a concept of care espouses: choice with regard to the place of one's dying; attention to the comfort of the individual; a consideration of spiritual, social, and psychological concerns, as well as the physiological and functional manifestations of the disease process; a focus on the family as well as on the patient; an emphasis on dying, death, and the bereavement that follows; the provision of interdisciplinary care (not simply the attention of professionals from multiple disciplines); and the implementation of coordinated care across settings. (Corless, 1995, p. 78)

As a program of care, hospice care is provided in a variety of settings, including the home, hospital, extended care facility, or designated hospice or palliative care beds. Hospice as a place for care is setting-defined and is either free-standing or part of another facility.

History

Arising from the research of Florence Wald and her colleagues (see Terminal Illness) and the model of St. Christopher's Hospice in England and inextricably bound to the death awareness movement, the first hospice programs developed in the United States in the late 1970s and early 1980s. Dame Cicely Saunders, nurse, social worker, and physician, was one of the founders of the modern hospice movement. She emphasized the importance of research as a part of hospice care. Her focus and that of Melzack, Ofiesh, and Mount (1976) was on the alleviation of pain. The concern with symptom control was part of the research focus of the Royal Victoria Hospital's Palliative Care Unit (PCU), founded by Balfour Mount and his colleagues.

The PCU's research team included Mary Vachon (Vachon, Lyall, & Freeman, 1978), who studied the stress that caring for the dying created for the caregiver. Vachon (1987) expanded her focus to examine the issue of occupational stress, discovering in her research that caring for the dying was not the major problem for caregivers. Rather, such issues as poor communication, lack of continuity, and conflicts between units were more significant sources of stress for caregivers.

Areas of Research

Support for caregivers and the prevention of burnout has continued to be of interest in hospice care but is not currently a primary area of research endeavors. Concerns about burnout have been superseded by an interest in spirituality, that of caregivers and of patients. Highfield and Cason (1983) investigated whether the spiritual needs of patients were being met. The paucity of attention to this area, in the United States, was likely due to the confluence of three factors. First, the emphasis in hospice care initially was on program development, referral of patients, and funding. Second, a number of the early hospice programs were started by psychiatrists or those with a psychosocial bent. Thus, psychiatrists were utilized both for patients and their families and to provide staff support. A third factor that had an influence is the historic division between church and state, a division not found in England. So devotions are incorporated in the life of St. Christopher's Hospice in a way that has not occurred in American hospices. That is not to say that the integration of spirituality is not an area of continuing concern for hospice programs.

Initially, however, most of the emphasis was on demonstrating the efficacy of the hospice intervention. The problems of effecting improvement in symptoms and quality of life in what is inevitably a downward trajectory, together with a concern about the research burden for dying persons and their family members, makes this a challenging area for investigators. Much of the more recent research has utilized hospice as a site for symptom control research rather than for evaluating whether hospice programs are more skilled in symptom management than nonhospice sites.

Economic and Regulatory Issues

The comparison of hospice programs with hospital and home care programs that served as controls was initiated by the federal government as a demonstration program to assess the cost savings of a hospice benefit. The benefit, however, was written into law prior to the completion of the research. As a result of the legislation and accompanying regulations, hospice funding is on a capitated basis rather than on a per visit basis. In addition, visits could be made by hospice personnel for psychosocial and other reasons that did not meet the "skilled care" requirements of traditional home care.

The emphasis in the regulations is on home care. Hospice programs are penalized if the yearly quota of home care is not met. This quota is determined by the 80/20 cap, which specifies that 80% of the care of hospice patients as a totality must be provided in the home if financial penalties are to be avoided. The hospice benefit provides for four levels of care: routine home care, continuous home care, inpatient respite care, and general inpatient care. The low level of reimbursement for respite care means that this approach to providing some rest for caregivers is not utilized. It would cost the hospice program more money to secure this care than they would receive in compensation from the government.

Reimbursement is dependent on level of care received but is also financially capped. The constraints of the financial cap and the 80/20 cap have limited both the amount of care provided and the type of person accepted into the program. Consequently, individuals without a caregiver may not be accepted in many hospice programs unless the program has some other mechanism for keeping a dying person safely at home.

The advent of HIV/AIDS (human immunodeficiency virus/acquired immunodeficiency syndrome) has resulted in a change in the federal hospice requirements for persons with HIV disease. The 80/20 cap is not applied to these individuals. Nonetheless, some hospice programs have been slow in opening their programs to HIV-infected persons. At the same time, hospice was not an option readily selected by individuals dying as result of AIDS. The emphasis on dying was not congenial to these individuals, who were still looking for further treatment. And appropriate treatment often could cure an illness resulting from an opportunistic pathogen; consequently, meaningful life was still an option. With the advent of the protease inhibitors many AIDS hospice patients have been discharged and are resuming their former activities.

Hospice programs have been challenged with the opening of beds for palliative care, a term popular in England and Canada. Palliative care focuses on symptom control as well as psychosocial care and is more acceptable as a consultation service to many physicians practicing in major medical centers. Hospice care also can be offered as a consultation service but has been identified with home care and limited inpatient beds as a result of the government's reimbursement mechanisms for hospice care. Another term, supportive care only, is used to indicate that care is no longer directed at cure or invasive procedures but at helping the patient be comfortable in the dying process. Supportive care and palliative care may incorporate hospice principles of care and thus meet the goal of the early hospice pioneers, namely, that mainstream medicine and nursing incorporate hospice principles in the care of all patients.

INGE B. CORLESS

See also:
CAREGIVER
PAIN ASSESSMENT
PAIN MANAGEMENT
TERMINAL ILLNESS

PHYSICAL RESTRAINTS

A physical restraint is attached to or adjacent to a person's body, cannot be removed easily, and restricts freedom of movement. Physical restraints are applied primarily for three reasons: fall risk, treatment interference, and other behaviors (e.g., restlessness, agitation, confusion, etc.). During the 1980s several nurses called attention to frequency of the practice, suggesting it was understudied, poorly understood, and a worthy area for nursing research. Because of the serious sequelae associated with restraint use for frail elders in hospitals and nursing homes and the authority of nurses to determine whether or not a restraint is used, research on use of physical restraints is an important concern as nurses seek evidence-based, best practices.

The first thorough review concerning use of physical restraint for the elderly was published by Evans and Strumpf (1989). At the time, incidence and prevalence of restraint varied depending on settings and studies but was reported as 7% to 22% in hospitals and 25% to 85% in nursing homes. Ten studies on the subject of physical restraint were identified in the review, and all were descriptive. Although prevention of injury to self or others was the most frequently cited rationale for use, no scientific basis for efficacy of restraints in safeguarding patients from injury was found.

Somewhat paradoxically, literature existed from the 1980s onward noting safety hazards associated with physical restraints, along with numerous physical, physiological, psychological, and behavioral consequences of restraint and immobilization. Since 1990, documentation of consequences has intensified. Physical restraints are implicated in serious injuries and death. The negative impact of physical restraints on functional capacity has been demonstrated and includes (a) development of complications, (b) dependency and morbidity, (c) biochemical and physiological effects, (d) altered perceptual and behavioral responses, and (e) emotional desolation.

The persistent use of physical restraints is troubling given a wealth of empiric evidence against the practice. The history and the culture of restraint use in the United States suggests a practice based more on myth than science. Reports from several European countries indicate that despite cross-cultural similarities in disability and illness between hospital patients and nursing home residents, there are pronounced differences in therapeutic belief and style and in the assumptions made about managing and controlling behavior (Strumpf & Tomes, 1993). One study compared the differences in prevalence in three American and two comparable European homes. Prevalence in the United States was nearly 40%, and in the Scottish and Swedish homes less than 10%. Scores on a measure of functional status showed the European residents to be even frailer than residents of U.S. homes (Evans et al., 1993). Remarkably contrasting practices with regard to restraint use can be attributed to differences in philosophy and cultural style, perceptions concerning legal liability, staff mix, availability of knowledgeable professionals, limitations on use of catheters and feeding tubes, nonavailability of restraining devices, and modifications in equipment and architectural environment.

In view of differences in American and European homes and with no empiric evidence for the therapeutic value of restraints, deep-seated myths explain the prominence of restraint use in the United States. The myths are based on the following beliefs about restraints: (a) they prevent falls and injuries, (b) they eliminate perceived harms associated with various behaviors, (c) they limit legal liability, (d) they do not bother the restrained person, (e) they substitute for inadequate staffing, and (f) they remain the only intervention available (Evans & Strumpf, 1990). Shifting the paradigm from a risk focus aimed at controlling behavior to an individualized focus aimed at restraint-free care is part of a significant debate occurring between researchers and clinicians. Arguments for individualized care are being bolstered by clinical intervention studies that dispel myths and demonstrate that restraint practices can be changed.

A recent and still small body of research on restraint reduction or elimination suggests that restraint-free care is a transitional process facilitated by understanding and applying change theory to guide a program of education, policy change, and procedural innovation for all levels of staff. Changing the traditional and habitual practice of physical restraint depends on altering beliefs and increasing knowledge about appropriate practices and standards of care.

Although hundreds of articles have been written on the subject of physical restraints, the only research studies to emerge in the past decade have focused on compliance with regulations or efforts at reduction and elimination. In one clinical trial on restraint reduction in nursing homes (Evans et al., 1997), three homes were randomly assigned to restraint education (RE), restraint education with consultation (REC), or control. The RE and REC homes received intensive education by a master's-prepared gerontological nurse to increase staff awareness of restraint hazards and knowledge about assessing and responding to resident behaviors likely to lead to use of restraints. In addition, one nursing home also received 12 hours per week of unit-based nursing consultation to facilitate restraint reduction for residents with more complex conditions. Only the home receiving REC had a statistically significant reduction in restraint prevalence. This was achieved without increased staff, psychoactive drugs, or serious fall-related injuries, dispelling several of the above-mentioned myths that have plagued progress in restraint reduction.

Although education is useful, a far greater effect is achieved when education is combined with consultation to assist staff in providing individualized, high-quality care for clinically challenging patients and residents. In addition, a continuing focus on individualized care is necessary if changes in practice are to be implemented, maintained, and appropriately modified over time. The success of consultation and other "best practice" models supports the use of advanced practice nurses to improve quality of care and outcomes for frail older adults in nursing homes and other settings. Recently, interest in restraint reduction has intensified in hospitals, driven in part by warnings of restraint hazards by the Food and Drug Administration and guidelines from the Joint Commission on Accreditation of Healthcare Organizations (Sullivan-Marx & Strumpf, 1996).

Given the state of the science on restraint use, restraint reduction, and the emergence of restraint-free care as the standard of practice, ethical debate on the subject of physical restraints has also shifted. Until recently, this debate has been framed as the classic moral conflict between caregiver determinations of beneficence versus individual autonomy. Although physical restraint has long been viewed as an infringement of personal rights, the ethics literature has focused on three basic concerns: (a) mental competence, (b) patient wishes and duties of staff to protect from harm, and (c) the benefit-to-burden ratio. In these formulations, however, the choice to restrain is always an option. Protection of the patient, preventing harm to others, and the benefits of preventing a fall, keeping a tube in place, or controlling behavior outweigh any burdens.

Today an expanding empiric base and practices guided by a philosophy of individualized care are transforming our understanding of beneficent and autonomous care for frail elders. Beneficent care requires empirical knowledge, along with an appreciation of its uncertainties, and commitment to evidence-based practice. Autonomy means enabling independent function to the fullest extent possible given the circumstances, including frailty and physical and cognitive impairment. Thus, the classic beneficence and autonomy conflict has new meaning. Care that adheres to the principles of both beneficence and autonomy, in light of existing knowledge of physical restraints, must be restraint-free. Even if restraint-free care remains merely a goal or is held out as a gold standard, on purely ethical grounds, care without restraints is what patients and residents should expect and what professionals should provide.

In 1994 a priority expert panel report for the National Institute of Nursing Research included physical restraints in its research agenda for long-term care for older adults. The recommendations were to determine reasons for restraint use and clarify decision making; investigate care needs of the restrained patient; examine ethics, values, and attitudes as they affect use of restraints and quality of patient care; establish and evaluate standards of care; and test and evaluate alternative approaches with a view toward reducing or eliminating restraint use. Substantial knowledge now exists in all but the last of these areas. As no therapeutic value for physical restraints has been determined, the devices should be eliminated; the research clearly indicates this can be done safely and with positive outcomes. The emphasis for future research should be enhancement of care protocols for those behaviors and situations that have, in the past, resulted in the application of physical restraints. This means research directed toward specific nursing interventions aimed at minimizing falls and serious injuries, enhancing delivery of technological care (when necessary), and individualizing care approaches for a range of behaviors associated with cognitive impairment.

NEVILLE E. STRUMPF
LOIS K. EVANS

See also:
ACTIVITIES OF DAILY LIVING
CAREGIVER
ELDER ABUSE
FALLS
FUNCTIONAL HEALTH
MOBILITY

RESPITE CARE

As the population continues to age, the percentage of older adults with chronic illnesses and disabilities requiring care also increases (Administration on Aging, 1998). In *A Profile of Older Americans: 1998* (Administration on Aging, 1998), it is reported that 14% (4.4 million) of persons aged 65 or over receive assistance with activities of daily living (in particular personal hygiene and mobility tasks). Previous epidemiological studies indicate that more than 11% of older adults living outside of institutions may suffer from underlying Alzheimer's disease (Carnoni-Huntley et al., 1985; Pfeffer, Afifi, & Chance, 1987). Families provide the bulk of care to noninstitutionalized older adults, including those with Alzheimer's disease: personal care (bathing, dressing, feeding), instrumental services (shopping, transportation, household maintenance), medically related care (such as injections and medications), continuous supervision, and emotional support (Stone, Cafferata, & Sangl, 1987). As the population of very old adults increases in our nation, the demands on family caregivers are also expected to increase.

It is well documented in the literature (Brody, 1981; Shanas, 1979) that families committed to caring for elderly family members at home often shoulder tremendous emotional, physical, and financial costs. Even beyond the point where a substantial toll has already been wrought, most families have no choice but to provide care to their elderly relatives, while simultaneously carrying on with their already hectic lifestyles. This results in varying degrees of stress, also referred to as caregiver burden, strain, or burnout (Baldwin, 1990). As a consequence, the caregivers themselves ultimately require help which is often overlooked in our society. This help may be in the form of respite care, in other words, care for the caregiver.

Respite care was first specifically named and developed in Europe by gerontologists and researchers as one approach to giving needed support to family caregivers (Baldwin, 1990; Cohen, S., 1982; Kosloski & Montgomery, 1993). The development and legitimization of respite care as a specific type of formal services for the elderly did not occur in the United States until the mid to late seventies when a number of articles on the topic of respite care were published in the scientific literature (Toner, 1993). The increased concern regarding the role of the family in caring for the chronically ill elderly led to the early studies of family caregiving characteristics (Shanas, 1979). This, in turn, led to the early studies of the effect of caregiver burden (Lebowitz, 1978) and work on old age and family functioning (Fengler & Goodrich, 1979). Ultimately studies of how formal services might reduce caregiver stress by providing relief from caregiving responsibilities were conducted (Rathbone-McCuan, 1976). The acknowledgement from health providers and policymakers of the critical role that families play in the long-term care of their older family members and their need for formal services to supplement the care they deliver, eventually led to the development of formal respite services (Montgomery, R., 1986; Toner, 1993). It just so happened that about the late 1970s and early 1980s, adult day-care programs began to emerge as a long-term care option. Although not originally conceived of as a respite service, adult day care has evolved as a legitimate form of respite care.

Respite care includes a wide range of physical, emotional, and social services provided to a dependent person by someone other than the primary caregiver in order to provide the latter with a temporary reprieve from caregiving tasks and duties (Weber & Schneider, 1993). The term respite care normally covers the following services: in-home respite care, adult day care, and short-term periods of institutionalization (Feinberg & Kelly, 1995; Jones & Peter, 1992; Larkin & Hopcroft, 1993). Although there is no generally accepted definition for this service, the United States Department of Health and Human Services describes it as "short term inpatient or outpatient care delivered to an elderly person in lieu of his or her regular support" (U.S. Department of Health and Human Services, January, 1981).

Nowadays the primary caregiver is more likely to be an elderly spouse; approximately 50% of caregivers are elderly females who simultaneously must confront their own aging, lack of stamina, and multiple health problems (Ryan, 1993). Adult daughters, daughters-in-law, nieces, friends, and sons comprise, in that order, the remaining caregiver cohort (Ryan, 1993). Caregiving of an elderly person may result in strained or shattered marriages, rebellions on the part of the caregiver, and in some instances elder abuse (Kiecolt-Glaser, 1987). In spite of the fact that caregiver studies routinely report high levels of caregiver stress related to the burden of providing care, families often wish to continue with their role of providing care (Grant & Nolan, 1994). There are many reasons given by family caregivers as to why they continue to endure the stress of providing care. These include guilt, obligation, satisfaction, gratification, appreciation, affection, positive family and intergenerational relations, expectations, reciprocity, desire to avoid institutional or nursing home placements at all costs, and filial responsibility (Brody, 1981; Cohen &Warren, 1985; Flint, 1995; Jansson, Almberg, Grafstrom, & Winblad, 1998).

Respite care has been identified as the single most important service that can be provided to families (Baldwin, 1990). It is unique in that it provides services to those who care as well as to those who receive care. In the study done by Braithwaite (1998), respite use is expected to be high when caregivers report high need and when they are predisposed to use support to take a break from caregiving. Considering the facts that: (a) the potential for institutionalization increases with advancing age; (b) caregivers experience more severe overall problems and greater stress levels than the general population; and (c) respite care is considerably less expensive than institutionalization, it is surprising that respite care is still underutilized. Surveys done by Segall and Wykle (1988–89) indicate that caregivers long for respite services. However, studies reveal that eligible persons are often reluctant to use respite care (Gwyther, Ballard, & Hinman-Smith, 1990; Montgomery, 1988; Montgomery & Borgatta, 1989). According to Lawton and associates (1989), one of the reasons for this may be that caregivers appear hesitant to use respite services, require education and even encouragement before using them, and wait until crises occur before taking advantage of respite care.

Findings from Duke University's respite care demonstration indicated that the benefits in caregiver well-being were modest although satisfaction was high (Gwyther et al., 1990). Similarly, participants in the Philadelphia demonstration project reported high satisfaction with the service although it had no noticeable effect on their mental health (Lawton, Brody, & Saperstein, 1989). In another project, users claimed to be satisfied although there were no noticeable reductions in their levels of burden or stress (Burdz, Eaton, & Bond, 1988).

More recent studies have been able to document the effects of respite services on caregivers. Caregivers in the Michigan model respite program experienced both increased morale and decreases in their subjective burden (Kosloski & Montgomery, 1995). In addition, findings from the Seattle respite study (Kosloski & Montgomery, 1995) revealed that the increased use of respite decreased the likelihood of nursing home placement.

Although researchers have yielded mixed results thus far as well as uncertainty over the effectiveness of respite programs for caregivers, two findings have held firm. First, caregivers are satisfied, for the most part, with respite programs and ask that more be available (Braithwaite, 1986, 1998; Gallagher, Lovett, & Zeiss, 1989; Lawton et al., 1989). Second, services often are not utilized fully, with many elders who are regarded as the most in need not taking advantage of the opportunities available (Lawton et al., 1989; Montgomery & Borgatta, 1989; Oktay & Volland, 1990).

According to Fortinsky and Hathaway (1990), challenges in elder care are twofold: (1) to link caregivers with available services in order to preserve their own health and well-being; and (2) to continue to develop appropriate services for caregivers as well as for care recipients. Therefore, it is imperative that future studies explore both caregiver motivation for service use and the expected and actual benefits of respite services. In addition, future research needs to focus on finding ways of establishing how best to reach caregivers who are most in need of respite care.

In view of expectations by various experts that the percentage of elderly people will increase in the future and the subsequent physical and psychological demands placed on home-based caregivers will increase commensurately, the nurse, as the family's primary contact throughout the care of older adults, is instrumental in providing needed assistance and referrals to the caregiver so that care of older adults can be optimized. However, respite care receives little emphasis in nursing literature as a significant component of routine nursing integrated holistic assessment of older clients which includes attention to caregiver's needs. Nurses are in a very favorable position to reach caregivers and make recommendations for early interventions and to institute appropriate respite care. Therefore, nurses working with older adults must ensure that a holistic need assessment is performed, which includes assessment of caregivers' needs.

OPHELIA EMPLEO-FRAZIER

See also:
CAREGIVER
ADULT FOSTER CARE

TEAMS

Initially developed in fields such as mental health and rehabilitation, the popularity of healthcare teams has waxed and waned over the past 80 years

(Ducanis & Golin, 1979). Today, interdisciplinary healthcare teams are flourishing, amidst rudimentary scientific data related to team behaviors, team effectiveness, and patient outcomes. Patients with complex problems, such as geriatric patients, present health professionals with a tremendous challenge. Typical geriatric syndromes associated with multiple illnesses, polypharmacy, increased social problems, and fragmented care require skills that no one individual possesses. These patients are best cared for utilizing the team approach. Increased life expectancy, and the proportion of older adults over the age of 80, will increase the demand for comprehensive geriatric care.

As healthcare progressed and changed over the years, the literature reflects the works of Martin Cherkasky from Montefiore Hospital, considered to be the originator of healthcare teams in the 1950s (Cherkasky, 1949). Comprehensive care at home demanded the participation of various disciplines, which ultimately developed into the first organized healthcare team seen in the literature (Tsukuda, 1998). Pioneering efforts in team work shifted when George Silver developed the Family Health Maintenance and Demonstration Program (Silver, 1958). It is here that the first references are made to delineating roles and responsibilities, relative to the team process.

The literature on healthcare teams over the past 30 years has focused on describing the meaning of healthcare teams, and their particular role and function within a specific discipline or institution. Another focus of the team literature relates to education of healthcare professionals and the utilization of an interdisciplinary student experience. Beginning in the early 1970s, nursing educators realized the need for interdisciplinary team training. Based on the assumption that students needed practical experience, The University of Wisconsin Family Health Service offered students an opportunity to participate in a comprehensive community-based team that included nurses, social workers, physicians, and family health counselors to provide an array of health services to children (Aradine & Hansen, 1970). It is also recognized that interdisciplinary education requires an increased level of commitment from clinical educators, who may need additional preparation in the interdisciplinary perspective (Strumpf & Whitney, 1994).

Nursing educators committed to interdisciplinary models of education recognize that differences among the cultures and philosophies of the disciplines involved in interdisciplinary team training present a challenge for nursing and other disciplines involved (Evans, L. K., 1994). The disciplines engaged in interdisciplinary care, including nursing, medicine, and social work, all have unique characteristics and distinct cultures. Discipline-specific behaviors including dress codes, jargon, schedules, and salaries all contribute to defining the culture of a discipline and the way in which they function on a team (Tsukuda, 1998).

Models of interdisciplinary care have been reported in the nursing literature, focusing on specialized interdisciplinary teams such as hospice (Eng, 1993) and surgical care (McHugh et al., 1996). Today, much of the literature on healthcare teams focuses on care specific to the geriatric population. The Department of Veterans Affairs (VA) developed an extensive effort aimed at providing team care for the elderly. The commitment to provide team care is evident in all areas of service provided by the VA. An Interdisciplinary Team Training Program in Geriatrics (ITTG) was developed to enhance research education and the clinical programs dedicated to the care of the elderly (Tsukuda, 1990, 1998).

Despite repeated reports in the literature as to the need for teams of professionals from different disciplines to work together, little consensus exists with regard to conflict and communication. The approach to interdisciplinary care by experts is influenced by modes of communication, value-related dimensions of professional practice, and the socialization of professionals into differing systems of care (Clark, 1995). Expert clinicians in geriatrics, recognized for their leadership skills and knowledge, may not have expert skills in team dynamics. Significant differences exist in leadership styles of experts. The characteristics of certain leadership styles, which enable effective academic and managerial leadership, may not be consistent with expert team skills (Drinka, 1999).

Research which has focused on relationships among teams members, specifically physician-nurse relationships, has resulted in the Collaborative Practice Scales. These scales, which have been tested for reliability and validity, enable researchers to examine constructs such as avoidance, accommodation, compromise, competition, and collaboration. Based on a theoretical frame of reference, this instrument enables further research into relationships of team members and their potential impact on patient care (Weiss & Davis, 1985).

In 1995, recognizing the need to prepare healthcare trainees to be members of teams in geriatrics, The John A. Hartford Foundation supported the Geriatric Interdisciplinary Team Training (GITT) project. Evaluation focuses on the trainees within the GITT project. Measuring the effectiveness of these training programs challenged researchers to create new mechanisms to quantify the success of these training models. Core measures aimed at assessing students' attitudes toward teams, knowledge of geriatric care, and knowledge of team dynamics were created based upon research done on team skills or team dynamics. Over the 3 years of implementation funds (1996–1999), the GITT is expected to train 2,633 student trainees and 173 practicing health professionals in geriatric interdisciplinary team training. This $10-million commitment to a national, multicenter Geriatric Interdisciplinary Team Training Program will significantly enhance the current base of knowledge regarding the critical factors that lead to the success of interdisciplinary care team training (Hyer, 1998).

Additional ongoing research focusing on the evaluation of interdisciplinary teams has resulted in the development of an Attitudes Toward Health Care Teams Scale. This measure, which has demonstrated reliability and validity, has potential for use as a research tool and as a pre- and posttest tool for educational interventions with teams and for evaluating clinically based team training programs for medical and health professions students (Heinemann, Schmitt, Farrell, & Brallier, 1999).

The challenges presented by the changing healthcare system of today will enable further research on interdisciplinary teams. Ongoing research related to measuring team effectiveness, discipline-specific behaviors and cultures, and outcomes research related to team effectiveness will significantly broaden the knowledge base of interdisciplinary teams.

Ellen Flaherty

See also:
CERTIFICATION IN GERONTOLOGICAL NURSING
GERONTOLOGICAL CARE
GERONTOLOGICAL NURSING: ADVANCED PRACTICE

WANDERING

Nurses who care for the elderly generally agree that wandering is a common behavior, especially among cognitively impaired people. Caregivers are concerned about three possible negative consequences of wandering: potential injury to the wanderer, the risk of the wanderer becoming lost, and the invasion of privacy of (or injury to) others. Families often identify wandering as a factor that influences their decisions regarding nursing home placements. In institutional settings, extensive nursing time is consumed by the management of wandering.

In 1980, Burnside expressed dismay at the lack of a suitable definition of wandering, as well as the lack of nursing articles or research on the topic. She was able to cite only five published articles on wandering between 1941 and 1978. Since that time, a renewed interest in wandering has spawned various definitions and numerous articles and research studies.

Two elements common to most definitions in the 1970s and 1980s were aimless locomotion and cognitive impairment (Monsour & Robb, 1982; Hussian, 1981, 1982; Snyder, Rupprecht, Pyrek, Brekhus, & Moss, 1978). An early definition of wandering was "a tendency to move about, either in a seemingly aimless or disoriented fashion, or in pursuit of an indefinable or unobtainable goal" (Snyder et al., 1978, p. 272).

Wandering can also be viewed as a form of agenda behavior, meaning it is a manifestation of an effort to fulfill felt needs (Rader, Doan, & Schwab, 1985). From this perspective, wandering may not be aimless, although the aim may not be apparent to others. Cohen-Mansfield (1996) asserts that wandering could be both adaptive and appropriate for the cognitively impaired elder. Wandering probably has physical and psychosocial benefits, but positive aspects have received less attention than have the negative consequences.

Algase, who has studied wandering for a decade, treats it as a rhythm—an approach that lends itself to the precise measurement required for valid and reliable research. She defines wandering as "movement that changes over time and, thus, is a nonlinear ultradian rhythm, with locomoting and nonlocomoting phases" (Algase, 1992a, p. 29).

These varying definitions suggest that there are several types of wanderers. Snyder and colleagues (1978) classified different types of wandering behavior as overtly goal directed/searching, overtly goal-directed/industrious, and apparently nongoal-directed behavior. Thomas categorized wanderers as either continuous or sporadic. Continuous wanderers were defined as "ambulating more than 50% of their wakeful-time," whereas sporadic wanderers were those who "move about less than half of their wakeful time" (1995, p. 35). Acello (1998) recognized the categories of exit seeking, modeling, akathesia, aimless, purposeful, and precarious wandering.

The characteristics of wanderers, and possible influential variables in the physical and social environment, have received considerable attention. Snyder and colleagues (1978) studied the characteristics of wanderers and nonwanderers and used behavior-mapping to record their patterns of activity and possible underlying influences. Individuals identified as wanderers by staff did spend more time in motion than those labeled nonwanderers. Wanderers were found to have lower mental status scores, and more problems with memory, orientation, and verbal responses. In other studies comparing wanderers to nonwanderers, wanderers were found to be more cognitively impaired, especially in relation to language (Algase, 1992b). They were also found to have more spatial skills deficits (deLeon, 1984), and to have been more extroverted prior to illness (Thomas, D. W., 1997).

Some studies have examined wandering as an expression of personality continuity and/or previous lifestyle. Thomas (1997) investigated the relationship between wandering and premorbid personality, as reported by family members. In his study, wanderers rated higher in warmth, gregariousness, activity, positive emotion, and altruism. This is consistent with the conclusions of Monsour and Robb (1982) who reported that wanderers previously had participated in high levels of social and leisure activities, had experienced high levels of stress, and used physical activity to cope with stress. Beck, Rossby, and Baldwin (1991) found positive correlations between premorbid personality and disruptive behavior. Based on a review of the social history of wanderers, Snyder et al. (1978) concluded that life-long patterns of coping with stress, previous work roles, and a search for security may all induce wandering.

In contrast, Cohen-Mansfield, Marx, and Rosenthal (1989) found no relation between past leisure activities and agitated behavior. Linton, Matteson, and Byers (1997) used direct observation to assess the activity levels of wanderers and questionnaires were sent to family members to assess premorbid leisure activities, hobbies, exercise, stress management, types of employment, and social interactions. There were no significant correlations between these variables and the amount of time spent standing, walking, and pacing.

During the 1980s, the emphasis of research was on describing and preventing wandering. Physical and chemical restraints were commonly used. The passage of the Omnibus Budget Reconciliation Act (OBRA) in 1987 mandated the use of the least restrictive interventions necessary to address behavioral problems, and efforts have shifted toward making wandering safer. Initial efforts focused on the environment. Cohen-Mansfield and Werner (1998b) assessed the impact of an enhanced environment on pacing, exit seeking, agitation, and mood. The enhanced environment consisted of pleasant visual, auditory, and olfactory stimuli in selected hallways. Wanderers were found to spend significantly more time in the enhanced areas. Although agitation decreased, the change was not statistically significant. Pleasurable responses to the enhanced environment (as perceived by observers) improved significantly. Matteson and Linton (1996) observed patient activity and concluded that the behaviors of dementia patients in a special care unit appeared to be related to activities in the environment, with quiet behavior at night and more active behavior during the day.

Special care units for cognitively impaired people were designed to permit maximal independence, while lessening the risk of unsupervised departure. A variety of strategies to reduce the risk of patient exits have been implemented. These most often include perimeter devices and visual illusions to disguise exits. Perimeter devices may be simple alarms that sound when doors are opened, or more complex sensors that sound when patients wearing special devices move beyond a designated area. The nursing literature describes these systems (McConnell, 1998; Wagner, 1996), but presents little research regarding their effectiveness. Melillo and Futrell (1998) surveyed caregivers (of dementia patients) who identified wandering as a source of worry. The researchers showed that they indicated an interest in some type of technological device that could locate lost patients.

Visual illusions to discourage wandering beyond certain limits have been widely used, but have been studied infrequently and with inconsistent results. Namazi, Rosner, and Calkins (1989) concealed doorknobs in several ways, and used two different types of tape grids near fire-door exits to study the effects on patient-exit attempts. They were successful in discouraging patients from opening the door by disguising the doorknob with cloth. Tape grids on the floor did not discourage exits. In contrast, Hewawasam (1996) found horizontal lines to be an effective barrier for patients with Alzheimer's disease, but not for patients with other types of dementia. Based on the premise that wandering represented a need for more physical activity, Holmberg (1997) implemented an evening walking plan for nursing home patients with dementia. On the evenings that the patients walked, there was a 30% reduction in aggressive events on the part of those patients.

Wandering research continues to focus on defining the nature of the problem. Intervention studies have produced inconsistent results. Comparisons of these results are complicated by varied definitions, classifications, and theoretical perspectives. The tendency to identify wanderers for study based on staff recommendations may have led to underestimation of the phenomenon and inaccurate identification of correlates. As the number of individuals requiring long-term care continues to grow, wandering will remain an important area of nursing study. Suggested topics for future research are: (a) patterns of wandering, and/or patient correlates that create risk; (b) unmet needs that trigger wandering and interventions to meet those needs; (c) benefits of wandering; and (d) interventions that preserve the benefits of wandering while minimizing hazards.

ADRIANNE LINTON

See also:
ALZHEIMER'S DISEASE
ALZHEIMER'S DISEASE: SPECIAL CARE UNITS IN LONG-TERM CARE
COGNITIVE DISORDERS
COGNITIVE IMPAIRMENT
COGNITIVE INTERVENTIONS
PET THERAPY
PHYSICAL RESTRAINTS

Part IV

GERIATRIC EMOTIONAL HEALTH

INTRODUCTION

It is generally believed that older adults no longer develop emotionally or physically in their final years. Although it is true that physical decline exceeds the rate of physical growth in the older adult, there is no evidence that emotional development is reduced in any way. In fact, Erickson's theory of development illustrates that older adults must pass through developmental stages just as infants, children, and younger adults do (Erickson, 1982).

Ego Integrity versus despair is the developmental stage associated with aging (Erickson, 1982). The attribute associated with triumphant passage of this stage is integrity, defined as an honest acceptance of the life that has passed and the stage of life that is currently being lived. Individuals who have successfully reached this stage are said to be at peace with themselves. Inability to reach this stage leads to fear of death and despair that life has been lived in vain (Erickson, 1982). Aggressive behavior, as discussed in this section, may be a result of unsuccessful development in later life.

Nurses working in all environments of care are called upon to assist older adults in their emotional development through interventions such as reminiscence. Studies have shown that residents who were recognized as possessing integrity by the nursing staff often withdrew from the daily liveliness of the long-term care facility to sit alone and contemplate how they and other individuals behaved, think about alternatives for life, and appraise situations. Promoting "cogiation" among older adults may be an effectual method to promote ego integrity in this population (Nystrom, 1995). Pet and music therapies, also reviewed in this section are additional methods by which to help the older adult progress through final emotional development

The common stresses of older age present many challenges to development. Nurses caring for older adults may be very helpful in the coping process. Moos and Billings have identified three ways in which the older individual may cope with the stress they are currently experiencing (Moos & Billings, 1986). These are: (a) appraisal-focused coping, which concerns defining the meaning of the situation; (b) problem-focused coping, which focuses on dealing with the reality of the situation by modifying the source of the threat, handling the consequences of the problem, or changing the individual self impacted upon; and (c) emotion-focused coping, which is aimed at the management of the emotions aroused by an event. After evaluating the most effective method by which the individual desires to cope with the situation, the nurse may help to create an appropriate environment for coping with the stresses of aging.

The incidence of depression increases sharply among older adults. The cause of this rise is not completely understood. The abundant losses experienced by older adults may be somewhat to blame for the appearance of depression among older adults. Depression may also be related to physiological changes in the aging body. Depression has been the subject of detailed study and is featured as an entry within this section of the digest. Estimates of depression range from 15% to 60% of elders over 65 years old, depending upon the sample (Timiras, 1988). While it seems that depression impacts elders in much the same way it affects younger people, symptom patterns, as well as the older adult's overall susceptibility, are markedly different from those of younger individuals. Some of the behaviors frequently displayed in depression include: sullen affect, decreased participation in activities of daily living and social activities, and suicidal ideation. Nurses are integral in helping to diagnose and treat depression in older adults. The Geriatric Depression Scale, discussed in this section, may facilitate the assessment of depression in all environments of care. Once diagnosed, treatment may include antidepressant medications and psychosocial therapy.

Data found by Casey (1991) indicate that suicide rates are greater in the elderly than in any other age group. The rationale for the great number of suicides among older adults is unknown. The increased rate of depression as discussed in this section provides insight into the motive behind many older adults' suicide. Serious medical illnesses also provide a partial explanation behind the desire to take one's life. Risk factors for suicide include: social isolation, alcohol abuse, psychosis, bereavement, serious medical illness, and depression (Casey, 1991). It is reported that as a final call for help, older adults may visit healthcare providers with a somatic concern prior to the suicide attempt. Nurses working with older adults should be cognizant of the prevalent rate of suicide in this population and alert for the risk factors. Suicide threats should be taken seriously and interventions should be implemented to maintain the safety of the older adult.

Although it is commonly believed that emotional growth and development cease prior to older adulthood, this is not the case. Older adults face many stressors and must continue to develop emotionally through their last stage of life. Many interventions are available for nurses to use to help proceed through these stages. The following section provides rich information on the emotional health of older adults and how nurses can best foster further emotional development.

Meredith Wallace

AGGRESSIVE BEHAVIOR IN COGNITIVELY IMPAIRED ELDERS

The behavioral changes that accompany cognitive impairment are of great concern to caregivers of elders residing in community, acute-care, and long-term-care settings. The behavior of most concern to direct caregivers is aggressive behavior. Aggressive behavior has been identified as one of the key risk factors for institutionalization of community-based cognitively impaired elders (Steeman, Abraham, & Godderis, 1997). It is also cited as one of the most difficult behaviors to manage for certified nursing assistants (CNAs) in long-term care, resulting in job stress, burnout, and turnover (Burgio, Jones, Butler, & Engel, 1988).

Definition

Aggressive behavior has been defined as hostile actions directed toward oneself, other persons, or objects (Ryden, 1988). Kolanowski (1995) defined the concepts of aggressive psychomotor behavior (defined as an increase in gross motor movement that has the effect of harming or repelling another) and verbally aggressive behavior (defined as vocalizations that have the effect of repelling others). These definitions evolved from the five most disturbing behaviors characteristic of dementia.

Researchers conducting work in the mid-1980s developed instruments to measure behavioral changes with dementia. These instruments measure aggressive behavior as: (1) the main tool concept with subscales for physically, verbally, and sexually aggressive behaviors (e.g., Ryden Aggression Scale (RAS) or Overt Aggression Scale (OAS)); (2) a subscale on a scale with other behavior changes or items (e.g., Cohen-Mansfield Agitation Inventory (CMAI) or Behavioral Pathology in Alzheimer's disease (BE-HAVE-AD)); or (3) one or several items on a scale of behavior changes (e.g., Dementia Behavior Disturbance Scale (DBD); Behavior Rating Scale of Dementia of the Consortium to Establish a Registry for Alzheimer's Disease (CERAD-Behavior Scale); or The Caretaker Obstreperous Behavior Rating Assessment (COBRA)) (Baumgarten, Becker, & Gauthier, 1990; Cohen-Mansfield, 1986; Drachman, Swearer, O'Donnell, Mitchell, & Maloon, 1992; Reisberg et al., 1987; Ryden, Bossenmaier, & McLachlan, 1991; Tariot et al., 1995; Yudofsky, Silver, & Hales, 1995).

Conceptual Models

Several models for understanding the origins of dysfunctional behavior in older adults have been proposed by nurse researchers. These models share many similar components. Lanza's (1983) model of the origins of aggressive behavior was modified by Ryden and colleagues (1991) to explain aggressive behavior in cognitively impaired populations. This model identifies internal factors (instinct, physical or chemical changes, genetic components, and learned responses) and environmental interaction factors (familial, social, and physical elements) that interact to bring about the potential for aggression.

Hall and Buckwalter (1987) proposed the Progressively Lowered Stress Threshold (PLST) model derived from psychological theories of stress, adaptation, coping, behavioral and physiological research on Alzheimer's disease. The PLST model proposes that cognitive losses, affective or personality changes, cognitive or planning losses, and loss of the stress threshold produce the changes in behavior seen in dementia patients. The model identified five common stressors which produce dysfunctional behavior including: (a) fatigue; (b) change of environment, routine, or caregiver; (c) misleading stimuli; (d) internal or external demands to achieve that exceed functional capacity; and (e) physical stressors such as pain, discomfort, infection, acute illness, and depression.

Recently researchers have reconceptualized the behaviors of physical aggression, wandering, and problematic vocalizations as "Need-driven behaviors" in an effort to focus nursing care away from the specific behavior toward an approach that identifies the need underlying the behavior (Algase et al., 1996). Similar to the Lanza and PLST models, background factors and proximal factors are operative across all dementia-related behaviors. The background factors (dementia-compromised functions, health state, and psychosocial variables) are the characteristics that shape the more enduring patterns of behavior. Proximal factors (physiological need state, psychosocial need state, physical environment, and social environment) are factors which precipitate dementia-related behaviors.

In addition to the above models, Hutchinson and Wilson (1998) have evaluated the midrange Theory of Unpleasant Symptoms as an explanatory model for behaviors in Alzheimer's disease. This model emphasizes the complexity and interaction of symptoms as well as the interrelationships among symptoms, the influencing factors, and the symptom consequences or performance outcomes (Lenz, Pugh, Milligan, Gift, & Suppe, 1997). The Theory of Unpleasant Symptoms identifies influencing factors (physiologic, psychologic, and situational) that affect the occurrence, intensity, timing, distress level, and quality of symptoms. In the case of Alzheimer's disease, behaviors are the symptoms that present in complex and interacting ways.

A model based on Piaget's cognitive developmental stages has also been tested (Matteson, Linton, Cleary, Barnes, & Lichtenstein, 1997). In this model, the behavioral symptoms of middle to late stage Alzheimer's disease are correlated with the sensorimotor, preoperational, and concrete stages hypothesized by Piaget. Use of this model determines consistent behavioral and environmental intervention for persons at all stages of cognitive decline.

Research on Aggressive Behavior

Prevalence.   Prevalence rates of aggressive behavior for community-based persons with dementia range from 12% to 52% (Aarsland, Cummings, Yenner, & Miller, 1996; Chemerinski et al., 1998; Gibbons, Gannon, & Wrigley, 1997; Eastley & Wilcock, 1997; Lyketsos et al., 1999) In institutionalized elders the prevalence of aggressive behavior in persons with Alzheimer's disease ranges from 19% to 66% of residents studied; prevalence variations have been noted based on location on a special care unit and type of nursing home (Cohen-Mansfield, Werner, Culpepper, Wofson, & Bickel, 1996; Rudman, Alverno, Matteson, 1993; Ryden et al., 1991).

Precipitants and Correlates.   Physical aggression has been linked to male gender, longer duration of illness, dyspraxia, and more severe cognitive impairment (Chemerinski et al., 1998; Eastley & Wilcock, 1997; Kunik et al., 1998). Dementia severity accounted for 16% of the variance in physical aggression and 5% of the variance of verbal aggression in one study (Kunik et al., 1998). Physically aggressive behavior has also been found to be significantly correlated with psychotic symptoms, thought disturbances, irritability, impairment in activities of daily living, premorbid personality, and depressive symptoms (Aarsland et al., 1996; Chemerinski et al., 1998; Kolanowski, Strand, & Whall, 1997; Kunik et al., 1998; Lyketsos et al., 1999). Kolanowski and colleagues (1994) found that personal characteristics of the resident and a staff composed of fewer licensed personnel explained 22% of the variance in aggressive behaviors. Significantly higher aggression scores were found in persons with two or more pain-related diagnoses (Feldt, Warne, & Ryden, 1998). In a recent study by Ryden and colleagues (1999), four variables accounted for 23% of the variance in physical aggression scores for cognitively impaired institutionalized elders. These were: location on a secured unit, not receiving an antidepressant, being restrained, and the number of psychotropic or anxiolytic medications administered. Over half of the episodes of aggressiveness in long-term care residents occurs within the context of caregiving activities (Bridges-Parlet, Knopman & Thompson, 1994; Ryden et al., 1991; Swanson, Maas, & Buckwalter, 1993). Verbal aggression has been correlated with female gender, shorter duration of illness (Chemerinski et al., 1998), depression (Kunik et al., 1998), and delusional ideation (Aarsland et al., 1996).

Interventions. Research on nursing interventions to modify or reduce behavior problems associated with dementia have included the following strategies: staff education, behavioral approaches, environmental approaches, and alternatives to physical and chemical restraints.

Several researchers have tested the effect of educational interventions for caregiving staff on behavior changes in both staff and patients. In one study, 75% of CNAs caring for cognitively impaired older veterans identified physical aggression as the most difficult behavior to manage prior to the educational intervention. This dropped significantly (to 56%) following the training sessions (Palmer & Withee, 1996). Significant reductions in "combative behaviors" were found in another population of veterans with dementia after CNA and nursing staff received an intensive educational program that included didactic, empathy, and skill training (Williams, Wood, & Moorleghen, 1994). Similar significant reductions in aggressive behaviors have been reported by other researchers who have tested the effects of training licensed and unlicensed staff on care of residents during specific activities of daily living (Hagen & Sayers, 1995; Hoeffer, Rader, McKenzie, Lavelle, & Stewart 1997; Maxfield, Lewis, & Cannon, 1996).

Woods and Ashley (1995) tested simulated presence therapy (SPT) to reduce problem behaviors in cognitively impaired nursing home residents. Fifteen minute personalized audiotape messages from a family member (reminiscence of family anecdotes or cherished memories) were played for residents when they displayed problem behaviors. The SPT approach was most effective in improving social isolation. Although only two subjects demonstrated physically aggressive behavior, one of the subjects with aggressive behavior became noticeably more calm. The SPT approach was effective in reducing verbal aggression 91% of the time. Vaccaro (1988) demonstrated a 70% decrease in physically aggressive behavior and a 70% decrease in verbally aggressive behavior for a small sample of six institutionalized elderly men. She used a combination of positive differential reinforcement of nonaggressive behavior, time-out, and social skills training in her study. Other behavioral approaches that have shown reductions in aggressive behavior during care activities include use of bird songs, sounds of babbling brooks, food, and music (Clark, Lipe, & Bilbrey, 1998; Whall et al., 1997).

Although research on special care units to reduce aggressive behavior has brought mixed results, restricted environments have been recommended to reduce environmental overstimulation and stress for cognitively impaired elders (Hall, Kirschling, & Todd, 1986). Testing of a multimodal approach, including environmental modifications and behavioral interventions based on Piaget's model of cognitive development, demonstrated a significant reduction in disruptive behaviors including aggression (Matteson et al., 1997).

Pharmacological intervention studies indicate that treatment of depression may reduce verbally aggressive behavior. Furthermore, treatment of psychotic symptoms, particularly suspicion, is effective in reducing physically aggressive behavior (Kunik et al., 1998). Pharmacological treatment of pain was shown to markedly reduce the number of aggressive incidents in one study. However, the sample size was small and significance was not reported (Middleton, Richardson, & Berman, 1997).

Summary and Recommendations

Aggressive behavior in cognitively impaired elders arises from complex interactions of intrapersonal, interpersonal, and environmental factors. Empowering caregivers with education, whether community- or institutionally-based, may improve understanding and skill in providing care to this vulnerable population (Beck, Ortigara, Mercer, & Shue, 1999). Future research should focus on multifaceted approaches (educational, behavioral, and pharmacological) to this complex problem.

KAREN S. FELDT

See also:
ALZHEIMER'S DISEASE
CERTIFIED NURSE ASSISTANTS
COGNITIVE DISORDERS
COGNITIVE IMPAIRMENT
MUSIC THERAPY

DEATH AND DYING

Nursing research on death and dying began to appear in the literature in the 1960s. Prior to the 1960s, most reports centered on technical activities associated with care of the dying (Quint, 1967). The beginnings of formal research on death and dying in the late 1960s and early 1970s was influenced by nurses studying for doctorates in other fields, such as sociology and anthropology. Benoliel (1983), in a comprehensive review of nursing research on death and dying from 1969 to 1984, noted that most studies by nurses were diverse in conceptualization, lacked a central paradigm, and were descriptive in approach. Studies were conducted in hospitals, and focused on nurses' attitudes toward death and dying, family responses, and the influence of social structure and environment on patient and family coping with death and dying. Benoliel concluded that although the stressful nature of death and dying was well documented, little is known about the nature of support that is helpful to patients and families, and the influences of other variables, such as age and culture.

Hospice studies began to be reported in the literature in the 1980s. Coreless (1994) reviewed hospice studies from 1983 to 1992 and noted that these studies mainly examined the impact of the hospice as an innovation, rather than studying discrete symptom-control interventions. Studies also explored familial perceptions of hospice care, the coping strategies of families in hospice home care, and the resulting satisfaction with hospice care. The approaches used were primarily case studies, Q-sort techniques, and retrospective medical-record analysis. Coreless concluded that research is needed on the precipitating factors for reinstitutionalization, the effectiveness of transdermal patches for pain control, approaches to the care of persons with dementia and other cognitive impairments, patient values and their impact on individualizing care, and quality of life.

In summary, the early studies of death and dying called attention to the need to study the nature of social support that is helpful to dying patients and their families in this life transition, to the impact of values on end-of-life care, and to approaches to the care of persons with illnesses other than cancer, such as dementia. These factors are important considering that people are living longer with chronic and progressive illnesses.

Nursing research on death and dying that is specific to older adults was reviewed for the period of January 1989–July 1999. The search was conducted using CINHAL with the subject headings terminal care, death, and aged and was limited to journals published in English. The paucity of studies by nurses on death and dying in older adults is of concern. Research has focused on broad areas including hospice home care, bereavement, interventions, and approaches to care for special populations.

Hospice-based home-care studies comprise the largest group of studies with a specific emphasis on the needs of primary caregivers (Bramwell, MacKenzie, Laschinger, & Camerson, 1995; Decker & Young, 1991; Masters & Shontz, 1989; Stelle & Fitch, 1996b), caregiver coping strategies (Hull, 1992; Stelle & Fitch, 1996; Wilson, 1992), quality of life of family caregivers and patients with cancer (McMillan, 1996; McMillan & Mahon, 1994), and concerns about pain and use of analgesics (McMillan, 1996; Ward, Berry, & Misiewicz, 1996). Studies of the needs of caregivers are descriptive, with small samples; therefore the results cannot be generalized. Common themes in these studies include the need for rest, adequate sleep, and social and professional support. One study identified the fact that the sample was comprised entirely of Caucasian families as a limitation (Steele & Fitch, 1996).

Knowing how families cope with caregiving is essential to the designing of interventions. Hull (1992) described coping techniques utilized by families as "windows of time," social comparison, cognitive reformulation, avoidance, and "taking a day at a time." Keeping busy, thinking positively, and talking the problem over with friends and family were all described as effective coping strategies by Steele and Fitch (1996a). Wilson (1992) described the support of hospice staff and 24-hour availability of staff, as well as finding meaning in caregiving, as effective coping strategies. The above studies were limited to cancer patients, and some sample biases were introduced as the hospice selected families for participation and avoided those families who were too busy or too stressed. The quality-of-life (QOL) of patients and primary caregivers was the focus of two studies using the Hospice Quality-of-Life Index and Caregiver Quality-of-Life Index (McMillan, 1996; McMillan & Mahon, 1994). Patients scored highest on social/spiritual aspects of quality of life, and lowest on the physical-functional scale. A positive correlation was found between caregivers' QOL and their estimates of the patients' QOL. The findings suggest the need to design interventions with a focus on physical/functional aspects of care.

Although one of the major emphases of hospices is pain management, problems do occur with pain relief, and patients and families express concerns about analgesic use and addiction (McMillan, 1996; Ward, Berry, & Misiewicz, 1996). Patients' and caregivers' expectations of pain management need to be clarified, and continuing education on pain management is needed for nurses and physicians.

Studies of nursing interventions explored the use of slow-stroke back massage, therapeutic touch, and fostering hope in dying patients. Therapeutic touch was effective in promoting well-being in patients with cancer and slow-stroke back massage (SSBM) promoted relaxation evidenced by changes in vital signs (Giasson & Bouchard, 1998; Meek, 1993). It is not possible to determine from these studies if SSBM is more effective than other types of interventions using touch. Herth (1990b) explored the meaning of hope, and identified strategies that foster and threaten hope in a convenience sample of hospice patients. The findings support the importance of hope in patients facing death. The most frequently reported sources of hope were family, friends, and God. Threats to hope were abandonment, uncontrolled pain, and the devaluation of personhood. This study has practical implications for nurses as they further develop and examine interventions intended to foster hope.

Studies of bereavement have focused on the well-being of caregivers and their grief experiences (Denham, 1999; Diamond, Caserta, & Lund, 1994; Jacob, 1996). Few studies have examined how specific illness characteristics influence the grief experience. Alzheimer's disease (AD) affects over four million Americans; however little attention has been given to family perspectives' about how dementia care influences bereavement (Collins, Liken, King, & Kokinakis, 1993; NIH, 1995). In a longitudinal study of family caregivers of relatives with dementia, Collins et al. (1993) reported that primary caregivers' well-being improved during the year following death. This is contrary to the findings of most bereavement literature—that individuals who experience loss have increased psychological distress. Family caregivers of relatives with dementia experience multiple losses before death (and the relief of caregiver burdens) actually occurs. Male caregivers experienced an increase in depression following their relatives' death (Collins, Stommel, Wang, & Given, 1994). Nurses need to address the multiple losses faced by these caregivers.

Few studies have examined environments where older adults reside. Older adults residing in a nursing home with end-stage dementia do not meet the requirements for hospice care. To test whether hospice concepts could be applied to long-term care, Kovach, Wilson, and Noonan (1996) conducted an experimental study to determine the effects of hospice interventions on behavior, discomfort, and the physical complications of end-stage-dementia clients residing in a nursing home. A multidisciplinary approach was used to design interventions focusing on comfort, quality-of-life, and dignity. The study results showed a significant difference in comfort in the treatment and control groups, with the treatment group experiencing less discomfort.

Focus groups conducted with staff and administrators in nursing homes explored the learning needs of staff in caring for dying residents (Wilson & Daley, 1998). The following staff learning needs were identified: how to communicate with dying residents, how to address spiritual needs, pain management, and how to support families when coping with the loss of a relative. Ersek, Kraybill, and Hansberry (1999), in preliminary studies of the educational needs of staff providing end-of-life care in nursing homes, reported findings similar to those of Wilson and Daley.

Death touches the lives of older people more than any other age category (Atchey, 1991). Over 75% of the people who will die in the United States this year are over the age of 65 (IOM, 1997). The fastest growing age group in the United States is that of 85 years and older; this group will reach nearly five million by the year 2000. Among older adults, death occurs in institutions more often than at home among family and friends. Older adults have a right to expect that care in the final stages of life will be directed toward promoting quality-of-life and death with dignity.

Research on end-of-life care for older adults is an area where nurses can make a difference in the lives of older adults and their caregivers (Moody, 1999). The National Institute of Nursing Research, National Institute on

Aging, National Cancer Institute, and the Agency for Health Care Policy and Research have identified research on end-of-life care as a national priority.

Research on end-of-life care is an area where nurses can make a difference. Little is known about how older adults die, the environment in which they die, and how caregivers can be supported in the caregiving experience. Few studies have examined dying in a nursing home, yet this is where many older adults die. Other areas for research on end-of-life care include: what kind of support is needed by caregivers to prevent institutionalization and caregiver exhaustion; and the manner in which culture influences dying. Nurses in clinical practice and research have an obligation to improve the care of all persons regardless of disease and prognosis.

SARA WILSON

See also:
   GRIEF
   HOSPICE
   SUICIDE
   TERMINAL ILLNESS
   WIDOWS AND WIDOWERS

DEPRESSION

The most common mental health disorder in late life is depression. It is often manifested as a recurrent illness or as a comorbid condition occurring with chronic health disease. Among older adults living in the community, 3% have a major depression and 10% to 14% have depressive symptoms. Depression has a wide severity and morbidity range and is conceptualized as an abnormal mood state, a pattern of symptoms, or a clinical syndrome ranging from sadness to major depression.

As a mood state, depression is a universal human condition. In general, persons of all ages who experience a lowering of mood or transient feelings of sadness claim to be depressed. Clinically, the concept of depression is used to indicate a collection of symptoms, such as sadness, reduced ability to experience pleasure, pessimism, inhibition, retardation of action, and a variety of physical complaints. Symptoms of depression have been classified into types: physical, emotional, cognitive, and motivational (Beck, 1978).

Emotional symptoms of depression include sadness, dejection, anxiety, irritability, distress, disappointment, frustration, extreme negativity, overt hostility, intense anger, and inability to derive pleasure from previously satisfying activities. Cognitive symptoms include pessimism, negative self-evaluation, expectation of failure, self-blame, learned helplessness, disturbance in thought processes, inability to concentrate, and impaired decision making. The inability to complete even simple tasks, lack of initiative to perform daily activities, procrastination, avoidance of responsibility, and psychomotor retardation or agitation are referred to as motivational disturbances. Physical symptoms of depression are loss of appetite, sleep disturbances, loss of libido, and diffuse aches and pains. Psychosomatic complaints are more dominant in older individuals than in younger persons. Older persons also have a tendency to mask sad moods. Finally, interpersonal aspects of depression are likely to include withdrawal from social activities, increased dependency, acquiescence, dysfunctional communication patterns, and proneness to interpersonal tension and conflict.

Generally, a nursing diagnosis of a major depression is made if five of the following symptoms have been present for at least 2 weeks: changes in appetite, weight loss or gain, agitation, fatigue and loss of energy, feelings of hopelessness and guilt, and suicidal ideation. Be aware that cognitive impairment symptoms may be marked in the older person with depressive illness and may be mistaken for dementia. Differentiation between dementia and depression is a critical part of the nurses' assessment.

As a clinical syndrome, depression is usually qualified by an adjective to specify a particular type or form. Clinically, forms of depression include reactive, agitated, and psychotic. In addition, depression has been classified as endogenous (due to internal processes) or exogenous (due to external factors), terms that refer specifically to etiology. Moreover, depression is called primary when not preceded by any physical or psychiatric condition and secondary when preceded by another physical or psychiatric disorder. Finally, depression has been classified as acute (less than 2 years duration) or chronic (more than 2 years).

As a clinical entity, depression comprises attributes and characteristic signs and symptoms, including a definitive type of onset, course, duration, and outcome. The *Diagnostic and Statistical Manual of Mental Disorders* (DSM IV; American Psychiatric Association, 1994) classifies clinical depression into major, minor, and dysthymic subtypes. Major depression refers to a clinical depression that meets specific diagnostic criteria as to duration, impairment of functioning, and presence of a cluster of physiological and psychological symptoms. Minor depression includes fewer depressive symptoms than does major depression. Dysthymia consists of fewer symptoms than are expressed in major depression but more than in minor depression, and it is more chronic.

Many theories of depression have been presented through the years. The earliest discussions of depression are in the psychoanalytic literature, where depression is viewed as mourning or melancholia (Freud, 1957). According to this perspective, loss, which may be conscious or unconscious, is central to both mourning and melancholia. Mourning is qualitatively different from melancholia in that the external world becomes impoverished and empty in mourning, and the internal world, including one's ego, feels the loss in melancholia. Psychoanalysts believe that the person experiences ambivalent feelings toward the lost object, which results from high dependency needs. Because the expression of dependency needs has the potential for destroying relationships with others, feelings of dependency, frustration, and hostility are repressed. When the loss of the loved object occurs, negative feelings of anger and hostility are unleashed against oneself.

Peplau's interpersonal theory in nursing describes depression as a painful experience occurring as a way of managing anxiety when an individual's self-esteem is threatened. The energy of anxiety is displayed as anger turned inward toward the self, and the individual experiences feelings of overwhelming guilt, hopelessness, and suicidal ideation. Thus, depression can be a life-threatening illness and a serious concern for health care providers for older adults because of the potential for suicide.

Behavioral theories of depression emphasize social learning and environmental responses or stimuli that cause or maintain feelings of sadness. For learning theorists, the concept of reduction in reinforcement is central. Reinforcement is defined by the quality of one's interactions with the environment so that, when one is faced with a loss, behaviors previously reinforced by the lost object or person decrease. This theory is relative for elderly persons, who suffer a multitude of losses in their later years. Depression therefore is attributed to a reduction in activity due to a decrease in positive reinforcement that comes from significant others. Feelings of depression are elicited when a behavior receives little or no reinforcement. In addition, lower levels of behavioral activity result in a further reduction of positive reinforcement from the environment. Therefore, both activities and rewards decrease. Behavior theorists believe that changing a person's behavior directly through positive social interactions is the best way of reducing depressive symptoms.

The self-control model of depression is a behavioral perspective from which people are viewed as capable of exercising control over their behavior (Rehm, 1997): they do not merely react to external influences but exert control over the environment. This theory of depression includes cognitive aspects because depressed persons are believed to have deficits in self-monitoring (reflected in pessimism and hopelessness), self-evaluation (reflected in low self-esteem), and self-reinforcement (reflected in excessive self-punishment and negative self-statements).

Cognitive theories of depression postulate that depressive symptoms are experienced because of disturbances in thinking that lead to false beliefs and ideas. Cognitive and behavioral theories of depression are sometimes closely related, especially when thought processes are instrumental in self-reinforcing and self-evaluating activities. The original learned helplessness theory of depression postulated that the belief that one has no control over outcomes in one's life is the basis for depression (Seligman, 1975).

The attributional theory is similar to Beck's cognitive theory of depression, which proposes that depression is primarily a result of the tendency to view the self, the future, and the world in an unrealistically negative manner. This distorted, negative view of self, world, and future has been referred to as the "negative cognitive triad" (Beck, 1978). According to this theory, depressed persons regard themselves as unworthy, incapable, and undesirable; they expect failure, rejection, and dissatisfaction and perceive most experiences as confirming these negative expectations. The major symptoms of depression (affective, behavioral, somatic, and motivational) are viewed as direct consequences of this negative cognitive set.

Most recently, biochemical theories of depression have emerged and attained credibility. Electrolyte disturbances, including increases in intracellular sodium and decreases in intracellular potassium, have been reported to occur with depression. In addition, neurophysiological alterations have been identified through electrophysiological studies of evoked potential and electroencephalography, demonstrating increased right hemisphere activity and decreased left hemisphere activity in the brain of depressed persons. Hormonal or neuroendocrine factors also have been related to depression, including decreases in estrogen, hypothyroidism, and hyperadrenalism. Finally, the neurochemical changes in the neurotransmitters, especially in the biogenic amines that act as central nervous system and peripheral neurotransmitters, have been documented in cases of depression. The biogenic amines, including catecholamines (dopamine, norepinephrine, and epinephrine), serotonin, and acetylcholine, have been hypothesized to be causally related to depression.

Specific biochemical theories have been proposed. The catecholamine hypothesis states that some, if not all, depressions are associated with an absolute or relative deficiency of catecholamines, particularly norepinephrine, at functionally important receptor sites in the brain. A competing explanation for the etiology of depression lies in the serotonin hypothesis, which specifies that there is a deficiency in serotonin in persons with depression. Empirical evidence of deficits in either norepinephrine or serotonin or both has provided an important rationale for the usefulness of antidepressant medications that are specifically designed to increase the concentration of norepinephrine, serotonin, or both, in the brain.

However, the precise etiology of depression remains unknown; that is, no single theoretical explanation is sufficient from a holistic nursing perspective. In fact, there is mounting evidence that there is probably multiple causation, including genetic, biochemical, and psychosocial factors that contribute to one's vulnerability to depression. Evidence for this model of depression lies in the success of multimodal treatment approaches for depression that may include antidepressant medication, psychotherapy, diet therapy, light therapy, and electroconvulsive therapy.

Depression severely affects quality of life in older persons because of the nature of the symptoms, which can lead to total inability of the individual to care for self and to relate to others. There is a potential for persons with depression to negatively affect family members and others around them. Not surprisingly, only 2% to 4% of elders in the community seek mental health services. Most depressed elders are seen by general practitioners for psychosomatic complaints. Part of the symptomatology of depression is a focus on physical problems and requires the practitioners to carefully assess for depressive symptoms. Suicide is a factor in the depressed older adult. The suicidal rate for individuals aged 80 and over is twice that of the general population and is particularly high in older White males. Interestingly, most suicidal elders had recently visited a general practitioner prior to their suicidal act. Direct assessment of suicidal potential should be a routine part of any assessment of dementia in elders.

Although depression follows a finite course and will eventually dissipate unless the person commits suicide, the life of the individual can be particularly miserable. For some time there was reluctance on the part of psychiatric practitioners to treat depression aggressively in older adults. This attitude was partially based on Freud's notion that individuals could not benefit from psychotherapy after age 50. However, we have learned that older adults will respond favorably to antidepressant medications and the psychotherapies. Electroconvulsive therapy, once disregarded because of the crude method of application, is now seen more favorably as a mode of treatment for depressed older adults who do not respond to medications. Due to modern technology electroconvulsion therapy is believed to be a safe and effective treatment for depression in older adults when other therapies fail. Additional therapies that are found to be useful by nurses are life review, guided imagery, and family and group therapy.

Research in depression among older adults has been ignored in the past and is a neglected area, where much more nursing research is needed. It is critical that nurses assume a leadership role in disseminating information about the outcomes of a variety of treatments that can be used for depression in later life. There is a particular need to examine suicide in late life and to develop better assessment instruments for the purpose of detecting sources of suicide ideation in elders.

MAY L. WYKLE
JACLENE ZAUSZNIEWSKI

See also:
DEPRESSION AS A CARDIOVASCULAR RISK FACTOR
GERIATRIC DEPRESSION SCALE
SUICIDE

FATIGUE

Fatigue is a universal symptom associated with most acute and chronic illnesses. It also is a common complaint among otherwise healthy persons and is cited as one of the most prevalent presenting symptoms in primary care practices. Defining fatigue, however, has challenged scientists for years. To date, no biological marker of fatigue has been identified. Because nursing is interested in symptoms and symptom management, fatigue is of major concern for nurse researchers and clinicians. Fatigue was named one of the top four symptoms for study by an expert panel on symptom management convened by the National Institute of Nursing Research.

The North American Nursing Diagnosis Association (NANDA, 1994) defines fatigue as "an overwhelming sustained sense of exhaustion and decreased capacity for physical and mental work" (p. 62). A number of nurse researchers have studied fatigue and have offered various proposals for categorizing it. Researchers at the Center for Biobehavioral Studies of Fatigue Management at the University of Kansas School of Nursing offer an alternative view of fatigue: "The awareness of a decreased capacity for physical and/or mental activity due to an imbalance in the availability, utilization, and/or restoration of resources needed to perform an activity" (Aaronson et al., in press). This definition is not inconsistent with the NANDA definition. However, it adds a generic understanding of potential causes of fatigue, which may vary in different situations, to facilitate studying the mechanisms of fatigue in different clinical conditions. This addition also allows for a clearer conception of fatigue as a biobehavioral phenomenon.

Investigators who have focused on categorizing fatigue generally distinguish acute fatigue from chronic fatigue. Piper (1989) identifies acute fatigue as protective, linked to a single cause, of short duration, with a rapid onset, perceived as normal, generally occurring in basically healthy persons, with minimal impact on the person and usually relieved by rest.

On the other hand, chronic fatigue is perceived as abnormal, has no known function or purpose, occurs in clinical populations, may have many causes, is not particularly related to exertion, persists over time, has an insidious onset, is not usually relieved by rest, and has a major impact on the person (see Potempa, 1993, for a review of chronic fatigue).

In the research and clinical literature, fatigue related to childbearing (see Milligan & Pugh, 1994, for a review) and fatigue related to cancer (see Irvine, Vincent, Bubela, Thompson, & Graydon, 1991; Smets, Garssen, Schuster-Uitterhoeve, & de Haes, 1993; Winningham et al., 1994, for reviews) have received the most attention. However, even these areas remain largely understudied and poorly understood. Although fatigue has been studied in a number of chronic illnesses, such as multiple sclerosis and rheumatoid arthritis, cancer-related fatigue is somewhat unique in that it is often associated with the treatment for cancer (both radiation and chemotherapy) that is most troublesome to the individual. In fact, fatigue associated with cancer treatment has been cited as a major reason for prematurely discontinuing treatment.

One of the more puzzling manifestations of fatigue is what is currently called chronic fatigue syndrome (CFS). Chronic fatigue syndrome is a diagnosis used for cases of severe and persistent fatigue for which no specific cause has been identified (see Fukuda et al., 1994, for the current full-case definition of CFS). Under varying names (e.g., neurasthenia, myalgic encephalomyelitis, postinfectious or postviral syndrome) a similar syndrome of unexplained, chronic, persistent fatigue has been documented in the literature since the late 19th century. Preliminary evidence from controlled studies and extensive clinical descriptions point to both a hypo-thalamic-pituitary-adrenal disorder (Demitrack et al., 1991) and an immune system disregulation (Bearn & Wessley, 1994) as likely central mechanisms operating in CFS.

Difficulty in studying, understanding, and treating fatigue is largely due to its ubiquitous nature and the unknown, multiple causes of fatigue. Moreover, untangling the relationship between fatigue and depression further confounds investigations of fatigue. Although fatigue is an identified symptom of depression as identified by the American Psychiatric Association, long-standing chronic fatigue, unrelated to an existing affective disorder, may precipitate depression. Further, although the hypothalamic-pituitary-adrenal axis is implicated in both CFS and depression, some evidence suggests a different pattern of neuroendocrine disturbance in CFS from that seen in depression (Ray, 1991).

A lack of consistent, valid, and reliable measures of fatigue also contributes to problems studying and understanding fatigue. Early work on fatigue in the workplace was conducted by industrial psychologists, hygienists, and the military. Consequently, these measures focused on healthy individuals and fatigue experienced at the time of measurement. More recent concern about the debilitating and distressing health effects of fatigue in clinical populations has led to the development of other measures, targeting fatigue in ill persons.

However, because there is no known biochemical test or marker for fatigue and because fatigue is first and foremost a subjective symptom, most measures of fatigue in healthy or ill populations rely on self-reports. Although a number of different self-report measures of fatigue can be found in the current literature, each taps a different aspect of fatigue or assesses fatigue in a specific clinical condition. When different measures of fatigue are used in different studies, it is difficult to know if discrepant findings result from substantive differences in fatigue or simply to the differences in the measures.

In sum, although there may be many causes of fatigue, each may ultimately be traced to a disruption in either the hypothalamic-pituitary-adrenal axis, the immune system, or both. If so, then continued investigations into CFS may lead to a better understanding of fatigue in other, clearly diagnosed clinical problems. Until work is done that suggests specific treatments for fatigue, nursing intervention studies that target ameliorating fatigue in different clinical populations must continue. Although rest generally alleviates acute fatigue, currently there are no known methods to eliminate the fatigue that plagues persons with various chronic illnesses or those whose fatigue is secondary to the treatments for their chronic illness. Using standardized measures, fatigue is a fertile area for nursing research.

LAUREN S. AARONSON

See also:
CAREGIVER
CHRONIC ILLNESS
DYSPNEA

GERIATRIC DEPRESSION SCALE

Declining health status, secondary to multiple chronic illnesses, is one factor which contributes to the masking of the symptoms of depression in older adults. Healthcare providers often resolve that depression is a normal occurrence in older adults with social and economic problems in addition to numerous health problems (NIH Consensus Development Panel, 1992). Undertreated depression may lead to an increase in isolation, anorexia, sleep disorders, and cognitive impairment, all resulting in a diminished quality of life. However, compelling evidence demonstrates a high degree of reversibility in certain patients through safe effective treatments. Therefore, the ability to diagnose depression in older adults is an essential component to a comprehensive assessment of an older adult. The frequently used Geriatric Depression Scale (GDS) is an effective screening tool for depression (Yesavage et al., 1983). This useful instrument has been tested and used extensively in both clinical practice and in research.

The GDS is a 30-item verbal questionnaire with a yes or no response required. Respondents are asked to choose the best answer for how they have felt over the last week. The instrument includes simple questions such as: (a) Are you hopeful for the future?; (b) Do you enjoy getting up in the morning?; and (c) Do you worry a lot about the past? Scores of 1 to 10 are considered normal, 11 to 20 indicate mild depression, and 21 to 30 indicate severe depression (Yesavage et al., 1983). The GDS-S is a shortened version of the GDS, consisting of 15 questions.

Nurse researchers studying depression in older adults have consistently found the GDS to be effective. The GDS was found to have 92% sensitivity and 89% specificity when evaluated against diagnostic criteria. The validity and reliability of the tool have been demonstrated through both clinical practice and research (Parmelee, Lawton, & Katz, 1989; Snowden, 1990; Yesavage et al., 1983).

A comparison of the Center for Epidemiologic Studies-Depression Scale and the GDS was conducted by Lyness and colleagues (1997). One hundred and thirty patients 60 years or older, attending three primary care internists' practices, participated in the study. Two screening scales were used: the Center for Epidemiologic Studies-Depression Scale (CES-D) and the Geriatric Depression Scale (GDS). The Structured Clinical Interview for the Diagnostic and Statistical Manual of Mental Disorders, Third Edition, Revised, (DSM-III[R]) was used to establish "gold standard" diagnoses including major and minor depressive disorders. The results demonstrated that both the CES-D and the GDS had excellent properties in screening for major depression. The optimum cutoff point for the CES-D was 21, yielding a sensitivity of 92% and a specificity of 87%. The optimum cutoff point for the GDS was 10, yielding a sensitivity of 100% and a specificity of 84%. A shorter version of the GDS had a sensitivity of 92% and a specificity of 81% using a cutoff point of 5. All scales lost accuracy when used to detect minor depression or the presence of any depressive diagnosis. Lyness et al. (1997) concluded that because of the GDS's yes or no format it has increased ease of administration.

The limitations of the GDS reported in the literature include cautionary statements regarding the use of the GDS as a diagnostic tool rather than the screening tool it is intended to be. Some controversy exists over the use of the GDS with patients with dementia (Burke, Housten, & Boust, 1989). Some studies have brought into question the difficulties with the GDS when differentiating between dementia and depression (Christensen & Dysken, 1990). However, other studies defend the use of the GDS with dementia patients, and attribute confounding results to the use of a written form of the GDS and not the verbal instrument (Parmelee & Katz, 1990).

Parmelee, Katz, and Lawton (1991) conducted a 1-year longitudinal study examining the incidence and persistence of depression among nursing home and congregate apartment residents. Depression was assessed using: (a) the GDS, and (b) a structured interview for psychiatric symptoms, based on cues from the Schedule for Affective Disorders and Schizophrenia, that included items tapping all subjective and vegetative symptoms of depression identified by the DSM-III[R]. These two measures were used to generate research diagnoses using DSM-III[R] criteria. The diagnosis of possible major depression was defined as presence of significant dysphoria, as indicated by either a positive response to the checklist "dysphoria" item or a score of 11 or more on the GDS, plus four additional depressive symptoms as listed by DSM-III[R]. Dysphoria without the four additional depressive symptoms was labeled minor depression, and persons without dysphoria were considered nondepressed. Fifteen respondents completed the GDS but failed to provide complete checklist data. In these cases, cutoffs of 17 for possible major depression and 11 for minor depression were used.

An additional study utilizing the GDS (Parmelee, Kleban, Lawton, & Katz, 1991) investigated the interrelations between depression using the GDS and cognitive impairment using the Blessed test. Participants included 201 nursing home and congregate apartment residents in a 2-year, two-wave study. Analyses indicated that the relation of depression to subsequent cognitive status was strongest among persons with borderline (versus impaired or intact) cognitive status.

In another study using the GDS, the prevalence of depression among nursing home residents was estimated by screening a group of residents selected from a random sample on the basis of cognitive status (Katz, Lesher, Kleban, Jethanandani, & Parmelee, 1989). Although individual patients changed over a 6-month period, depression, as assessed by the GDS, was constant. Major depression was clinically confirmed in 8 of 10 patients identified in the screening.

The relationship between pain and depression among institutionalized elderly was investigated by Parmelee, Katz, and Lawton (1991). Depression was assessed on the basis of a DSM-III[R] symptom checklist and categorized into possible major, minor, or no depression. The GDS and the Profile of Mood States (POMS) scales were also administered. The results revealed that possible major depressives reported more intense pain and a greater number of localized pain complaints than did minor depressives. Nondepressed individuals reported the least intense pain and fewest localized complaints. The effect remained strong even when functional disability and health status were controlled statistically.

The short form of the GDS (GDS-SF) has also been validated. A high correlation was found between the 15-item GDS when compared to the original 30-item version. The GDS-SF and the GDS-LF were shown to have high sensitivity rates. The specificity rates for both forms were similar, but lower than desirable (Lesher & Berryhill, 1994).

In conclusion, the GDS has been shown to be reliable and valid in older adults. Ease of administration, especially with the GDS-SF, enables its use in clinical practice and research. The GDS is not a substitute for further clinical diagnostics performed by mental-health professionals, and should only be used as a screening tool. Verbal administration of the tool has demonstrated consistency and validity with older adults with cognitive impairments. Simple screening tools, such as the GDS, are necessary components of a comprehensive assessment of an older adult. Screening patients for potentially treatable conditions such as depression may prevent the devastating effects of depression in late life.

Ellen Flaherty

See also:
DEPRESSION AMONG OLDER ADULTS
SUICIDE

GRIEF

Definitions

Grief is the characteristic pattern of psychological and physiological responses a person experiences after the loss of a significant person, object, belief, relationship, body part, or body function. Grief includes the entire range of physical, psychological, cognitive, and behavioral responses to a loss. It is characterized by intense mental anguish and varies in duration from a few weeks to many years. Two major types of normal grief have been identified: conventional grief, which occurs after a loss, and anticipatory grief, which occurs in anticipation of a loss. Anticipatory grief is the characteristic pattern of psychological and physiological responses a person makes to an impending loss. Although there is little agreement on the exact nature of anticipatory grief, there is general agreement that anticipatory grief facilitates coping with a loss when the loss actually occurs.

Three terms related to grief should be defined: *loss, bereavement,* and *mourning.* Loss is defined as the experience of parting with an object, person, belief, or relationship that is valued; the loss necessitates a reorganization of one or more aspects of the person's life. Losses range from minor ones, such as the loss of a wallet, which necessitates only minor adjustments, to major ones, such as the death of a loved one, which necessitates major adjustments. Bereavement is the state of having experienced a loss, particularly the death of a significant other. Bereavement is usually but not always accompanied by grief. Mourning encompasses the socially prescribed behaviors after the death of a significant other. Such behaviors vary from culture to culture. Mourning behaviors are symbols or conventional outward signs of grief that are socially constructed and do not necessarily indicate the presence or absence of grief. Examples include wearing black clothing or a black veil or armband.

Throughout time nurses have had key roles in dealing with grief. Nurses in diverse settings are especially involved in dealing with anticipatory grief; however, little nursing research was conducted on grief until the late 1980s.

Researchers and Major Studies

Jeanne Quint Benoliel (1983) presented a review of nursing research on death, dying, and terminal illness at a time when few nurses were conducting research in those areas. Since then research on grief and bereavement has proliferated. Demi and Miles (1986) published a review of research on bereavement, and subsequently Opie (1992) published one on childhood and adolescent bereavement. Nursing interest in grief and bereavement flourished during the 1980s and 1990s and extended to grief and anticipatory grief related to hospice care. Martinson (1995) reviewed research on pediatric hospice care and addressed both anticipatory grief and grief following the death of a pediatric hospice patient; Corless (1994) in her critique of research on symptom control within hospice care reviewed research on coping with dying, strategies, and needs. All these reviews can be located in the specific *Annual Review of Nursing Research* volume, edited by J. J. Fitzpatrick et al. and published by Springer Publishing. A number of nurses developed research programs focused on grief, including J.Q. Benoliel, R. Constantino, A. Demi, M. Diamond, M. Miles, J. Saunders, and M. Vachon.

Researchers have used both quantitative and qualitative approaches to study grief. Standardized instruments such as the Texas Inventory of Grief, the Grief Experience Inventory, and the Bereavement Experience Questionnaire have been used to assess grief manifestations. The emotional distress that accompanies grief was often measured with instruments such as the Brief Symptom Inventory, the Profile of Mood States, the Impact of Events Questionnaire, or a depression scale such as the Beck's or Hamilton's. Children's and adolescents' grief was often measured by the Child Behavior Checklist.

Much nursing research on bereavement has been directed at describing the manifestations of grief among diverse samples: bereaved parents, children, siblings, and widows; suicide survivors; and people facing a life-threatening or terminal illness. Other researchers have described bereaved persons' responses to events such as the loss of a home by fire and a spontaneous or elective abortion. Still other researchers have focused on describing nurses' responses to caring for the dying or the bereaved. These descriptive studies have used diverse methods, including grounded theory, phenomenology, participant observation, semistructured interviews, survey questionnaires, structured instruments, and q-sort techniques. For example, Jacobs (1996) used grounded theory to describe the grief experience of older women whose husbands received hospice care during their final illness; Grossman, Clark, Gross, Halstead, and Pennington (1995) used interviews to describe children's bereavement process after paternal suicide; Feldstein and Gemma (1995) used the Grief Experience Inventory to describe oncology nurses' responses to caring for dying patients; McCowan and Davies (1995) used the Child Behavior Checklist to assess patterns of grief in young children following the death of a sibling; and Kerr (1994) used a qualitative approach to assess the meanings adult daughters attach to a parent's death.

Some nursing research on bereavement has focused on comparing different modes of bereavement (suicide vs. accident, expected vs. unexpected) or comparing bereaved persons with a nonbereaved group. For example, Kovarsky (1989) compared loneliness and grief manifestations of parents whose child died by suicide with those whose chid died accidentally.

A number of nursing studies have investigated variables related to bereavement outcomes. For example: self-blame was associated with poorer outcomes after the death of a loved one (Weinberg, 1995); coping process was related to social support and adaptational outcomes in widows (Robinson, 1995); and a significant relationship was found between effective grief resolution and hope, coping styles, and death within a hospice setting among the elderly widowed (Herth, 1990).

A few studies have used quasi-experimental designs to investigate the effects of specific interventions to help the bereaved or to help nurses to better meet the needs of the bereaved. For example, researchers have studied the effect of a support group on bereaved parents whose child died from cancer, the effect of a support group on bereaved children and adolescents, and the effect of a grief workshop for pediatric oncology nurses.

Strengths and Limitations of the Studies

The descriptive studies have contributed greatly to our understanding of the grief process and the many forms it may take. The comparative and correlational studies have provided insight into variables related to good and poor bereavement outcomes. However, very little research has been done to assess the effects of bereavement interventions. More attention needs to be paid to intervention studies that address what helps people deal with anticipatory grief and grief due to a loss that has already occurred. Further, most of the participants in the studies reviewed were White Americans. With increasing cultural diversity in the United States, it is important that research address bereavement responses among diverse cultural groups. In addition, researchers should work on developing culturally relevant instruments to assess bereavement outcomes.

Ethical Issues

Grieving people are vulnerable and need special attention to protect them from studies that could increase their vulnerability. Although many grieving people find that participating in research that focuses on their grief provides them an opportunity to express their thoughts and feelings to a nonjudgmental researcher, there is the potential of increasing the participant's pain and distress. The researcher must have the skills to provide immediate support if this occurs and also should be prepared to refer participants for counseling if they need further support at a later time.

ALICE S. DEMI

See also:
   COPING
   DEATH AND DYING
   HOSPICE
   SUICIDE
   TERMINAL ILLNESS
   WIDOWS AND WIDOWERS

MUSIC THERAPY

Music therapy is the use of a musical intervention to improve physiological and psychological health and well-being. For music to be therapeutic, there must be an interaction between the music and the person who desires a health outcome (Meyer, 1956). Music therapy may be provided by a registered music therapist; however, any member of the health care team may suggest to patients that music can be helpful for stress, pain, mood, or exercise. Nurses can assess musical preferences, offer a choice of selections, and encourage patient involvement in the music with the goal of achieving specific health outcomes.

Throughout history, music has been used for a variety of therapeutic purposes by primitive people—ancient Egyptians, Persians, Hebrews, Greeks, and Romans. Music has been used to ward off evil spirits, prevent or cure illnesses, relieve depression, modify emotions, and achieve inner harmony. Early cultures had little means to treat disease, so music and spirituality were used to provide comfort and help people cope. During the Renaissance, physicians became interested in the scientific basis of healing. Because many physicians were also musicians, they believed in the therapeutic value of music and incorporated it in their training and practice. From the 17th century onward, physicians studied the effect of music on physiology and psychology. During this time there was debate over the need to focus on what type of music was effective versus what type of person responded positively to music. At the beginning of the 20th century, the first laboratory studies of the physiological effects of music were conducted on animals and humans. These experiments demonstrated changes in vital signs and body secretions related to various types of music, but they are rejected by most investigators today because of the poor quality of measurement, analysis, and control. In the 1930s music began to be used in patients' hospital rooms, in surgery prior to general anesthesia, and during local anesthesia. It was used in obstetrics and gynecology to reduce the side effects of inhalation anesthetics. During the past 50 years music has been used to (a) reduce acute, chronic, and cancer pain; (b) reduce stress and anxiety; (c) potentiate the effects of analgesic medications in patients during and after surgery and during labor and delivery; and (d) promote exercise.

Music can stimulate, soothe, encourage, or give pleasure to patients. Music has been found to reduce muscle tension, reduce pain and anxiety, raise levels of beta-endorphins, and lower adrenocorticotropic stress hormones. Nursing reviews of research on the effect of music on health outcomes can be found in chapters by Buckwalter, Hartsock, and Gaffney (1985), Cook (1981), Guzzetta (1988), and Chlan (1998). The *Journal of*

Music Therapy is another resource. Music has been found to improve the immune system, salivary cortisol, and cardiac autonomic balance. It has also been investigated for its effect on sleep disturbances, cancer pain, and acute and chronic pain during stressful or painful procedures (e.g., injections and lumbar punctures). Music has been generally found to reduce anxiety before and during surgery, with injections, in chronically ill patients, in intensive care patients, and after myocardial infarction. It has been studied in agitated elderly or psychiatric patients, in critically ill patients, and in those who are comatose or dying.

Music has been categorized into stimulative and sedative types. Stimulative music has strong rhythms, volume, dissonance, and disconnected notes, whereas sedative music has a sustained melody without strong rhythmic or percussive elements. Stimulative music enhances bodily action and stimulates skeletal muscles, emotions, and subcortical reactions in humans. Sedative music results in physical sedation and responses of an intellectual and contemplative nature (Gaston, 1951). Precategorization by the nurse, however, does not consider the kind of subject response.

To choose music that is therapeutic, the nurse should consider the nature of the music, the patient preferences and the health state. Variations in the music include the type of music and the intensity, tempo, rhythm, pitch, tone, timbre, blending, complexity, melody, familiarity, length, variety, and novelty. Variations in the patient include age, sex, cultural background, musical preferences, music training, participation in music, degree of auditory discrepancy, time available, and most of all, degree of liking for the music under consideration. Variations in the nature of the health state determine whether music is needed to cheer, encourage, and soothe or will be used to relax, distract the mind, stimulate exercise, or evoke emotions of joy, triumph, resolve, or peace.

Music is economical for patient use. Tapes, compact discs., and players are relatively inexpensive, and a small library can be maintained on any nursing unit. Music piped into patients' rooms also may be available. Nurses can suggest that patients and their families bring in favorite music from home that is likely to invoke healthy responses. They can refer patients to a music therapist if one is available.

Future research in music may include studies that determine the kinds of music that are effective for health outcomes in countries around the world, between cultures in each country. More work on comparing symptomatic response with physiological response is needed to generate theories of conditions in which music is effective, how it affects body processes, and what effect it has on recovery, immune function, and health.

Music brings an air of normalcy, entertainment, pleasure, and escape into a world where illness is often the enemy and both patients and caregivers are fighting back. Music is an integral part of most people's normal lives and should not be forgotten when they go to hospitals and other health care facilities. With the increased reliance on technology in health care today, music can add a humanistic touch. But beyond the humanistic value of music is the therapeutic value in reducing stress, pain, anxiety, and depression and promoting movement, socialization, and sleep.

MARION GOOD

See also:
ALZHEIMER'S DISEASE
COGNITIVE DISORDERS
COGNITIVE IMPAIRMENT
COGNITIVE INTERVENTIONS
REMINISCENCE

PET THERAPY

As advances in healthcare technologies contribute to longer life spans and the burgeoning numbers of chronically ill older adults, time-honored modalities known to contribute to wellness are regaining interest. Among these health-enhancing modalities is the therapeutic use of animals in healthcare settings. Although animals have been used for domestic purposes and as companions to humans for thousands of years, the therapeutic use of animals in healthcare is more recent. Seventeenth-century Quaker asylums used small animals as part of their social milieu to rehabilitate psychiatric patients. Florence Nightingale, in *Notes on Nursing* (1860/1969), advocated that animals serve as companions to people with confining or long-term illnesses. In this century, successes have been reported in the psychiatric treatment of children when animals were included in the therapeutic regimen. Programs using horses in treating a wide range of physical disabilities have spread to the United States from Europe (Willis, 1997). Such programs are fostering an increased awareness of, and interest in, the multifaceted ways that people with psychiatric or physical needs can benefit from animals as a part of their treatment.

Animals are being used in a variety of healthcare settings and in a variety of ways. Diverse and overlapping terms are used to describe these programs, such as animal therapy, assistance animals, pet therapy, and animal-assisted therapy. The program models range from simple to complex. The simplest model is pet visitation in which individuals or animals shelters bring their animals for visits in healthcare settings. Typically, the animals are not trained, and the rules of visitation are governed by local healthcare regulations and institutional policies. These visits are used to provide socialization opportunities for institutionalized or homebound people and their visitors. Often, trainers of service dogs will use such visits to socialize the animal.

A model that is more structured than pet visitation is animal-assisted therapy (AAT). AAT programs are more goal-oriented than are the visitation models, and they view the human/animal bond and the interactions it promotes as therapeutic. AAT programs provide protocols outlining the goals and implementation process for a specific program. Persons (often called handlers) escorting the animals are given training, and the animals are screened and certified for health, obedience, sociability, and temperament. AAT teams are typically asked to volunteer for specified periods of time, and often the human member of the AAT team is a healthcare professional. Delta Society, a nonprofit international organization, is one of many groups providing referral information for agencies or individuals interested in initiating or participating in AAT programs.

In both visitation and AAT models, particular animal characteristics are desired. Breed is not as important a criterion as some other qualities. The animal should be friendly, tolerant, and well mannered, and its energy level should be compatible with the healthcare environment in which the team will work. Although dogs are commonly used in animal-assisted therapies, many other species are also used—such as cats, birds, pigs, fish, horses, dolphins, llamas, and even snakes. Each AAT team has specific goals, and animals are chosen for their ability to assist in accomplishing those psychosocial or physical therapeutic goals. AAT teams have been active in healthcare settings for decades, and concerns about allergies and zoonoses (diseases communicable from animal to human) have not been substantiated in the existing literature.

The most complex model uses highly trained, and legally defined, animals called "service animals." The American Disabilities Act of 1990, a federal civil-rights law, defines a service animal as any animal individually trained to do work or perform tasks for the benefit of a person with a disability. The tasks that service dogs are able to perform include guiding people with impaired vision, alerting people with hearing impairments to various sounds, pulling wheelchairs, pulling a person into a lying or sitting position, turning switches on or off, retrieving objects, and summoning help. Certain dogs can even sense an impending seizure, and can alert their owners before the seizure occurs.

Much of the research exploring the therapeutic effects of animals in healthcare is anecdotal. In one of the few randomized, controlled trials exploring the use of service dogs with people who have physical disabilities,

Allen and Blascovich (1996) found that all participants showed significant improvements in self-esteem, internal locus of control, and psychological well-being within six months of receiving their service dogs. The participants improved in community integration and showed increases in school attendance and/or part-time employment. Dramatic decreases in the number of paid and unpaid assistance hours were also demonstrated.

Studies most commonly cited in the literature explored pet ownership or visitation and its effect on physiological or psychological indexes of stress, such as blood pressure and pulse. Friedmann, Katcher, Lynch, and Thomas (1980) reported a positive correlation between pet ownership and cardiovascular health. Since then, other studies have reported decreases in physiologic indexes of stress (blood pressure and heart rate) and, lower anxiety when participants were tested with animals nearby, or while petting the animals (Baun, Bergtrom, Langston, & Thoma, 1984; Harris, Rinehart, & Gerstman, 1993). Raina, Walter-Toews, Bonnett, Woodward, and Abernathy (1999b) reported that the physical health of older adults without pets (as assessed by their ability to perform Activities of Daily Living) deteriorated more on average than did that of older adults with pets. An association between pet ownership and owner well-being was not found, but Raina and colleagues suggest that researching the relationship between pet ownership and owner well-being is complex. Other researchers have postulated that it is the relationship and interaction with the pet, not simply ownership, that may be associated with greater well-being in pet owners (Tucker, Friedman, Tsai, & Martin, 1995).

Findings in most studies have been limited by small sample sizes, convenience samples, or the lack of a control group. Nurses, however, have been foremost in initiating pet visitation and AAT programs in home-care, acute-care, and long-term-care settings. Many benefits have been suggested or demonstrated—for example, feelings of improved well-being reported by participants (Francis, 1991), improved emotional health of families (Cain, 1991), decreased staff stress (Carmack & Fila, 1989), increased sense of connection (Dossey, 1997), and improved communication skills of withdrawn or isolated persons (Barba, 1995).

As the number of older adults increases, the number of elderly patients with chronic, debilitating illnesses will continue to rise. Many will live for decades with chronic physical and psychiatric conditions, including loneliness. Treatments that benefit the individual or family will depend on their unique needs, as well as the availability of health-enhancing services. There is increasing evidence that the human/animal bond is a crucial part of wellness for many individuals and families. The use of service animals is a vast area of untapped research for the elderly. Projects using monkeys to assist quadriplegics, and pilot studies exploring service dogs to minimize unsafe wandering of older persons with Alzheimer's disease (Shelkey, Sherman, Edwards, & Lantz, 1996) are only a beginning.

MARY SHELKEY

See also:
ALZHEIMER'S DISEASE
ALZHEIMER'S DISEASE—SPECIAL CARE UNITS IN LONG TERM CARE
COGNITIVE INTERVENTIONS
FALLS
LONG-TERM CARE DEMENTIA
WANDERING

REMINISCENCE

Reminiscence is defined as thinking about or relating past experiences, especially those personally significant (McMahon & Rhudick, 1961). It is regarded as a successful method with which to assist older adults, at all cognitive levels, to reach Erickson's (1982) developmental stage of ego integrity versus despair (Nugent, 1995). In a concept analysis, Burnside and Haight (1992) report that the ordinary uses of reminiscence include: providing a basis for other groups, increasing interactions with peers, focusing on conversation, and finding commonalities.

Reminiscence may be facilitated by asking an older adult about his/her memories of certain events, smells, or photographs. Early exploration into reminiscence reveals the following suggestions for stimulating reminiscence: writing about or tape recording memories of past events, developing a family tree, and encouraging the older adult to write to old friends (Butler, 1963).

Research on the use and effectiveness of reminiscence is limited. Although the concept has been used since the 1960s, little scientific research is available to support the use of this popular and unique nursing intervention. Two studies explored the themes resulting from reminiscence. Watters (1995) used a qualitative semistructured interview approach in a sample of 21 women aged 75 and over residing in a retirement community. Eight themes about reminiscence resulted from the data collection: nurturing family, source of strength, hard times, resilience, goal directness, sense of accomplishment, regrets/opportunities to learn, and legacy. Male reminiscing styles was the subject of another study of 6 community-dwelling males aged 76 to 84. Subjects were interviewed regarding the content of reminiscence sessions on two occasions. Themes resulting from the interviews included: joys, social connections, difficulties, choices, and control (Kovach, 1993).

The outcomes of reminiscence have been the subject of several experimental and quasiexperimental studies. McMahon and Rhudick (1961), in their classic study of the concept, determined that reminiscence is positively correlated with self-esteem, identity, and mastery. Burnside and Haight (1992) reported positive behavioral responses, change in affect, increased exchange of information between nurse and client and between group members, improvement in communication skills, and thinking about things to share in the future. However, these outcomes have not all been demonstrated empirically.

In an experimental study of 36 individuals with chronic renal failure and their significant others, a pretest-posttest experimental design was used to examine the impact of participation in six reminiscence therapy sessions on family coping. The sample was randomly selected from three outpatient hemodialysis centers and included 18 elderly individuals (65 years of age or older). The results indicated that there was a statistically significant increase in coping after the completion of the six reminiscence sessions (Comana, Brown, & Thomas, 1998).

Two studies have been conducted to explore the relationship between reminiscence and depression. Youssef (1990) examined a sample of 60 female subjects, aged 65 years and older. Subjects were randomly assigned to one of two experimental groups or one control group. The experimental groups received group reminiscence therapy. The results revealed a statistically significant improvement in level of depression in the younger subjects (aged 65 to 74) receiving the reminiscence treatment, but not in the older subjects. Another study of 34 female nursing home residents aged 65–88 utilized a similar experimental method (Taylor-Price, 1995). The experimental group received reminiscence group therapy twice a week for 60 minutes per session over a 6-week period. This group again showed a significant improvement in level of depression, as well as a significant increase in psychological well-being.

Although most of the outcome research is focused on patients, Puentes (1999) conducted a study to measure the effectiveness of reminiscence training on Registered Nurses' attitudes and empathy levels. An experimental design was again employed. The intervention consisted of a 1-hour didactic program and a 3-week period that was composed of didactic presentation and data collection in which the experimental group implemented the techniques acquired during the didactic training. The results revealed a statistically significant increase in both empathy and attitudes of RNs participating in the reminiscence training.

Reminiscence therapy is a popular, widely accepted nursing intervention. It is a process of assisting the older adult to recall past events in order for further development to occur. Despite the widespread use of this intervention, little research is available to describe or support it. Several descriptive studies have revealed the major themes that evolve from reminiscence. Other studies have explored the outcomes of the concept. Further research is needed in all areas of reminiscence.

MEREDITH WALLACE

See also:
MUSIC THERAPY

SUICIDE

Suicide is defined as a death that is the result of an intentional self-destructive act. Nurses have demonstrated a great deal of clinical and theoretical interest in suicide, suicide attempts, attitudes toward suicide, and assisted suicide but have conducted very little research on these topics. A related topic that has been studied fairly extensively by nurses is suicide survivors, those family members and significant others who are bereaved by a suicide.

Suicide, Suicide Attempts, and Suicidal Thoughts

Few studies have addressed suicide specifically. Using a qualitative methodology, messages of psychiatric patients who attempted or committed suicide were compared by Valente (1994). She found that clear suicidal messages were sent by most psychiatric patients and that the messages of suicide completers and suicide attempters could be differentiated. Demi, Bakeman, Sowell, Moneyham, and Seals (1996) studied suicidality in HIV-infected women and found that suicidal thoughts were common among the women and that family cohesion moderated the effect of HIV-related symptoms on emotional distress. They also found that there were clear differences between women who neither thought about nor attempted suicide and those who thought about or attempted suicide, but there were no significant differences between those who thought about suicide and those who attempted it. Grabbe, Demi, Camann, and Potter (1997) used a national data base to assess suicidal risk factors among the elderly during their last year of life; and using logistic regression, they confirmed the traditional risk factors of age, race, gender, alcohol use, and mental illness and provided preliminary evidence that cancer is also a risk factor among the elderly.

Two studies addressed adolescent suicide. Burge, Felts, Chenier, and Parrillo (1995), using a national data base, studied suicidal behaviors among U.S. high school students and found a significant positive relationship between cocaine use and severity of outcomes of suicide attempts. They also found a significant but less strong relationship between marijuana use, alcohol use, sexual activity, and suicide attempts. Conrad (1992) explored adolescents' beliefs about the causes of adolescent suicide and found that teens identified "too much pressure" as the major cause of teen suicide.

Attitudes Toward Suicide

Several studies by nurses have investigated attitudes toward suicide in diverse groups, four studies addressed nurses' attitudes, and one studied elderly persons' attitudes. Oncology nurses' knowledge and misconceptions about suicide were explored through use of a vignette depicting a suicidal cancer patient (Valente, Saunders, & Grant, 1994). Although the nurses correctly identified a number of risk factors, few knew that race, age, and gender were risk factors. Further, few nurses assessed whether patients had a specific suicide plan, and less than one third identified appropriate interventions to prevent suicide in an at-risk patient. A second study compared nurses' attitudes toward suicide based on their clinical specialty, age, and highest degrees; they found no significant differences on any of the subscales based on clinical specialty, although age and degrees were significant on only the right to die subscale (Alston & Robinson, 1992).

When Irish casualty nurses' attitudes toward attempted suicide were assessed, older and more experienced nurses had better attitudes toward suicide attempters than did younger, less experienced nurses (McLaughlin, 1994). Positive attitudes toward suicide attempters were found among psychiatric nurses working in an acute psychiatric ward (Long & Reid, 1996). The only study of nonnurses explored attitudes toward suicide among low-income, elderly, inner city residents and compared attitudes toward suicide of men and women, African Americans and Whites, finding no significant differences. The researchers suggested that social class and place of residence may be better predictors of attitudes toward suicide in the elderly than race and gender (Parker, Cantrell, & Demi, 1997).

Suicide Survivors

Many studies have been conducted on suicide survivors, including parents, spouses, children, siblings, and therapists. Most of the studies of suicide survivors have been descriptive and have found that a death by suicide produces extreme distress in the survivors, with evidence of increased guilt, stigma, and resentment and a continuing questioning of "why" the suicide occurred. Several studies have compared those bereaved by suicide with those bereaved by other modes of death and have reported conflicting findings. Recently, an attempt was made to use a quasi-experimental design to study the effects of two group interventions on outcomes among spouse survivors of suicide (Constantino & Bricker, 1996). The researchers found that participants in both the social group intervention and the bereavement intervention experienced an overall reduction in distress; however, the bereavement intervention group experienced significantly lower levels of anger or hostility and guilt.

Future Directions

The suicide rates for the elderly are rising. At the same time, there is increased interest in euthanasia and assisted suicide. Nurses are intimately involved with elderly and terminally ill patients who are contemplating suicide and assisted suicide. At the same time, suicide rates among adolescents and young adults are rising. Much more research attention should be directed to this topic. Researchers should move beyond describing attitudes toward suicide and effects of suicide on survivors and toward studying interventions to prevent suicide and to assist those coping with a death by suicide.

ALICE S. DEMI

See also:
   ALCOHOLISM
   DEPRESSION AMONG OLDER ADULTS
   TERMINAL ILLNESS

Part V

PATHOLOGICAL CONDITIONS OF AGING

INTRODUCTION

The current standard of living, nutrition, prevention and treatment of infectious diseases, and progress in medical care have sharply increased the survival rate for persons born in the United States. However, despite these challenges there remains a prevalence of pathological illness among older adults. In fact theories of aging postulate that pathological illness rather than old age is usually the cause of mortality. Disease, death, and loss of function among older adults is generally linked to four major causes: inadequacies of the healthcare system, lifestyle, environment, and biology (Lalonde, 1974).

Although illness is not a normal change of aging, years of environmental assault, poor health behaviors, and stress have placed the older adult at a high risk for developing illness. In general, health deteriorates with aging through an accumulation of chronic disorders and disabilities. Although heredity and genetics were once regarded as major factors in the length of time an individual lives, their influence on aging is not currently strongly regarded. Currently, heredity and genetics are only considered to be part of a larger picture influencing the aging process. Mitchell, Gingrich, and Jones (1994) reported that aging is influenced by heredity, lifestyle, behavior, nutrition, and education level.

Thirty million Americans have some dysfunction attributable to chronic disease, and 33% of these individuals are over 65 years old. The experience of illness among older adults is often accompanied by fatigue, pain, and sadness, impairing the quality of life of older adults. In addition, the experience often impairs an individual's capacity and motivation to learn new health-promoting behaviors.

The top ten pathological conditions resulting in death in those age 65 and older are: (1) heart disease; (2) malignant neoplasms; (3) cerebrovascular disease; (4) chronic obstructive pulmonary disease; (5) pneumonia and influenza; (6) diabetes mellitus; (7) accidents; (8) kidney disease; (9) atherosclerosis; and (10) septicemia (NCHS, 1998). Furthermore, 13% of the total elderly population are from minority groups. Some of the common health problems of the African-American minority group include higher incidence of strokes, cancer, diabetes, obesity, and hypertension. Hispanic Americans have higher rates of hypertension, cancer, diabetes, arthritis, and high cholesterol than their Caucasian counterparts. In the American Indian population there is a higher rate of diabetes and alcoholism leading to accidents and cirrhosis of the liver. Asian Americans and Pacific Islanders battle with a higher incidence of cancer (Keating, 1995).

Many pathological conditions common to the aging adult are contained within this section. The section contains reviews of the nursing research pertinent to 27 pathological diseases ranging from alcoholism to urinary incontinence. Several entries are devoted to the top three causes of mortality among older adults, specifically, heart disease, cancer, and cerebrovascular disease.

Cardiovascular diseases are major contributors to mortality and morbidity in the elderly. This group of diseases includes stroke, hypertension (HTN), arrhythmias, coronary heart disease (CHD), and congestive heart failure (CHF).

Although only 12% of the population are considered older adults, greater than 50% of total cancers diagnosed are found in the older adult population. The reason for the large proportion of cancer in this country is not known. Theories that have been postulated include longer exposure to carcinogens, increased susceptibility to cancer in the older body, decreased cellular healing ability, loss of tumor-suppressing genes, and decreased immune function. Although the exact cause cannot be determined, it is clear that cancer is a large problem for older adults in the United States. The most common type of cancers are breast cancer for aging women and prostate cancer for aging men (Boyle et al., 1992). Both these cancers are included in this section. In addition, this section includes entries on cancer chemotherapy—a common treatment for the disease, and cancer survivorship.

Although premature mortality related to pathological illness is of great concern to nurses, living with chronic illness is also paramount. Hall (1997) reports that the principal causes of severe, chronic disability among older adults are not the same as those illnesses that result in death. The top eight pathological chronic conditions in those age 65 and older (by order of frequency) are: arthritis, high blood pressure, hearing impairment, heart disease, orthopedic impairment, chronic sinusitis, diabetes, and visual impairment (Hampton, 1992). This section covers a variety of such chronic illnesses and pathological conditions.

The pathological conditions common to aging contained in this chapter may assist nurses in understanding why research evidence is so paramount to nursing care delivery. The research illustrates how clearly each pathological condition discussed affects the quality of life of older adults and their caregivers. Furthermore, the discussion of the pathological conditions provides an impetus for developing new research questions, on which future clinical practice may be based.

MEREDITH WALLACE

ALCOHOLISM

The DSM-IV diagnostic category of alcohol dependence is commonly called alcoholism. Alcohol dependence is a disease characterized by abnormal alcohol-seeking behavior that leads to impaired control over drinking (NIAAA, 1993). A diagnosis of alcohol abuse refers to a pattern of use that results in detrimental effects on health or social life that may eventually lead to alcohol dependence.

Alcohol dependence (alcoholism) is a primary, chronic disease with genetic, psychosocial, and environmental factors that influence its development and manifestations. Alcoholism results after prolonged, continuous or periodic use of alcohol. Alcoholism is noted when control over drinking is impaired, when preoccupation with alcohol occurs, and when use continues despite adverse consequences. The disease often is progressive and fatal. Distortions in thinking, most notably denial, result (Sullivan, 1995).

Alcohol is a depressant drug and is the most commonly used and abused substance of addiction. It is widely available, can be legally acquired by persons over 21 (in most states), and is relatively inexpensive.

Prolonged use of alcohol results in numerous physiological and psychological effects. Alcohol is metabolized by the liver; women may metabolize alcohol less efficiently than men. Liver damage often occurs as a result of prolonged use. Alcohol-induced cardiovascular injury, immune system impairment, and neurological disorders also can occur. Alcohol withdrawal syndrome is usually mild and self-limiting but in about 5% of cases can result in delirium tremens, which can be potentially fatal.

In contrast with other health problems, there is no definitive physical finding or laboratory test for alcoholism. Tests for liver function reveal end-stage organ damage; they do not detect the primary disorder.

Alcohol use has occurred throughout recorded history. Alcoholism has often been considered a moral failing caused by the availability of alcohol. The temperance movement and Prohibition were attempts to control alcoholism. The establishment of Alcoholics Anonymous in the early 1930s and the acceptance of alcoholism as a medical condition in the mid-1950s were more therapeutic efforts to address alcoholism.

Reflecting absence of societal interest and the health care community's lack of understanding, research and clinical reports about alcoholism have been sparse in the nursing literature and in nursing science. Prior to 1989, studies of alcohol abuse or alcoholism were often descriptive, addressed nurses' attitudes toward clients with alcohol problems, or studied nurses who were recovering from alcoholism (Naegle, 1995). Nurse researchers who have contributed to the early literature on alcoholism include Haack, Hughes, Naegle, and Sullivan, among others.

In fact, information about alcoholism has been scant in nursing curricula. Thus, nursing students and presumably future clinicians and scientists were not aware of the extent of alcoholism as a health problem, and few studies of this serious illness were pursued. Nurses, however, care for clients with alcoholism regularly. It has been estimated that 30% of hospitalized patients have disorders secondary to alcohol abuse, such as trauma, falls, cirrhosis, pancreatitis, or cardiovascular disease (NIAAA, 1993). Further, 15% to 20% of clients seen in primary care settings are estimated to have alcohol disorders (Fleming & Barry, 1992).

Recent initiatives by the federal government have attempted to ameliorate the lack of content and expertise in nursing education. Beginning in 1989, the National Institute on Alcohol Abuse and Alcoholism (NIAAA), the National Institute on Drug Abuse (NIDA), and the Office of Substance Abuse Prevention (now the Center for Substance Abuse Prevention) established initiatives to improve substance abuse education in schools of nursing through model curriculum projects and faculty development programs. Three curriculum models are now available, and more than 60 faculty fellows from 13 schools of nursing have been prepared through the federal faculty development grants; some have now received funding for alcohol research from NIAAA. Reports of this work, however, are in progress and not yet available in the literature. However, empirically based studies examining clinical interventions are beginning to appear in the literature (Mudd, Boyd, Brower, Young, & Blow, 1994; Wing & Thompson, 1995).

The potential for improved access to information about alcoholism exists through the curriculum models and the expertise of faculty, some of whom will continue alcohol research efforts and will encourage alcohol research among their students. It must be noted, however, that most schools of nursing do not have faculty trained in these projects and must rely on individual initiative to develop or enhance alcohol-related content.

Alcohol remains the most widely used and abused drug in America. Nurses will continue to encounter the consequences of alcohol abuse and dependence among their clients. It is essential that nurses be cognizant of the dire results of excessive alcohol consumption and be participants in the efforts to rehabilitate alcoholic clients. Although past research has focused on such issues as alcohol abuse content in nursing education or nurses with alcohol problems—both important topics—nonetheless, future research must target intervention strategies to improve the care of clients with alcohol disorders. The health of millions of clients with alcohol problems depends on it.

ELEANOR J. SULLIVAN

See also:
COGNITIVE DISORDERS

ANGINA

In women aged 70 to 84, the prevalence of angina is 19%, and this increases to 24.7% in those 85 and older. In men aged 70 and older the prevalence is 27.3%. Thus, angina is an important problem to the elderly population. Although angina usually indicates underlying coronary heart disease (CHD), myocardial ischemia can result from any variety of conditions that lead to an imbalance between oxygen supply and demand. Examples include left ventricular hypertrophy and aortic valve stenosis. Myocardial ischemia, however, frequently occurs in the absence of angina or its equivalents (jaw pain, numbness, dyspnea, fatigue, or other nonspecific symptoms related to transient left ventricular dysfunction). This shows that angina is neither a reliable nor sensitive marker of myocardial ischemia. Many elderly people have atypical findings, or have totally asymptomatic CHD. Nursing research must be directed at CHD which is symptomatic and that which is asymptomatic.

Despite the limitations of using angina as the sole marker of CHD, the presence of angina supports the diagnosis of CHD and is useful in assessing disease progression and the efficacy of medical management. Nursing has played an important role in studying the dissemination—and resulting adoption—of specific guidelines for secondary prevention. These were established by the American Heart Association (AHA) to inform the elderly as well as their healthcare providers (AHA, 1995). According to the guidelines, careful attention should be paid to the use of aspirin, the encouragement of physical activity, and the control of lipids, HTN, obesity, and smoking, as well as the side effects associated with these interventions. Consideration of psychosocial factors that are specific to the elderly and that influence CHD management is also warranted.

Psychosocial (social support and interactions and relationships between persons managing the condition), personal (self-efficacy, denial, lack of motivation, educational, lifestyle, beliefs, and past experience with management), environmental, as well as cultural influences may contribute to CHD management. Quality of life may also be affected by controlling CHD, yet this has not been widely studied in the elderly population. In contrast, depression and the importance of social support have been well documented in the elderly (Berkman & Syme, 1979; Seeman et al., 1987), as well as in individuals with CHD (Berkman, Leo-Summers, & Horowitz, 1992; Friedman, 1993; Frasure-Smith, 1993), but few interventional studies have extended these findings. Psychosocial and educational factors have been linked to how individuals perceive their own health status and manage chronic illness (Hubbard et al., 1984; Kaplan et al., 1983; Mossey et al., 1982; Robinson, 1988; Thorne & Robinson, 1988). These require further study within the elderly population with CHD, as does the influence of other comorbid conditions commonly affecting the elderly (Fried et al., 1998).

Atypical manifestations of CHD include nontypical chest, shoulder, or back pain; dyspnea; pulmonary edema; and cardiac arrhythmias. Atypical symptoms, or absence of symptoms, may not only lead to underdiagnosis of CHD, but in the setting of acute myocardial infarction (MI), it may cause delays in seeking treatment and in diagnosis (Turi, 1986; Meischke, 1993). This may contribute to higher morbidity and mortality (Kannel & Abbott, 1984; Uretsy, 1977). Atypical presentation of MI is common in the elderly, and the prevalence increases with age (Appelgate, Graves, Collins, Zwaag, & Akins, 1984; Bayer, Chadha, Farag, & Pathy, 1986; Muller et al., 1990; Solomon et al., 1989). The presence of chest pain with MI may occur in as few as 19% of the elderly (Pathy, 1967). Differentiation of atypical symptoms from other chronic conditions can be difficult, and MI may not even be suspected. Individuals may often present with dyspnea, gastrointestinal (GI) symptoms, syncope, stroke, confusion, faintness, giddiness, weakness, or restlessness (Aronow, 1987; Bayer et al., 1986; Konu, 1977; Lusiani et al., 1994; MacDonald, 1984; Tinker, 1981; Tresch, 1987). The individual who has suffered an unrecognized MI, whether a few days or weeks prior, may in fact present to the hospital in congestive heart failure (CHF), or with recurrent angina. MI may also be the result of other primary processes causing an increase in demand or a decrease in flow, such as intercurrent illness, GI bleed, or CHF. Since prompt recognition and treatment of MI is crucial to limiting infarct size and preserving myocardial function, it is vital that nursing research address issues central to atypical presentation (Dracup & Moser, 1991; Johnson et al., 1995; Reilly et al., 1994). These include identification of anginal equivalents; factors that delay decision to seek treatment (perception of symptoms and expectations); caregiver reactions to symptoms; healthcare provider recognition; assessment strategies specific to the elderly; and educational interventions aimed at reducing delay in seeking treatment.

Myocardial ischemia and infarction can also exist in the absence of signs and symptoms, and thus unrecognized MI is common in the elderly (Kannel & Abbott, 1984). Individuals with asymptomatic ischemia tend to have a higher incidence of asymptomatic MI, underscoring the importance of detecting ischemia early in its course. Silent episodes outnumber symptomatic episodes in patients with chronic stable angina or unstable angina, and in asymptomatic patients following MI (Pepine, 1986). Silent ischemia is present in 50,000 to 100,000 persons following MI, and in 3 million persons with angina. Symptomatic ischemia during daily activities, the extent of CHD, the degree of left ventricular dysfunction, and unstable angina are associated with an adverse prognosis (Nadelman et al., 1990). Asymptomatic ischemia may also occur in the absence of known CHD, and is frequently found in individuals with lower-extremity arterial disease and diabetes (Barzilay & Kronmal, 1998). Widespread screening of the elderly for asymptomatic CHD, however, has not been accomplished, so the true prevalence in the elderly is not known, although it could be expected to be high.

Nursing must play an important role in determining the prevalence of asymptomatic ischemia in the elderly with or without known CHD. ST-segment monitoring, although shown to be a reliable measure of myocardial ischemia following thrombolytic therapy or coronary angioplasty, is not widely used to monitor the elderly in the acute-care setting. Most contemporary monitoring systems provide the capability to monitor ST-segment changes without extra costs to the individual and with minimal time commitment on the part of nursing professionals. Nursing, therefore, has a unique opportunity to detect ongoing myocardial ischemia in the elderly, as well as to correlate asymptomatic episodes with precipitating factors, psychosocial factors, response to medications, and adverse outcomes.

Nursing also should share the responsibility for expanding our knowledge base regarding the timing and circadian variation of silent episodes, and the psychosocial, environmental, cultural, and pathologic factors that influence an individual's response to pain (Droste & Roskamm, 1983; Glazier et al., 1986). Although research is limited in the area, certain personality traits—lower on levels of nervousness, dominance, and excitability, and higher on the masculinity scale—have been associated with silent ischemia (Droste & Roskamm, 1983). Further research is warranted, utilizing personality characteristics not only to identify asymptomatic individuals, but as a basis for patient education. Patient coping, management of ischemic episodes, and psychosocial adjustment to asymptomatic disease are important nursing considerations, yet these have not been widely studied (Cohn & Cohn, 1983; Cohn, 1986).

Pain prompts individuals to modify their activities and help them assess the effects of cardiac risk factor modification and medications. When dealing with silent ischemia this opportunity is lost, and individuals must be provided with other strategies for controlling the underlying condition. An absence of symptoms may contribute to denial and a lack of motivation on the part of the patient in following the management scheme. Identifying ischemia triggers, such as daily activities and mental stress (Rozanski et al., 1988), and helping patients recognize other vague symptoms associated with ischemia may allow more aggressive management of the condition. Quality of life may be affected through fear of activity, yet it has not been widely studied in this elderly population. With recent technological advances in myocardial perfusion imaging and more aggressive screening for asymptomatic disease in high-risk individuals, the prevalence of individuals with known asymptomatic disease is likely to increase. Nursing must be prepared to implement educational interventions, document their efficacy, and play an active role in assisting the individual in recognizing and managing asymptomatic disease.

DEBORAH CHYUN

See also:
CARDIOVASCULAR DISEASE
DEPRESSION AND CARDIAC DISEASE
OBESITY AS A CARDIOVASCULAR RISK FACTOR
SMOKING AS A CARDIOVASCULAR RISK FACTOR

APHASIA

The term "aphasia" refers to a neurological condition that is always due to injury to the brain. In older adults, the most common cause of aphasia is stroke. The National Institutes of Health have estimated that 85,000 new cases of aphasia occur every year in the United States, leaving more than a million persons to cope with this seriously handicapping condition (American Heart Association, 1994). Within minutes, the lives of aphasic victims (and their families) can change drastically. Individuals stricken with aphasia lose, in part or whole, the ability to communicate effectively. The aphasia renders them unable to comprehend and exchange thoughts and feelings (Chapey, 1994). In addition to spoken language impairment, aphasic individuals usually have difficulty reading and/or writing, and may be affected in the way they approach tasks, solve problems, respond to stimuli, monitor their performance, interact with others, and view themselves (Brookshire, 1997). The ability to communicate is so basic to a person's integrity that reducing or eliminating language skills places strain on nearly every aspect of a person's being (Piotrowski, 1978).

Researchers have attempted to describe the alterations in language demonstrated by aphasic patients, and to relate these changes to both the neuroanatomy of the disorder and the cognitive status of the person. Technological advances in the latter half of the twentieth century provided researchers with an unprecedented opportunity to test models of the brain and of language (Benton & Anderson, 1998). The rapid evolution of brain imaging techniques, specifically CT and MRI, have enabled researchers to significantly advance their understanding of the correlation between focal brain damage and language deficits. By studying this information in relation to clinical data, researchers and aphasia therapists are hoping to improve language intervention strategies while reducing the overall time and cost associated with long-term rehabilitation (Frumkin, Palumbo, & Naeser, 1994).

Much of the aphasia research in the past 20 years has focused on the consequences of strokes and various degenerative neurological disorders. Considerable knowledge has been gained in terms of how the brain changes with age, and of the neuropathologies often associated with normal aging. It is now known that several components of language function deteriorate by virtue of the aging process itself in the absence of disease, and that these components change at different rates. The most common complaint among elderly people, in terms of changes in language function, is the increased frequency of word-retrieval difficulties. Discourse production appears to be largely preserved with advanced age, although there may be some subtle changes, such as the use of simpler syntactic constructions (i.e., the way in which words are put together in a sentence to convey meaning) (Kynette & Kemper, 1986). Language comprehension appears to be an area in which older adults are especially vulnerable to a decline in performance. Although some loss of comprehension may be attributed to a decline in hearing acuity, recent research has concluded that there are consistent age-related differences in comprehension which may be explained by an impaired short-term memory, a reduced ability to inhibit irrelevant information, and the slowing of cognitive processing. It has also been proposed that these deficits may be related to problems with syntactic processing (i.e., the mental operations that govern the ability to translate between formal sentence structure and its underlying meaning) (Nicholas, Connor, Obler, & Albert, 1998).

Because of the advancements in the use of CT and MRI, much information has been gained regarding the neuroanatomy of language dysfunction in aphasia. Within the past 10 years, research has shown that anatomical changes in the language-related areas of the brain, deterioration of function and structure in the auditory system, and neurochemical changes are all features of the neurology of normal aging, all of which may interact to produce the major age-related changes of language (Nicholas et al., 1998).

Historically, aphasia has been defined from two different viewpoints. The anatomic approach emphasizes neuropathology in order to describe the cause of aphasia based on brain-lesion site. The functional or behavioral viewpoint has focused on describing the disturbances that occur in communication, as well as other behavioral changes. Researchers have developed a variety of systems for categorizing aphasia, in order to correlate neuropathology with the associated communication and behavioral changes that are observed. The two major types of aphasia that have most frequently been described in the literature refer to the historical distinction between fluent (i.e., Wernicke's aphasia) and nonfluent (i.e., Broca's aphasia) (Piotrowski, 1978). Current aphasia research describes very similar language patterns across aphasia types, without regard to the fluency of speech. For general clinical purposes, aphasia is best described as being primarily expressive (i.e., language formulation and use are impaired), primarily receptive (understanding of spoken and/or written language is impaired), or mixed (comprehension, formulation, and use of language are impaired).

Recovery from aphasia is a complex process, affected by the interaction between initial severity of language impairment, the premorbid level of language functioning, the concomitant medical and cognitive disabilities, the amount and type of treatment, etc. A critical reality in aphasia rehabilitation is the fact that, once the condition stabilizes, few patients recover fully and regain normal communication function (Sarno, 1998). Rehabilitation must be viewed as a process of patient management, with the focus being on assisting the aphasic individual, their families, and significant others to facilitate communication, enhance social interaction, develop compensatory communication strategies, and adjust to the alterations and intervention process. The most effective results are obtained with a truly interdisciplinary approach, with participation from nursing, medicine, physical and occupational therapy, psychology, social work, and other members of the rehabilitation team.

No single therapeutic technique has been found to be effective for all aphasic patients. The ideal approach to language intervention is based on individualized assessment, and is tailored to each patient. There are excellent resources available for informational and educational purposes. The American Heart Association has published several pamphlets, including *Caring for a Person with Aphasia* (1994) and *How Stroke Affects Behavior* (1994). Other appropriate booklets include: *Adult Aphasia: Understanding the Disability* (Jacob, 1994), and *Understanding Aphasia: A Guide for Family and Friends* (Sarno, 1986). An Internet search using the keyword "aphasia" also offers a wealth of information, and the address, *www.aphasia.org.NAAreadings.html* provides many additional references that are appropriate for aphasic individuals and their families.

Future considerations for improving the treatment of aphasia and developing more sophisticated intervention techniques lies in: continued research into language processing, the development of cost-effective, user-friendly alternative/augmentative communication systems, new applications of computer technology, and research into the psychosocial sequelae and pharmacological management of depression following stroke and the acquisition of aphasia (Sarno, 1998).

BARBARA A. RITGERT
MARIANNE SHAUGHESSEY

See also:
  CEREBROVASCULAR DISEASE
  DYSPHAGIA

BREAST CANCER

Breast cancer is a major health problem in the United States, affecting approximately 181,600 women, or 30% of new cancer cases in women in 1997. Research in breast cancer is highly relevant to women's health research and has been a major interest of several nurse researchers over a period of time. Breast cancer research is targeted as a high research priority of the National Cancer Institute (NCI) and the National Institute of Nursing Research (NINR). For instance, NCI funding for breast cancer research increased to nearly $450 million in 1994. In addition, NINR has supported studies to improve women's knowledge of and behavior in breast cancer prevention and detection and funded research that will lead to effective nursing interventions.

A review of breast cancer studies conducted by nurses from the early 1970s to the 1990s demonstrated four focused areas of research: early detection through breast self-examination (BSE), management of symptoms during treatment, psychosocial response of patient and family, and issues in long-term cancer survivorship. The major theoretical frameworks used in nursing research in breast cancer include the health belief model, the Roy adaptation model, and Orem's self-care deficit theory.

Screening and Early Detection Research

Nurse researchers have made significant contributions to our knowledge of early detection through BSE practice and the factors influencing the patient's ability to perform BSE (Champion, 1991). Early studies emphasized BSE rather than mammography, presumably because teaching and education were prime areas for nursing intervention. Mammography use has increased exponentially in this country, and nurses now aim their research toward predictors of mammography usage. In addition, nurse researchers must expand their focus to the triad of breast cancer screening modalities: BSE, mammography, and clinical breast examination (CBE).

Nurse scientists have also targeted screening and early detection activities for high-risk groups such as African Americans (Nemcek, 1989), Hispanics (Longman, Saint-Germain, & Modiano, 1992), rural populations, and older women (Lierman, Kasprzyk, & Benoliel, 1991). Nurse researchers continue to develop intervention studies addressing the reduction of barriers to breast cancer screening, particularly among the underserved and elderly populations (Ansell, Lacey, Whitman, Chen, & Phillips, 1994).

Diagnosis and Symptom Management

The second major contribution by nurses in breast cancer research pertains to issues in diagnosis and symptom management. Nurse researchers have improved our understanding of anxiety, critical thinking, decision making, care-seeking behavior, and preferential choice in treatment for breast cancer (Lauver, 1992; Lierman, 1988). Another cluster of studies focused on symptom management during treatment; they include hair loss, nausea and vomiting, fatigue, and pain in advanced cancer.

Intervention Studies to Manage Symptoms

Three notable areas of intervention by several nurse researchers included exercise as a means to improve well-being and fatigue (Mock et al., 1997), the use of a coach or partner to enhance adaptation to breast cancer (Samarel & Fawcett, 1992) and attentional fatigue (Cimprich, 1992).

Early investigations by Winningham and colleagues (Winningham et al., 1989) evaluated the effects of aerobic interval training in improving the functional capacity of breast cancer patients on adjuvant chemotherapy. This led to an increase in the number of intervention studies examining the effectiveness of exercise. In the most recent analysis, Mock and colleagues (1997) used an experimental design to test the hypothesis that women who participated in a walking exercise program during radiation therapy treatment for breast cancer would demonstrate more adaptive responses, as evidenced by higher levels of physical functioning and lower levels of symptom intensity, than would women who did not participate. Women in the exercise group maintained an individualized, self-paced, home-based walking exercise program, and the comparison group received usual care. Results showed significant differences between the two groups on the outcome measures. The walking exercise group scored higher on physical functioning and lower on symptom intensity, particularly on measures of fatigue, anxiety, and difficulty sleeping. Implications were that a nurse-prescribed and monitored exercise activity was an effective, convenient, and low-cost self-care activity to help reduce symptoms of breast cancer treatment.

Psychosocial Response

The third major area of breast cancer studies focused on psychosocial response. Researchers have examined adjustment of patients, spouses, children, and family to the impact of breast cancer over time, concerns about quality of life, threat of cancer recurrence, issues in self-transcendence, and improvements in emotional and spiritual well-being. Northouse (1995) conducted several studies evaluating the impact of women's cancer on the family. In a review of the literature, the consensus from studies on the emotional impact of breast cancer on spouses is an increase in number of reported psychosomatic concerns, increased feelings of anxiety and depression, and high distress levels. The strongest predictor of adjustment was the level of concurrent stress in the marital relationship. Northouse also found few studies of the impact of breast cancer on children and directed attention to developing future studies in this regard.

Future Directions

Nursing research in breast cancer has improved our understanding of response to chronic illness tremendously. In the future, nurse researchers will continue to develop programs of research in breast cancer, work collaboratively with other disciplines, and use their expertise in setting national health policy and helping to direct a national research agenda.

KAREN HASSEY DOW

See also:
BREAST CANCER SCREENING
CANCER CARE: CHEMOTHERAPY
CANCER SURVIVORSHIP

CANCER CARE: CHEMOTHERAPY

Definition and Overview of Chemotherapy

Chemotherapy is defined by the 1997 *Taber's Cyclopedic Medical Dictionary* (Thomas, 1997, p. 363) as "the application of chemical reagents that have a specific and toxic effect on the disease-causing microorganism." Chemotherapy is primarily associated with the treatment of cancer but can be used with other diseases. Historically, the overall goal of this treatment approach has been maximum cell kill with tolerable toxicity. The balance between these two approaches can result in life-threatening side effects.

The effects of chemotherapy are systemic and thus invaluable in the treatment of cancer, a disease characterized by micrometastatic spread. The purpose of chemotherapy can be cure, control, or palliation. Many cancers are cured by the administration of chemotherapy. Recent advances have resulted in extended disease-free intervals and prolonged survival in cancers that previously had poor prognoses. There are more than 50 chemotherapeutic agents in use, with new drugs being developed yearly. Despite the addition of new drugs to the armamentarium of agents that can be used to combat cancer, drug resistance remains a formidable problem.

Drug resistance can be temporary or permanent. Permanent, or phenotypic, drug resistance is genetically based and hypothesized to be the major factor in chemotherapy drug failure. Recent research indicates the existence of multidrug, or pleiotropic drug resistance. The strategies that have been developed to combat multidrug resistance include "(1) increasing intracellular drug concentration using high doses of drugs; (2) alternating noncross-resistant chemotherapy regimens; (3) use of monoclonal antibodies or conjugates to target P-glycoprotein; and (4) use of drugs to inhibit the function of P-glycoprotein" (Knobf & Durivage, 1993, p. 279).

Historical Perspectives. The first chemotherapeutic agents were hormones, estrogen and androgen, which were used in the 1940s in the treatment of breast and prostate cancer. Modern-day chemotherapy began with an accidental discovery during World War II of the toxic effects of poison gases, specifically exposure to mustard gas (nitrogen mustard). A derivative of this agent was used subsequently to treat patients with Hodgkin's disease; although not permanent, there was documented tumor regression. Nitrogen mustard is one of the oldest class of antineoplastic agents, titled alkylating agents. The next discovery, by Dr. Sydney Farber in the late 1940s, was that folic acid antagonists could be used successfully against acute leukemia in children. Folic acid antagonists constitute the plant alkaloids class of antineoplastic agents. In the 1950s, the chemotherapeutic classes of antitumor antibiotics and antimetabolites were introduced into the treatment of cancer.

Rationale for Use. Because cancer cells move through the five phases of the cell cycle as do normal cells, chemotherapeutic agents are classified according to the point in the cell cycle at which the agent's effect is exerted on the cancer cells. Chemotherapeutic agents affect both normal and malignant cells by altering cellular activity during one or more phases of the cell cycle. The two major classes of agents that have been established on the basis of their activity during the cell cycle are called cycle phase-specific and cell cycle phase-nonspecific. Cell cycle-specific drugs are those that are lethal only if the cell is dividing. Cell cycle-nonspecific are effective only against resting cells. There are some chemotherapeutic agents that are cell cycle-specific, phase-nonspecific. These are drugs that act on both resting and cycling cells.

Because chemotherapy drugs affect both cancer and normal cells, the cancer patient experiences many side effects during treatment. These include (a) nausea and vomiting, (b) diarrhea, (c) stomatitis, (d) fatigue, (e) anorexia, (f) bone marrow suppression, (g) organ toxicity (cardiac, neurological, hepatic), and (h) cystitis. Nursing research has focused on describing and designing interventions to lessen the side effects of the chemotherapy and on effective educational interventions to promote self-care.

Drug Development. Chemotherapeutic drugs enter the mainstream of clinical treatment through clinical trials. Implementation of clinical trials for new chemotherapy drugs is carried out by a multidisciplinary research team, including nurses serving in research and clinical roles. Clinical trials are the principal method for obtaining reliable evaluation of treatment effects and for examining the efficacy of new therapeutic drugs. There are four phases of clinical trials. Phase I studies the maximum tolerated dose for the delivery schedule of a specific chemotherapy drug. The purpose of Phase II studies is to determine the antitumor toxicity of the drug in a variety of cancers. Phase III studies define the role of a drug in a cancer treatment regimen, comparing the new drug with conventional treatments. Phase IV studies integrate a new agent into a proven treatment plan. At this point, the drug is known to be effective, but it is not authorized for widespread clinical use.

Initially, the primary role of the nurse in clinical trials was that of a data collector (data manager). The role of the nurse evolved to that of a research or protocol nurse, answering patient and family questions about the research study, providing education related to the study, accruing patients for the study, and observing patients' responses and toxicities. These research or protocol nurses were among the first nurses to participate as collaborators in cancer research. With the growth of oncology nursing master's and doctoral programs, the nursing role related to clinical trials has grown to be that of research collaborator and co-investigator. In this role the nurse is able to incorporate nursing issues into medical protocols. "Currently, oncology nurses enhance the care of patients with cancer through collaborative and independent nursing research that facilitates biomedical research outcomes, impacts severity of disease and treatment-related outcomes, and improves the patient's ability to live with a chronic illness such as cancer" (Jenkins, 1996, p. 4).

Evolving Role of Nursing in Chemotherapy

In 1991 and 1995 the Research Committee of the Oncology Nursing Society conducted a survey of the membership to determine the top nursing research priorities. In 1991 the top research priorities related to the administration of chemotherapy were quality of life, symptom management, outcome measures for interventions, and pain control; in 1995 they were pain control, quality of life, neutropenia, and patient education. In the past decade cancer nursing research has focused on documenting and describing the phenomenon of chemotherapy side effects. The focus has shifted to designing intervention studies that will provide direction for clinical decision making.

Nursing Research

Administration Issues. Considerable chemotherapy nursing research in the 1980s focused on the hazards to health professionals of administering chemotherapeutic drugs, a concern that developed after Falck's study (Falck et al., 1979) reported increased mutagenicity in the urine of chemotherapy nurses. Research studies during this period tended to assess the uptake of specific cytotoxic drugs in the urine of nurses handling these drugs or to look at the mutagenic changes that had occurred in their urine. Johnson and Gross (1982) were unable to find methotrexate in the blood and urine of nurses who administered this drug. The other focus of nursing research was to investigate compliance with Occupational Safety and Health Administration guidelines for the safe handling of cytotoxic drugs. Valanis and Shortridge (1987) investigated this area and documented inconsistent adherence to these guidelines. Although there was increased use of protective equipment among nurses, most nurses did not wear face protection when handling cytotoxic drugs except when cleaning up a spill.

Side Effect Issues. The side effects from the administration of chemotherapy affect all body systems and occur initially, throughout administration, and years later. The chemotherapy side effects that nursing research has focused on are nausea and vomiting, stomatitis, pain, and fatigue. Cotanch and Strum (1987) randomly assigned 60 patients who were beginning inpatient chemotherapy infusions to three groups: (a) experimental, (b) placebo, and (c) control. The patients who were taught progressive muscle relaxation had less frequency and duration of vomiting, less general anxiety, less physiological arousal, and greater caloric intake 48 hours following the drug infusion than those patients not taught progressive muscle relaxation.

Quality-of-Life Issues. Quality of life (QOL) became a critical outcome measure when the National Cancer Institute initiated a policy to include it as an outcome measure in all clinical trials. Cancer nursing has played a prominent role in encouraging clinical interest in QOL research. Nursing research in this area has been describing the phenomenon, developing instruments to measure it, and testing interventions to promote QOL. Many of the QOL nursing studies have investigated patient responses to treatment with cytotoxic drugs. Sarna (1989) described the effects of the initial cycle of chemotherapy on QOL and functional status in adults over 65 years of age with lung cancer.

Summary

The role of the nurse in relation to chemotherapy has changed dramatically over the past several decades. Initially, the research role of the nurse was that of a data collector assisting physicians involved in clinical trials. The research role of the nurse then evolved to conducting research independently of clinical trials and focusing on the hazards of administering cytotoxic drugs to patients and investigating the impact of nursing interventions on the side effects of the drugs. Nurses are now vital, equal participants and conduct their own studies within clinical trials. Quality-of-life nursing studies are frequently the vehicle with which nursing joins with physicians in seeking to improve the care of cancer patients.

MARILYN FRANK-STROMBORG

See also:
> **CANCER SURVIVORSHIP**
> **DEATH AND DYING**
> **GRIEF**
> **PAIN ASSESSMENT**
> **PAIN MANAGEMENT**
> **QUALITY OF LIFE**
> **WIDOWS AND WIDOWERS**

CANCER SURVIVORSHIP

Ten million cancer survivors are living in the United States today. The growing numbers are a result of improved cancer treatment, symptom management, and supportive care. A cancer survivor is defined as an individual who is living with, through, and beyond a diagnosis of cancer. Cancer survivors include individuals living through cancer treatment, those who are cancer-free, and those having intermittent recurrence or persistent or advanced disease. This definition differs from the traditional view of a cancer survivor as one who has lived at least 5 years after cancer diagnosis.

Cancer survivors have stressed the increased importance of and attention to quality-of-life (QOL) issues and have been instrumental in the growing debate in the larger political and health arenas on policy about cancer survivorship. The cancer survivorship philosophy reflects the personal experiences and wisdom of individuals who have "been there." The philosophy is based on the emergence of a more informed and assertive health care consumer having an optimistic expectation of survival.

The National Coalition for Cancer Survivorship (NCCS), which addresses concerns of cancer survivors, has grown from a grassroots organization to one having regional and national prominence. Major health policy issues on survivorship have continued to develop since the First National Congress on Cancer Survivorship in 1995 to the establishment of the Office of Cancer Survivorship at the National Cancer Institute in 1996. The purpose of the office is to explore critical research issues and consequences of cancer treatment through an interdisciplinary approach.

Studies of cancer survivors have focused primarily on the pediatric cancer survivor, but much research needs to be done with adult survivors. The concerns of cancer survivors can best be viewed through a QOL framework, which is a personal sense of well-being that encompasses a multidimensional perspective of physiological, psychological, social, and spiritual well-being. Changes in one area or domain of QOL can influence changes in other QOL domains.

Nurse researchers have contributed to our knowledge of the QOL concerns of cancer survivors. They have participated in clinical trials evaluating late physiological effects and have investigated high-incidence concerns of cancer survivors (Ferrell & Hassey Dow, 1997). Ferrell, Hassey Dow, Leigh, Ly, and Gulasekaram (1995) described the QOL in a study of long-term cancer survivors. They used a mailed survey of three instruments—a demographic tool, the QOL–Cancer Survivors tool, and the FACT-G—sent to 1,000 members of NCCS. The QOL instruments were designed to elicit concerns of cancer survivors in four areas, or domains: physical, psychological, social, and spiritual well-being. They received 687 returned surveys (57%). The mean age of the sample was 49.6 years; 81% were female, 72% college-educated, 63% married, 66% working full- or part-time. Results indicated that fatigue, aches and pains, and fertility were problematic physical late effects. Psychological concerns included the recall of distress at initial diagnosis and fear of recurrent, metastatic, or second cancers. Fear of future tests, anxiety, and depression were also problematic, as were family distress, sexuality, and financial burdens. In addition, hopefulness and purposefulness were positive outcomes of surviving cancer.

Nurse scientists continue to investigate late physical effects of pain, fatigue, dyspnea, functional changes (immobility, incontinence, and lymphedema), sexuality and intimacy issues, and cognitive impairments (Blesch et al., 1991) among cancer survivors. Physiological late effects where more research is needed include the development of secondary cancers, recurrent cancer, and late organ effects on the cardiovascular, pulmonary, reproductive, and endocrine systems.

Psychosocial late effects identified in descriptive studies of cancer survivors include the fear of recurrence, fear of testing procedures and medical surveillance, emotional distress, depression, uncertainty over the future, loneliness, and isolation (Mahon, 1991; Northouse, 1981). Uncertainty over the future and fear of recurrence have been identified as major areas targeted for interventions, although support groups have traditionally addressed some of these psychosocial issues.

Living with cancer may necessitate a change over time in the meaning of work and actual work practices. Nursing research in this area has identified work-related dilemmas such as overcoming bias in the workplace, disclosure, reentry concerns, breach of confidentiality, and lack of resources in the workplace (Berry & Catanzaro, 1992). Berry and Catanzaro described nursing interventions to help survivors return to the workplace. They divided the interventions into two categories: personal factors and environmental factors. Personal factors included collaborating with other health disciplines, addressing knowledge deficits about side effects and discrimination issues, and discussing the meaning of work. Environmental factors included the facilitation of reintegration of treatment with life activities and encouraging the worker to establish regular communication.

Spiritual distress characterized by loneliness, despair, grief, loss, and uncertainty has been identified in cancer survivors by nurse researchers (Kahn & Steeves, 1993). Positive life changes include risk taking, improved decision making, hope, and transcendence. These descriptive studies lay the groundwork for the development of interventions aimed at reducing such burdens. Interventions to help cancer survivors in the search for meaning are future areas of research (Ersek, Ferrell, Hassey Dow, & Melancon, 1997).

Future Areas of Research

Services needed by cancer survivors include access to long-term follow-up, development of guidelines and standards for long-term follow-up, expanded models of psychosocial and rehabilitative support, and education and health maintenance of cancer survivors. Nurse researchers have collaborated with advocacy and survivorship groups to describe the long-term needs of cancer survivors and have developed valid and reliable instruments to measure quality of life in this population (Hassey Dow, Ferrell, Leigh, & Melancon, in press). With the growing population of cancer survivors, survivorship research is a fruitful area for continued investigation in the future.

KAREN HASSEY DOW

See also:
   COPING
   DEATH AND DYING
   GRIEF
   QUALITY OF LIFE
   WIDOWS AND WIDOWERS

CARDIOVASCULAR DISEASE

Cardiovascular diseases (CVDs)—which include stroke, hypertension (HTN), arrhythmias, coronary heart disease (CHD), and congestive heart failure (CHF)—are major contributors to mortality and morbidity in the elderly. Although the most prevalent form of CVD is HTN, the majority of CVD deaths are attributed to CHD. The prevalence and incidence of CHD increase dramatically with age, and CHD is the leading cause of death in the elderly (American Heart Association [AHA], 1998). Angina, sudden death, and myocardial infarction (MI) are the major manifestations of CHD. Some 27% of men and 44% of women will die within one year of their MI (AHA, 1998). Although CHF may result from valvular dysfunction and other conditions, the majority of CHF cases are attributable to CHD. Despite the importance of CHD in the elderly, particularly elderly women, the prevention and management of CHD have not been widely studied in the elderly population. Rather, much of our current knowledge is based on studies conducted with nonelderly individuals; these findings may not necessarily be applicable to the elderly.

CHD and subsequent MI are potentially preventable conditions. Research aimed at prevention must address the importance of established risk factors in the elderly, as well as identifying new risk factors specific to the elderly population. Age-related differences exist between younger and elderly individuals with respect to cardiac risk factors, and the role of conventional cardiac risk factors remains controversial (Aronow et al., 1986; Krumholz et al., 1994; Seeman, Mendes de Leon, & Ostfeld, 1993). In addition, diabetes mellitus is prevalent in the elderly, and is an established risk factor not only for development of CHD but also for development of MI, and for mortality following MI. Yet knowledge of diabetes management in relation to the development of CHD and MI, as well as to long-term outcomes, is limited.

Although information on management of cardiac risk factors in the elderly is limited, recent trials of lipid-lowering agents have demonstrated a beneficial effect on morbidity and mortality (Dart et al., 1997). Therefore identification of other preventive interventions and evaluation of their efficacy specifically in the elderly population must be documented, along with individual characteristics that contribute to better risk-factor control. Nursing has an important role in studying the methods and adequacy of the dissemination of guidelines established by the AHA for primary prevention of CHD in the elderly, not only to the public but also to health-care providers (AHA, 1997). Levels of physical activity, as well as control of lipids, HTN, obesity, and smoking, need to be determined, along with the side effects of these interventions. Management of diet and exercise may pose special challenges to the elderly. Medications to treat hypertension and lipid abnormalities may not be well tolerated, and the potential for side effects and drug interactions is increased in the setting of polypharmacy. Finally, consideration of psychosocial factors is warranted. Neither psychosocial influences, which may contribute to the control of cardiac risk factors, nor quality of life, which may be affected by control of cardiac risk factors, have been widely studied in the elderly population.

Thirty-day mortality following MI in the elderly is currently estimated at 21% (Normand, Glickman, Sharma, & McNeil, 1996). Advanced age is known to be associated with an increased risk of in-hospital death following MI (Goldberg et al., 1989; Marcus et al., 1990; Rich, Bosner, Chung, Shen, & McKenzie, 1992), and we are beginning to understand prognostic factors for short-term mortality following MI (Chyun, 1998; Normand et al., 1996). Still to be studied are the efficacy of monitoring for complications, and the ways to prepare elderly patients and their caregivers for discharge, within a shortened hospital stay. Awareness of prognostic factors may help to identify patients at risk of short-term mortality and should result in improved assessment and nursing care targeted toward high-risk individuals.

Many of those who are eligible for aspirin (Krumholz et al., 1996) or beta-blocker therapy following MI (Gottlieb, McCarter, & Vogel, 1998) do not receive these medications upon discharge. Discrepancies between other medications known to have a survival benefit—such as ACE inhibitors and lipid-lowering agents—may also exist, and must be documented, along with reasons for the discrepancy. Although coronary revascularization procedures—angioplasty or bypass surgery—are being used more frequently in treating the elderly population, nursing research is needed to document postdischarge complications and long-term management of underlying CHD. Hospitalization for acute MI or revascularization may provide the only opportunity to maximize CHD management, as well as to link the individual to a cardiac rehabilitation program following discharge. Discovering the most effective ways to attain these outcomes requires further exploration.

Old age has consistently been associated with poorer long-term outcomes—death, recurrent MI, and CHF—following MI. Although acute MI-related prognostic factors are beginning to be identified (Chyun, 1998; Chung, Bosner, McKenzie, Shen, & Rich, 1995; Smith et al., 1990; Wong, Cupples, Ostfeld, Levy & Kannel, 1989), we still have insufficient information on postdischarge factors that may have contributed to these outcomes and to the use of healthcare services. Little is known about how patients manage their cardiac conditions and control specific cardiac risk factors, or whether they participate in cardiac rehabilitation. Additionally, it has not been determined what factors contribute to, or prevent, successful CHD management in the elderly. Psychosocial factors may contribute to long-term management of CHD and adverse outcomes, but data are not available on these possible influences. This information is crucial before beginning much-needed interventional studies aimed at decreasing the substantial mortality and morbidity rates associated with CHD and MI. Potential psychosocial factors that may contribute to poorer long-term outcomes in elderly individuals must be identified. Educational strategies directed specifically at the needs of the elderly and their caregivers also need to be identified and tested. In addition, factors specific to the elderly— such as functional status, which has been linked to mortality in the hospitalized elderly (Narain et al., 1988)—require further study in the elderly population with CHD.

Functional status has been shown to be an important prognostic factor in the elderly after MI (Mayer-Oakes, Oye, & Leake, 1991), even after adjustment for New York Heart Association class (Pernenkil et al., 1997). Yet it has not been widely studied, despite higher levels of functional disability in the elderly. Early functional limitations, or mild impairments that are not clinically evident, have been shown to predict subsequent functional dependence (Gill, Williams, Mendes de Leon, & Tinetti, 1997). Subjects at risk of functional decline may be identified early, prior to loss of function, so that interventions may be targeted. Physical performance and functional status may both influence a patient's participation in a cardiac rehabilitation program and the effectiveness of exercise rehabilitation.

Cardiac rehabilitation, including exercise rehabilitation, has been shown to improve exercise tolerance and to assist in the control of cardiac risk factors. However, few studies address these issues in the elderly (Ades & Grunvald, 1990; Lavie & Milani, 1995). Although physical activity is central to managing CHD in the elderly, the elderly, particularly women, are less frequently referred for physical therapy than are younger people and are enrolled less frequently even when they are referred (Ades, Waldmann, Polk, & Coflesky, 1992; Lavie & Milani, 1995). It is recommended that elderly men and women be strongly encouraged to participate in exercise-based cardiac rehabilitation, and special efforts should be made to overcome obstacles to entry and participation (U.S. Department of Health and Human Services [USDHHS], 1995). Even though exercise has been shown to improve functional status, anxiety, depression, mobility, healthcare resource consumption, and mortality (Lavie, Milanie, & Littman, 1993), 70% of older adults report having no regular exercise, and 60% report not having walked a mile in the past year (Kovar, Fitti, & Chyba, 1992; Wolinsky, Stump, & Clark, 1995). The reasons that individuals do not enroll in cardiac rehabilitation have not been well defined but probably relate to a combination of physical, psychosocial, and economic factors (Ades, Waldmann, McCann, & Weaver, 1992). Barriers to participation therefore must be explored, and strategies for improving access and maintaining participation must be tested.

Prevalence of CHF in the elderly increases with age; and following MI, old age has been shown to be related to the development of CHF despite normal systolic function (Pernenkil et al., 1997). Normal age-related changes in the elderly also appear to affect diastolic, rather than systolic, function (Lernfelt, Wikstrand, & Svanborg, 1991). CHF is associated with a lower quality of life and decreased functional capacity. Multidisciplinary teams focusing on coordination of inpatient, outpatient, and home care have demonstrated positive improvements in functional capacity, length of stay, readmission rates, self-care knowledge, patient satisfaction, and quality of life (Naylor et al., 1994; Rich et al., 1995; Venner & Solitro-Seelbinder, 1996), and prognostic factors for readmission have been identified (Vinson, Rich, Sperry, Shah, & McNamara, 1990), but CHF remains the leading cause of hospitalization in the elderly. Additional interventional studies are needed regarding the management of common problems in this population—monitoring for deterioration in clinical status, medication, dietary and fluid adjustment, social support, and noncompliance. Also awaiting further study are innovative strategies, such as the use of structured exercise programs, in CHF management (USDHHS, 1994).

DEBORAH CHYUN

See also:
ANGINA

DEPRESSION AND CARDIAC DISEASE
HYPERTENSION
OBESITY AS A CARDIOVASCULAR RISK FACTOR
PERIPHERAL VASCULAR DISEASE
SMOKING AS A CARDIOVASCULAR RISK FACTOR

CHRONIC GASTROINTESTINAL SYMPTOMS

Chronic gastrointestinal (GI) symptoms, including abdominal pain, bloating, constipation, dyspepsia, and diarrhea, affect approximately 8% to 22% of the U.S. population (Drossman et al., 1993; Longstreth & Wolde-Tsadik, 1993). Of those individuals who seek health care services for their symptoms, the majority are women of menstruating age (Drossman & Thompson, 1992). In many cases, the symptoms cannot be ascribed to a specific pathological or organic cause. The diagnosis of irritable bowel syndrome is applied to those individuals who experience abdominal pain and alterations in bowel function with no measurable pathology (Rome criteria). An outline of GI symptoms that characterize irritable bowel disease was developed by an international committee of experts who meet in Rome and has come to be known as the Rome criteria (Drossman et al., 1990). These criteria include (a) abdominal pain relieved by a bowel movement or associated with changes in stool consistency and (b) fewer or more frequent stools, harder or looser stools, straining, urgency, feeling of incomplete evacuation or passage of mucus, and bloating or feeling of abdominal distention (Talley, Phillips, Melton, Wiltgen, & Zinsmeister, 1989).

There are several etiological theories of irritable bowel syndrome. They include GI motility disorder, increased pain sensitivity, dietary factors such as intolerances (e.g., lactose) and low dietary fiber intake, autonomic nervous system imbalance, and psychiatric causes. The heterogeneity and chronicity of the problem, as well as the lack of a specific marker of irritable bowel syndrome, makes management particularly challenging. Nurses are frequently involved in the management of patients who experience GI problems, and thus empirical evidence is needed to determine etiological factors and mechanisms as well as interventions to alleviate symptom experiences and distress.

Research related to irritable bowel syndrome has been primarily conducted by medical researchers, in particular, gastroenterologists and psychiatrists and some basic scientists who have described GI motility patterns in symptomatic individuals. Researchers interested in symptoms and lifestyle factors have relied primarily on retrospective measures of symptom experiences as well as psychological state data. These studies have utilized patients recruited from tertiary care clinics who may represent one end of the continuum of patients with irritable bowel syndrome. In addition, although women predominate in studies of patients with irritable bowel syndrome, little or no attention is paid to menstrual cycle phase or menopausal status. Finally, there is limited study of ethnic variability in symptom experiences or health care seeking.

Recent nursing research utilizing both retrospective and prospective (daily diary) measures has focused on the relationships between chronic GI symptoms and the menstrual cycle (Heitkemper, Levy, Jarrett, & Bond, 1995), self-report of psychological distress (Jarrett et al., in press), self-report of stress (Levy, Jarrett, Cain, & Heitkemper, 1997) and physiological indicators of arousal (Heitkemper et al., 1996). In several of these studies, symptomatic women who sought health care for symptoms were compared with asymptomatic women as well as women with similar symptom levels who did not seek health care and thus did not have a formal diagnosis. These studies provided descriptive information about the fact that for some women GI symptoms are (a) closely linked with menstrual cycle phase (i.e., more symptoms in the late luteal phase compared to the follicular phase), (b) associated with higher self-report levels of psychological distress and stress, and (c) related to higher levels of urinary catecholamine and cortisol excretion.

Additional descriptive information collected in studies of both menstruating and midlife women indicate that dietary fiber is lower than the recommended daily intake in all groups of women. Preliminary data also suggest what has been found in the medical literature, that more women with irritable bowel syndrome report a history of or current experience with physical or sexual abuse, compared to nonsymptomatic women; however, additional work is needed.

Interventions for irritable bowel syndrome have included strategies to modify diet, produce relaxation, and pharmacologically manipulate motility or pain sensitivity. Intervention trials are plagued by the use of a heterogeneous sample, often including both diarrhea-prone and constipation-prone patients, the lack of a "gold standard" on which to measure improvement, reliance on retrospective symptom reporting for both sample selection and outcome measures, and a significant placebo effect in drug trials (Heitkemper et al., 1995). Well-designed clinical trials research examining multifaceted nonpharmacological therapies are needed to explore the benefits of dietary modification, relaxation techniques, education or reassurance on symptom experiences, health care seeking, and quality of life. It is unlikely that one therapy or therapeutic package will be beneficial for all patients. Therefore, studies must carefully describe symptoms as well as the biobehavioral characteristics of the samples prior to intervention. In this way, characteristics likely to be predictive of intervention success can be identified.

There are multiple opportunities for additional research in the area of chronic GI symptoms. More work is needed to understand the physiological basis, including motility and pain sensitivity, which may account for symptom occurrence. The interrelationships among other symptoms (e.g., insomnia, dysmenorrhea, and urinary incontinence) and irritable bowel syndrome should be clarified. Psychological factors such as psychiatric diagnoses, psychological distress, posttraumatic stress syndrome, and daily measures of stress must be further explored for their relationship to GI symptoms and bowel function. The natural course of functional GI symptoms is also poorly understood. For example, it is not certain whether children who experience chronic abdominal pain and constipation are more likely to manifest irritable bowel syndrome as adults. Finally, the outcomes of GI symptoms in terms of health care utilization, lost productivity, and impaired functional ability should be described in diverse samples of individuals.

MARGARET HEITKEMPER
MONICA E. JARRETT

See also:
   GASTROESOPHAGEAL REFLUX DISASE
   NUTRITION
   STRESS
   URINARY INCONTINENCE

CHRONIC ILLNESS

Chronic illness is a term used to denote clinical problems, particularly diseases of duration usually longer than 3 months that have frequent recurrences and that lack a cure (Clarke, 1994). Lubkin (1995), in a review of definitions of chronic illness, provided a definition that has a fit with nursing practice: "Chronic illness is the irreversible presence, accumulation, or latency of disease states or impairments that involve the total human environment for supportive care and self-care, maintenance of function, and prevention of further disability" (pp. 7–8). Nursing's focus on such chronic conditions as urinary incontinence constitutes an adjunct to these definitions and must be taken into consideration for completeness of chronic illness from nursing's perspective.

It is clear from these definitions that those who are chronically ill usually require long periods of care and observation to manage symptoms and the underlying pathology. A paradox of these conditions is that available therapies and strategies for control do not provide cure but are frequently vital for long-term survival. However, many patients have found adherence to some therapies and strategies difficult and stop using them, regardless of the potential danger of exacerbation of their illness. The complexity of factors involved in adherence to therapies probably is a multifactorial problem, involving physiological, behavioral, social, cultural, and economic factors that continue to require investigation.

Chronic illnesses can be placed in several groupings. For example, some chronic illnesses are life-threatening when there are treatments but no cures, and they require major life adjustments to maintain health, such as insulin-dependent diabetes mellitus (IDDM). Some are of uncertain origin and clinical pathway, may or may not be life-threatening, and there is no clear treatment, such as lupus and multiple sclerosis. Others have difficult clinical patterns and symptoms, usually affect functional ability but are not life-threatening, and treatment is symptomatic (e.g., osteoarthritis). Finally, some are not illnesses at all but chronic conditions that require clinical management; they occur frequently, have high health care costs, and are amenable to control (e.g., urinary incontinence).

Chronic illnesses also can be viewed from the perspectives of research foci. Considerable clinical nursing research has been carried out on aspects of chronic illness from the perspectives of prevention, adaptation, self-management, compliance and adherence, quality of life, function, symptom recognition and control/management, family involvement, cultural influences, and strategies for improved outcomes, such as patient education (Funk, Tornquist, Champagne, & Wiese, 1993; Gallo, Breitmayer, & Knafl, 1992; Lorig, Stewart, Ritter, et al., 1996; Roberson, 1992; University of California–San Francisco (UCSF) Symptom Management Faculty Group, 1992). Much of this work has been smaller-scale, limited-sample studies, but some represents strong programs of research (see Lorig, 1996).

There are a multiplicity of theoretical frameworks that can be used in chronic illness research. These come from a variety of nursing perspectives and are based in physiological, behavioral, social, cultural, and systems concepts. Corbin and Strauss (1991) proposed a chronic illness nursing management model based on a trajectory framework that several studies have used. Development and use of such models continue to be needed in nursing research.

Health care of chronically ill populations in the past has principally been managed from a disease-focused perspective, emphasizing acute care and control of exacerbations, and today it is managed from a more holistic, life-course, self-care, and community-based perspective. Chronicity of health problems leads people to seek nursing care for a variety of reasons; symptom control/management, assistance with coping, family adjustment, and educational needs are examples. One of the most important goals of care for those who have or are at risk for chronic illnesses is postponing the time of onset of chronic illness, symptoms, and associated disability and extending productive life. Self management and care are important goals of nursing practice and have been for some time (Connelly, 1987).

Chronic illness is an ongoing concern for health care providers and policymakers for a number of reasons; one is that increasing life expectancy presents the possibility of an associated increase in chronicity and disability, with an associated increase in health care costs. In the past, nursing research focused on chronic illness and chronicity as an important phenomenon in itself. Today nursing research is focusing increasingly on (a) specific conditions, such as cognitive impairment; (b) symptoms, such as pain; (c) adherence to specific disease treatments, such as blood glucose control for IDDM; and (d) intervention strategies, such as community-focused health care models. This change seems to be in response to new sources of research funding and other factors that are less clear. These new opportunities for research funding are important; however, developing conceptual coherence of the diverse aspects of chronicity is vital for increasing the scientific clarity of chronic illness research.

To strengthen chronic illness research, a cadre of nurse investigators continues to be needed, as there are a few nursing research centers but not many nurse scientists who are involved in this area. Examples of such centers are those at the University of Pittsburgh (chronic conditions), University of Michigan (cognitive impairment), University of California–San Francisco (symptom management), University of Pennsylvania (serious illness), and Stanford University (patient education). There are opportunities for substantial inquiry to be carried out in all aspects of chronic illness, particularly in the areas of primary and secondary prevention, assessment, symptom management, effectiveness of therapies and interventions, nursing-related outcomes, and costs.

It is also timely for nursing methodologies to include combined qualitative and quantitative designs, increased numbers of clinical trials, and inclusion of cost-effectiveness questions where feasible. Another aspect of scientific inquiry that it is timely for nursing research to continue to embrace is replication and substantiation. A hallmark of a scientific breakthrough is that a unique, cutting-edge finding can be replicated. It is this replication that leads to substantiation in which a clear scientific basis is developed for acceptance of the original results.

PATRICIA MORITZ

See also:
   ADHERENCE/COMPLIANCE
   ADVANCED DIRECTIVES
   DIABETES MELLITUS
   HYPERTENSION
   OSTEOARTHRITIS
   URINARY INCONTINENCE

DEPRESSION AND CARDIAC DISEASE

Studies using randomized experimental designs, large sample sizes, and advanced statistical analyses have documented a rate of approximately 15%–18% severe depression following a myocardial infarction (MI) (Ahern et al., 1990; Frasure-Smith, Lesperance, & Talajic, 1993). Depression is related to mortality, morbidity, and other psychosocial factors after an MI.

Relationship of Depression to Mortality

Severe depression is an independent predictor of mortality. Frasure-Smith et al. (1993) assessed 222 patients hospitalized post-MI, using the DSM-III-R psychiatric diagnosis of major depression (American Psychiatric Association, 1994). Sixteen percent of persons with an acute MI met the criteria for major depression. By 6 months, 17% of the 12 patients who later died were severely depressed.

In the Cardiac Arrhythmia Pilot Study of patients with significant ventricular arrhythmias (recorded 6–60 days after an MI), depression was a significant predictor of mortality or cardiac arrest within 1 year. The relationship of depression to mortality was significant even after controlling for history of prior MI, ejection fraction, beta-blocker or digitalis use, presence of transmural infarcts, and presence of runs of premature ventricular complexes on the 24-hour electrocardiogram at baseline (Ahern et al., 1990). The most frequent causes of death in severely depressed patients post-MI is reinfarction, arrthythmias, and congestive heart failure (Frasure-Smith et al., 1993). There has been a long-standing impression that symptoms of depression are common in patients with coronary artery disease.

Relationship of Other Psychosocial Factors to Depression

A history of major depression has been consistently reported as being established before the onset of the acute MI in 44%–56% of the cases who are depressed post-MI (Freedland, Carney, Lustman, Rich, & Jaffe, 1992). Other studies have found that nearly 66% of patients with MI have some psychosocial distress, other than depression, primarily anxiety. Although not completely studied, hypothetically, the psychosocial prognosis for severely depressed cardiac patients is poor, resulting in decreased quality of life, poorer social and physical functional status, perceived loss of energy, less likelihood to return to work, lack of initiative to perform optimal activities of daily living, and less likelihood for cardiovascular risk factor modification for health behaviors (Conn, Taylor, & Wiman, 1991). The mechanisms by which depression causes mortality and poorer clinical outcomes in cardiac patients is unknown; however, it may alter motivation for healthy behavioral modification (i.e., smoking cessation, exercise) and adherence to medication (Carney, Freedland, Rich, & Jaffe, 1995).

Biological Indices Related to Depression and Cardiac Disease

Plasma norepinephrine concentrations are increased in patients with severe depression (de Villiers et al., 1987). The evidence of increased norepinephrine concentrations suggests a potential mechanism for the effects of depression on mortality and ventricular arrhythmias in cardiac patients as an altered autonomic nervous system, resulting in increased sympathetic activity (Carney et al., 1995).

Heart rate variability, an index of the autonomic nervous system balance, can further describe altered autonomic function and mortality in cardiac patients. Kleiger et al. (1987) reported that low heart rate variability increased the risk of death by a factor of 5.3 in 850 persons followed for 31 months after an MI. Lombardi et al. (1987) reported increased sympathetic and decreased parasympathetic activity, as measured by heart rate variability, immediately after an MI. The heart rate variability "normalized" in most people within 6 months after the MI.

Sudden cardiac arrest survivors have low heart rate variability, specifically suggestive of a loss of parasympathetic activity (Cowan, Kogan, Burr, Hendershot, & Buchanan, 1991). Not many studies have investigated heart rate variability in cardiac patients with severe depression.

Cortisol is increased in 40%–60% of depressed patients. The hypothalamic-pituitary-adrenal (HPA) axis, along with the noradrenergic system, have been two of the most studied biological systems in relation to depression; both may coexist dysfunctionally in depressed patients (de Villiers et al., 1987). Arousal of the HPA axis, as manifested by increased cortisol secretion and resistance of plasma cortisol to suppression after dexamethasone administration, is common in major depressive disorders. Among depressed patients, norepinephrine measurements were significantly positively related to cortisol measurements in relation to dexamethasone administration (i.e., with the cortisol nonsuppressors).

Not many studies have reported on cortisol and norepinephrine levels in severely depressed cardiac patients. However, increased concentrations of cortisol have been found to occur within 72 hours of symptoms of acute MI. The magnitude of the cortisol response was positively correlated with infarct size as calculated by total creatinine kinase MB fraction enzyme release ($p < .0001$), and very high levels were predictive of mortality ($p < .05$) (Bain et al., 1992).

The serotonergic system has a role in the disturbed behaviors of depression, such as mood, sleep, sexual activity, and appetite (Meltzer, 1990). The brain concentration of serotonin (5-HT) is lowered in depressed subjects, and decreasing trytophan, the precursor of 5-HT, can induce severe depression in recovering depressed persons. Also, postmortem studies of suicide victims have indicated that brain 5-HT or its metabolite, 5-hydroxyindoleacetic acid (5-HIAA), is reduced. The most common measurement of serotonergic activity in depressed patients is the basal concentration of 5-HIAA in cerebrospinal fluid. Platelets have been used as a measurement of serotonergic mechanisms in severe depression because the processes of 5-HT uptake and binding sites in platelets are comparable to those in brain 5-HT sites (Meltzer, 1990). Plasma serotonin can potentially augment coronary vasospasm in coronary arteries with endothelial injury and/or augment intracoronary thrombosis contributing to an MI.

In summary, severe depression after acute MI is a predictor of mortality within 1 year. The most frequent causes of death are recurrent MIs, arrhythmias, and congestive heart failure. Severe depression is related to increased catecholamines, cortisol, and decreased serotonin.

MARIE J. COWAN

See also
CARDIOVASCULAR DISEASE
CORONARY ARTERY DISASE
DEPRESSION AMONG OLDER ADULTS
QUALITY OF LIFE

DIABETES MELLITUS

Diabetes mellitus is one of the most common chronic illnesses in the United States, with an estimated 16 million individuals who have diagnosed or undiagnosed diabetes, the majority having noninsulin-dependent diabetes (NIDDM). The total direct and indirect costs of diabetes are approximately $92 billion per year. Diabetes is responsible for about 400,000 deaths annually and was the seventh leading cause of death by disease in 1995. Diabetes is a leading cause of cardiovascular disease, stroke, hypertension, blindness, kidney disease, nerve disease, amputations, dental disease, and complications of pregnancy. Furthermore, these complications disproportionately affect minority populations for as yet unknown reasons. Several of the objectives of *Healthy People 2000* reflect the need to correct the substantial morbidity and mortality from this disease by vigorous case finding and management.

The recently released findings of the Diabetes Control and Complications Trial (DCCT) demonstrate the importance of nursing care for reducing the mortality and morbidity associated with diabetes (DCCT Research Group, 1993). The DCCT compared intensive with conventional diabetes therapy to determine the effects on the development and progression of early vascular and neurological complications of insulin-dependent diabetes (IDDM). In a cohort without retinopathy, the risk for developing retinopathy decreased 76% with intensive therapy, and in a secondary prevention cohort, the progression of retinopathy was slowed by 54%. Microalbuminuria was reduced by 39%, albuminuria by 54%, and clinical neuropathy by 60%. Although intensive therapy was associated with severe hypoglycemia and clinically significant weight gain, there were no differences between those in the intensive treatment group and those in the conventional group in mean total scores on a quality of life measure. On the basis of these findings, the researchers and the American Diabetes Association recommend *intensive treatment* for the care of patients with IDDM. Because nurses often are responsible for follow-up care of intensively treated patients, these recommendations point to the need for ongoing nursing research in diabetes care.

The majority (90%) of individuals with the NIDDM are obese; therefore, increases in rates of obesity and sedentary lifestyle will contribute to an increase in rates of NIDDM, as will the aging of the population and increased availability of screening to more groups. Increased age is associated with more obesity, and increased screening will find more latent cases. There has been a burgeoning of research in NIDDM, particularly in pharmacological treatment and exercise-diet interventions. Furthermore, because the relationship between poor glycemic control and diabetes complications appears to be the same for IDDM and NIDDM, the findings of the DCCT are being applied to management of NIDDM. The translation of these research findings to practice provides numerous opportunities for nursing research.

Traditionally, nursing has had a significant, key role in the multidisciplinary care and education of patients with diabetes. Management of diabetes requires that people with the disease significantly modify their lifestyle to adjust to a demanding treatment regimen. Long-term outcomes of avoiding or minimizing complications may be dependent on a complex series of interactions between biomedical and behavioral factors. Nursing research on the care of patients with diabetes has focused on four areas: descriptive studies dealing with *psychosocial adjustment* to diabetes; biobehavioral studies focusing on the relationship of various psychosocial parameters with metabolic control in diabetes; studies of the physiology of diabetes and its complications; and studies of diabetes care in the delivery of health care.

Studies of psychosocial adjustment to diabetes focus on either children and adolescents or adults. Dr. Margaret Grey's program of research examined the incidence of poorer adjustment in young children and the process of adjustment over time in children newly diagnosed with IDDM (Grey, Cameron, Lipman, & Thurber, 1995). Her work complements the work of other disciplines demonstrating that diabetes in childhood is associated with an increased risk of psychosocial difficulties. Similar work has been accomplished in adults, as summarized recently by Pollock (1993), who found in a number of studies that psychosocial functioning is associated with health-related hardiness and engagement in health promotion activities. Clearly, these problems are multifactoral and as such need a complex, multivariate approach.

Dr. Gail D'Eramo Melkus studied health care practices of African American women with NIDDM. The majority of studies examining these relationships used small samples obtained from one clinical site, examined simple bivariate relationships, and were not part of an overall theoretical approach to a program of research.

There are studies of the physiology of diabetes and its complications. Diabetes is a disease of relative or absolute lack of insulin secretion, which causes significant complications. Dr. Donna Hathaway at the University of Tennessee is the major nurse researcher whose program of research specifically deals with physiological aspects of diabetes care. She has been examining the relationship of quality of life to metabolic and physiological outcomes in patients with diabetes, and her work has focused on autonomic function and quality of life in adult kidney and pancreas-kidney transplant patients (Hathaway et al., 1993).

Finally, there are studies of diabetes care in health care delivery. Nurses have long been accepted as part of the diabetes care team, primarily as educators about diabetes. Dr. Sharon Brown conducted a number of meta-analyses of the diabetes education literature, concluding that patient teaching has positive outcomes in adults with diabetes. More recent work focused on the potential for interventions to affect knowledge as well as psychosocial adjustment and metabolic control (Brown & Hedges, 1994). Work on the impact of education on metabolic control in patients with NIDDM demonstrated that only minimal weight loss is necessary to improve metabolic control (D'Eramo-Melkus, Wylie-Rosett, & Hagan, 1992). Dr. Brown's most recent work on culturally sensitive management furthers the applicability of more general approaches to African American women with diabetes and the work of advanced practice nursing in caring for patients with diabetes. There have been few studies of the impact of other nursing interventions on patient outcomes specific to diabetes although there are several such studies currently in progress evaluating the impact of interventions such as coping skills training and culturally specific educational programs.

Some progress has been made in understanding these related and complex issues in the managements of patients with diabetes. A review of the chronic illness literature in pediatric nursing concluded that conceptually based interventions should be developed and appropriate outcomes measured. This conclusion is equally true of the literature on diabetes. The majority of the literature is descriptive and limited in scope to small clinical samples. Much research in diabetes is atheoretical, limiting the ability to develop theory and to apply findings across settings. There is much to be accomplished in studying diabetes care.

MARGARET GREY

See also:
> **ADHERENCE/COMPLIANCE**
> **CHRONIC ILLNESS**
> **OBESITY AS A CARDIOVASCULAR RISK FACTOR**

DIZZINESS

Dizziness is a common complaint of older adults, perplexing to them and their healthcare providers alike. The prevalence of dizziness has been reported at about one-third of the elderly, with a higher prevalence among women (Grimby & Rosenhall, 1995). The many presentations of the symptom, as well as multiple etiologies regarding it, make diagnosis and treatment difficult (Drachman, 1998; Isaacson & Rubin, 1999). Dizziness has been associated with falls, fear of falling, disability, and a decrease in quality of life (Boult, Murphy, Sloane, & Drone, 1991; Isaacson & Rubin, 1999; Kerber, Enrietto, Jacobson, & Baloh, 1998; Yardley, 1998). Despite these negative outcomes, complaints of dizziness are not always taken seriously and investigated thoroughly (Mendel, Lutzen, Bergenius, & Bjorvell, 1997). Research has contributed to our understanding of the phenomenon of dizziness, and to assisting individuals who suffer from it, but more nursing research is needed to find ways to prevent and manage this uncomfortable problem.

Descriptions of dizziness can range from a sensation of spinning or motion to lightheadedness, fainting or falling, or many variations and combinations of these. Balance—or the ability to maintain an upright position—results from visual, proprioceptive, and vestibular input to the brain and requires central integration and motor response. Dizziness results when there is a mismatch between the input and our position in space (Grimm, 1996). In addition, compromises in circulation, either local or through cardiovascular problems, can cause dizziness (Lawson, Fitzgerald, Birchall, Aldren, & Kenny, 1999). Aging can cause decreased efficiency of function in any or all of these balance mechanisms (Isaacson & Rubin, 1999), which may explain the increased incidence of dizziness with age. Because multiple disease processes can result in a feeling of dizziness, diagnosis and treatment are difficult, and even deciding which specialist to refer a patient to can be challenging.

Recent studies suggest appropriate methods for evaluating symptoms and making proper referrals, since most patients initially present their complaints to their primary physician. O'Mahoney and Foote (1998) assess a diagnostic algorithm for evaluating and diagnosing symptoms of dizziness, syncope, and falls in community-dwelling older adults. Lawson et al. (1999) explore diagnosis based on clinical characteristics of patients with symptoms of dizziness.

Most often, dizziness is related to vestibular and cardiovascular problems; Isaacson and Rubin (1999) report that over 80% of vestibular causes of dizziness can be determined. Benign positional vertigo (BPV) is related to movement and may be caused by displaced otoconal crystals in the inner ear. Acute labyrinthitis and Ménière's disease are also common peripheral vestibular causes. Vertebrobasolar insufficiency may interrupt blood flow to the vestibular system. Common cardiovascular causes of dizziness include orthostatic hypotension, arrhythmia, carotid sinus hypersensitivity, and vasovagal syncope. These are associated with lightheadedness or syncope more often than vertigo. Medication effects, anxiety, and neurological conditions should also be explored. Despite recent strides in diagnosing the causes of dizziness, the causes of approximately 22% of dizziness conditions still escape identification (Lawson et al., 1999).

Treatments for dizziness in elderly clients are based on the etiology of the symptom. Symptoms stemming from cardiovascular disorders are often resolved through medical management. Postural hypotension may necessitate ongoing safety measures to avoid dizziness, lightheadedness, or falls (Aaronson, Carlon-Wolf, & Schoener, 1991). Benign positional vertigo often responds to movement therapy designed to move the displaced otoconia, through a 360° rotation of the head (Lempert, Wolsey, Davies, Cresty, & Bronstein, 1997). Medication can lessen the symptoms of Ménière's disease. But despite medical strides, many continue to experience symptoms, which they must learn to live with.

A nurse-delivered educational program has been studied by Yardley and colleagues (Yardley, Beech, Zander, Evans, & Weinman, 1998). Patients with intractable dizziness were taught exercises designed to allow them to experience situations in which dizziness commonly occurs. This enabled them to learn to manage these situations; follow-up showed lessened anxiety, depression, and physical symptoms, and showed improvement in some balance testing. Further research is necessary to determine the best way to use the exercise program (Yardley & Beech, 1999).

The experience of dizziness has been documented by Mendel et al. (1997). According to Mendel, people feel vulnerable and insecure because of the unpredictable nature of dizziness, the possibility of experiencing exhaustion, nausea, or lack of balance. Dizziness impairs the ability to carry out normal activities and may cause people to depend on others for help. Because the problem cannot be seen, other people, such as healthcare providers, may misunderstand the symptoms and discount them. People may not be referred to specialists for diagnosis and treatment in a timely manner, and patients may have to work hard to convince healthcare professionals of the severity of the problem. Some of the coping techniques patients use to manage symptoms include distraction, denial, and relinquishing responsibility (Yardley et al., 1992). Appropriate assessment of the impact of dizziness on functional and psychological status is needed (Jacobson, 1998).

Dizziness has a negative impact on the quality of life for older adults. Grimby and Rosenhall (1995), in a representative survey of older adults in Sweden, found that those who experienced dizziness had more medical symptoms, such as unsteadiness, and falls, anxiety, memory problems, and depression. Others have found that an increase in falls (Kerber et al., 1998; Lawson et al., 1999), as well as a fear of falling, can lead to self-restriction of activity and resulting functional decline (Burker et al., 1995; Yardley, 1998).

Measures to explore the effects of dizziness have recently been developed. A vertigo symptoms scale was developed by Yardley, Masson, Verschuur, Haacke, and Luxon (1992) and used to examine the relationship between anxiety and vertigo. Questionnaires were completed by 127 patients at a specialty clinic. Factor analysis identified items for exploring symptoms of vertigo, anxiety, and somatization. The Inventory for Dizziness

(Hazlett, Tusa, & Waranch, 1995) measures symptoms, responses of significant others to the dizzy person, and activity levels. This instrument, an adaptation of a pain inventory, was administered to 184 patients presenting to a specialty dizziness clinic. Factor analysis was used for item selection and factor development, and support further investigation of the instrument.

The Dizziness Handicap Inventory (DHI5, Jacobson & Newman, 1990) was developed to explore the impact of dizziness on everyday life and includes 25 three-level items. Effects were grouped into three categories: functional, emotional and physical. The scale was applied to 63 patients who complained of dizziness, and findings indicated good test-retest reliability and homogeneity of the constructs. A short version was developed by Tesio, Alpini, Cesarani, and Perucca (1999) using item response methodology for item reduction. The original form was administered to 55 outpatients suffering from dizziness or imbalance. Rasch analysis was applied to remove items that did not fit, were redundant, or were off target, with a resulting 13-item, two-level form of the instrument. While not correlated with objective tests of dizziness, it is meant to provide information about the patient's perception of the severity of his/her symptoms.

Dizziness is receiving increased attention in the geriatric and nursing literature. The difficulties of diagnosis and treatment only increase the patient challenges in managing this uncomfortable symptom. Some measures have been developed to help understand the problem of dizziness and its impact, but further research is needed to fully explore the effects of dizziness, and to develop interventions to manage the symptoms. As new interventions become available, additional research will be needed regarding the best ways to disseminate this information to older adults who suffer from dizziness.

HELEN LACH

See also:
FALLS
MEDICATIONS IN THE ELDERLY
QUALITY OF LIFE

DYSPHAGIA

Dysphagia is characterized by an abnormality in transfer of a bolus from the mouth to the stomach (Groher, 1997). Dysphagia is a symptom with several causes: (a) myogenic—affecting smooth and striated muscles; (b) neurogenic—affecting the spinal, peripheral, or central nervous system;

(c) mechanical—related to an abnormality in the route from mouth to stomach; and (d) psychogenic (Amella, 1996). Because the symptom of dysphagia lies on a continuum from overt choking with occlusion of the airway to an occult problem that goes unrecognized, the nurse needs to make astute assessments while providing appropriate care.

The incidence of dysphagia varies by setting, diagnosis, and age of the patient with persons in nursing homes, those with multiple medical diagnoses, and those of advanced age being at higher risk (Fucile et al., 1998; Kayser-Jones & Pengilly, 1999; Langmore, Terpenning, & Schork, 1998). Estimates of dysphagia range from 16% of very old persons living in the community (Bloem et al., 1990), to 33% of persons with stroke (Smithard et al., 1997), to 44% of persons in nursing homes (Langmore et al., 1998). Although not a normal part of the aging process, loss of swallowing capacity has numerous negative consequences from aspiration to gradual weight loss resulting in increased mortality and morbidity (Fucile et al., 1998). For some individuals, dysphagia may be temporary and with aggressive rehabilitation may reverse, for example in the stroke victim (Logemann, 1995; Lugger, 1994; Smithard et al., 1997). However, for persons with progressive diseases such as dementia and Parkinson's disease, the goal of care is to maintain functional and safe swallowing for as long as possible.

Ethical Issues in Dysphagia

The ingestion of food and fluid is necessary to continue life. The assessment and treatment of dysphagia are not benign processes and range on a continuum from observational to intrusive (Evans, White, Wood, Hood, & Bailey, 1998; Kosta & Mitchell, 1998; Lambert & Gisel, 1996). For the older, frail person with multiple medical problems, functional decline, and/or cognitive impairment, the decision to thoroughly assess and treat dysphagia needs to be an interdisciplinary team decision based on projected goals, probable outcomes, and documented risks (Amella, 1999). At the end of the treatment continuum is the decision to use tube-feeding. This modality not only places the individual at high risk for aspiration, but it deprives him or her and caregivers the pleasure of eating in a culturally accepted way (Amella, 1998; Langmore et al., 1998). However, when compared to "comfort care" in persons with abnormal swallowing studies, the placement of a percutaneous endoscopic gastrostomy tube has been shown to lengthen life (Cowen, Simpson, & Vettese, 1997). Nurses also experience a range of beliefs concerning tube feedings and in a long-term-care setting, one qualitative study found the majority of experienced nurses preferred not to initiate tube-feeding in persons in the end stages of life (Wurzbach, 1996).

Predictors of Dysphagia

The prediction of dysphagia among older persons has recently seen a new category of individuals added to the "at risk" group. Kayser-Jones and Pengilly (1999) in a study of 82 nursing home residents who were described as "not eating well" by their caregivers, found that 55% had some degree of dysphagia with only 22% of that number referred by providers for further professional evaluation. Lack of recognition of dysphagia among those not eating well resulted in: (1) residents not being positioned properly; (2) residents being fed inappropriate food and liquids; (3) residents being fed too quickly; and (4) residents being labeled as uncooperative (p. 79).

While dysphagia has long been assumed to place an individual at risk for aspiration pneumonia with a consequent high rate of mortality, Langmore and colleagues (1998) found that the greatest predictor among outpatient, inpatient, and nursing home residents was dependence on another for feeding with odds ratio (OR) of 19.98. Tube-feeding (OR = 3.03), dependent for oral care (OR = 2.82), smoking (OR = 4.13), and number of medications (OR = 1.15) were the other most likely predictors of aspiration in this sample of 160 males who were followed for an average of 3.4 years.

In an attempt to determine prevalence of mealtime difficulties, 349 older nursing home residents had various attributes categorized into 14 domains (Steele, Greenwood, Ens, Robertson, & Seidman-Carlson, 1997). Of those screened, 87% had mealtime difficulties with 68% of those found to meet the criteria for dysphagia. Other indicators included poor oral intake (less that 75% of food offered was consumed), poor positioning, challenging behaviors, and eating problems such as drooling, spitting, and oral residue. This last category, eating problems, was most prevalent among persons with severe cognitive impairments. As such, nurses need to more carefully assess and, possibly refer for further dysphagia diagnostics, the individual who needs assistance with meals and is subjectively described as not eating well or having problems at meals.

Assessment of Dysphagia

The use of pulse oximetry to measure arterial oxygen saturation at mealtimes as an indirect measure of dysphagia was recently evaluated (Sherman, Nisenboum, Jesberger, Morrow, & Jesberger, 1999). By comparing results of Modified Barium Swallow exams with decrease in arterial oxygen saturation in 160 adult inpatients, a significant correlation was shown between persons who were aspirating and those who were desaturating, making pulse oximetry an excellent adjunct to the bedside swallow exam. The authors caution, however, that persons with high baseline saturation levels (95%–100%) did not demonstrate significant drops, although their oxygen partial pressure may have declined. Smithard and colleagues (1997) assert that swallowing capacity varies over time following recovery from an acute stroke and that longitudinal evaluation is necessary to determine problems. The instrumental swallowing exams (e.g., videoflurography and endoscopy) all require active participation on the part of the patient and therefore may not be appropriate for certain individuals (see Evans et al., 1998; Kosta & Mitchell, 1998; Lambert & Gisel, 1996, for full explanation of various tests). The nurse needs to advocate for those who may be needlessly put through the process and expense of an examination where results will not be meaningful (Amella, 1999).

Treatment

The SLP often generates a treatment plan for the person with dysphagia in concert with other members of the interdisciplinary team. Widely accepted techniques that facilitate meals for persons with dysphagia include: positioning upright with chin slightly tucked, good oral hygiene, nondistracting environment, food offered in small amounts with a delay between bites, altered food consistency, and assessing level of alertness before meals (Langmore & Miller, 1994). Miceli (1999) developed an interdisciplinary approach to care of the institutionalized individual with dysphagia based on severity of swallowing disorder, role of team members, strategies to promote independence, methods to change the environment, and monitoring of outcomes. Although no outcomes were reported, this program offers a practical institutional approach for staff training. O'Loughlin and Shanley (1998) developed a four-step training program that was taught to 15 registered nurses. At 3-month follow up, the nurses reported a significant improvement in assessment and management of swallowing problems. Because severity of dysphagia may change with time (Smithard et al., 1997), therapeutic treatments may also need to change. Of 212 persons who had received altered consistency diets (tube-feeding or puree) for dysphagia, 91% were found to be on diets that were below the recommended level for their needs when they were reevaluated after 30 days (Groher & McKaig, 1995). Therefore, nurses need to consider the possibility that persons on altered diets could be eating food of more appropriate and appealing textures, if they were reassessed. Appropriate referral and timely interventions may lead to a better quality of life for the person receiving "altered" food.

ELAINE J. AMELLA

See also:
APHASIA

ALZHEIMER'S DISEASE
CEREBROVASCULAR DISEASE
COGNITIVE DISORDERS
COGNITIVE IMPAIRMENT
NUTRITION

DYSPNEA

Definition

Dyspnea is the subjective sensation of difficult breathing. The origin of the word is the Greek *dys*, "abnormal or disordered," and *pnoia*, "breathing." Today it is a term used by clinicians to represent the subjective phenomena, with "shortness of breath" more often used to represent objective phenomena. The language used by patients regarding dyspnea has been factored into 19 descriptors (Simon et al., 1990), including such characteristics as "my breath does not go in all the way," "my breathing requires effort," "my chest feels tight," "I feel I am suffocating," "I feel that my breathing is rapid," and "I can't get enough air." Patients with a similar pathology are likely to use similar descriptors more often. For example, those with asthma tend to use the word *tight*. Healthy subjects also reliably report clusters of dyspnea descriptors.

Significance

Dyspnea is the most common reason for an emergency department visit by patients with asthma, chronic obstructive pulmonary disease (COPD), and heart failure. It also is associated with mortality and delayed weaning from mechanical ventilation. Some systems use dyspnea level as a criterion in determining disability. Millions of dollars are spent annually in symptom management and lost hours of work due to dyspnea.

The symptom of dyspnea may be acute, as in a tension pneumothorax; stimulus-related, as in exertional dyspnea; or chronic, as in emphysema. In acute states the symptom may be assistive in diagnosis. In episodic or chronic etiologies a common patient-initiated intervention is to decrease activity. Though the symptom severity may be reduced at first, the longer-range consequence may be deconditioning. Social interactions also may be reduced and depression increased. Quality of life is threatened as dyspnea frequency and intensity increase.

Mechanisms and Related Variables

Perceptual phenomena involve cerebral interpretation. The mechanisms and neural pathways that send messages to the brain for interpretation differ, however. Pain is a perceived phenomenon with specific pair receptors and a known neural pathway. Dyspnea lacks a common pathway but rather obtains messages from a number of peripheral and central receptors. Precise mechanisms for specific types of dyspnea continue to be investigated.

The brain stem is believed to be involved in some types of dyspnea, including but not limited to the chemoreceptor response to pH and CO_2. Oxygen level has very limited effect on dyspnea; many patients who are dyspneic have normal oxygenation levels, and those who are hypoxic generally have minimal improvement in dyspnea when normal oxygenation levels are reached. Oxygen cost has been moderately related to dyspnea but may have closer links to activity than to oxygen itself.

Ventilatory muscles, chest wall, lung, and airway receptors also have been identified as sources of information to make the interpretation of dyspnea. Stretch and irritation account for some stimuli. It has been proposed that a disproportional relationship between length and tension in the muscle spindle is also a stimulus. The theory has been expanded to involve a mismatch between outgoing motor signals to the respiratory muscles and incoming afferent signals.

Dyspnea is a multifactorial phenomena. Carrier, Janson-Bjerklie, and Jacobs (1984) developed a model to organize the variables related to dyspnea. The variables were grouped into personal, health status, situational, patient coping strategies and self-care behaviors, and therapeutic management strategies. Lung function values, work of breathing, fatigue, anxiety, and depression are often used covariates in dyspnea research.

Research

As with all subjective phenomena, the patient's report of the experience is considered valid. The similarity of dyspnea descriptors used by patients with similar pathologies supports the appropriateness of this assumption. The validity of many dyspnea measures today has been well established.

Reliability of dyspnea measures has been demonstrated by high correlations between the amount of resistive load added to the airway and the level of dyspnea intensity. Sensitivity was demonstrated when patients were able to discriminate between small changes in the resistive load added to the airway. Within-subject reliability regarding kinds of dyspnea remains to be examined.

Often the clinician is forced to rely on recall data regarding dyspnea. Because changing situational and personal variables can influence dyspnea over time, the question arises, how reliable is recall data? Meek and Lareau (1997) found that there was no statistical difference between actual and 2-week recall of average, greatest, and least dyspnea in males with severe COPD.

It has long been noted that patients with chronic dyspnea report lower levels of dyspnea than someone experiencing acutely the same level of physiological abnormality. It is proposed that developed coping strategies over the course of symptoms accounts for some of this difference. It is expected that we will better understand this difference as more is known about the mechanisms of dyspnea.

The cycle of dyspnea–inactivity–deconditioning–dyspnea also has been reported in numerous studies. Thompson (1990) showed that some patients could accurately predict how far they could walk before dyspnea would stop them, but some subjects underestimated their walking distance by as much as the distance of a football field during a 12-minute walk test. The fear of not being able to walk to the grocery or out to the mailbox because of predicted dyspnea can set up classic fear immobility. A major premise of pulmonary rehabilitation has been to break this inactivity cycle of dyspnea and to serve as a fear desensitization. Patients have reported reduced dyspnea and demonstrated greater walking distances and improved physical conditioning without direct improvements in pulmonary function after completing a pulmonary rehabilitation course.

A number of other effective coping strategies have been examined. Activity modification and energy conservation, symptom monitoring, relaxation techniques, education, and self-management of medication regimen have been effective. Positioning—sitting up, leaning forward, or resting their arms on their knees—decreases dyspnea for some. Abdominal breathing, paced breathing, or pursed-lip breathing are appropriate for some types of dyspnea.

Less nursing research has been conducted in the acute care setting. Gift, Moore, and Soeken (1992) examined the relationship of dyspnea, depression, and anxiety in asthma patients. Knebel, Janson-Bjerklie, Malley, Wilson, and Marini (1994) focused on dyspnea during weaning from mechanical ventilation. Thompson (1997) studied the pattern of dyspnea during tracheal suction of mechanically ventilated intensive care patients. The use of a fan blowing on the face of a patient with COPD has dramatic effects for some patients but not all—why? Many questions about dyspnea in the acute care population are yet to be examined. Within-subject comparison studies also are needed regarding dyspnea types and intensities and interventions for patients with acute exacerbations of chronic cardiopulmonary disease.

Future Directions

The search of mechanisms of dyspnea must continue in order to better understand this complex phenomenon. Much of the progress regarding dyspnea assessment and management can be attributed to the multidisciplinary community of scholars that meets annually and converses regularly. Such exchanges are vital to future advancement. Multidisciplinary as well as intradisciplinary efforts are encouraged in order to integrate the knowledge into practice decisions.

CAROL LYNN THOMPSON

See also:
CHRONIC ILLNESS
COPING
FATIGUE
PULMONARY CHANGES AGING
QUALITY OF LIFE
SMOKING AS A CARDIOVASCULAR RISK FACTORS

FAILURE TO THRIVE

Multiple, complex relationships between malnutrition, depression, dementia, and diminished functional status all contribute to the diagnosis of failure to thrive (FTT) in older adults. The Institute of Medicine described FTT late in life, or inanition, as a syndrome manifest by weight loss, decreased appetite, poor nutrition, and inactivity, often accompanied by dehydration, depressive symptoms, impaired immune function, and low cholesterol (Institute of Medicine, 1991).

An analysis of FTT by nurse researchers demonstrates the derivation of the concept from the analogous syndrome in children. Through concept derivation (Walker & Avant, 1983), a systematic evaluation of the differences and similarities between geriatrics and pediatric FTT was conducted. Characteristics frequently associated with FTT in both infants and older adults include alteration in body weight, delayed or impaired physical and cognitive function, and depression (Braun, Wykle, & Cowling, 1988). Newbern and Krowchuk (1994) completed a conceptual analysis of FTT in the elderly, drawing on the wider concept as applied to infants and young children.

In developing a diagnostic model for FTT, Groom (1993) also synthesized the geriatric literature with the infant model. The redefinition and alteration of terms from the infant model of FTT results in three categories of FTT in the elderly: (a) psychosocial, (b) predisposing, and (c) physical.

As the diagnosis of FTT is used with increased frequency, research has been conducted to determine the differential criteria used to make the diagnosis. An investigation into how physicians apply the term FTT in older adults was conducted by Hildebrand, Joos, and Lee (1997). The objective of this study was to describe the clinical presentation, underlying etiologies, diagnostic and therapeutic interventions, and discharge outcomes of veterans having the discharge diagnosis of FTT. Participants of this study included all veterans 65 and over whose coded discharge diagnoses included FTT (N = 132). A retrospective chart review was completed for a 3-year period. The results of the study revealed that 67% of the participants demonstrated weight loss; anemia was present in 55%; low cholesterol in 50%; and low albumin in 44%. Lymphopenia was seen in more than half of the participants (66%). Most patients were admitted from home (83%), and 36% were cognitively impaired. Only 46% of the subjects were discharged home, while 34% went to nursing homes. Fourteen percent of the participants died before they were discharged, 11% died within 30 days after discharge, and 11% died within 1 year after discharge. Hildebrand et al. concluded that FTT may constitute a discrete syndrome with diagnostic, therapeutic, and prognostic implications in older people. But in the absence of consensus about diagnostic criteria, there is great deal of subjective variation in how physicians apply the term.

Additional research related to how the diagnosis of FTT was applied to the geriatric population in the acute-care setting revealed a lack of specificity in the diagnosis and treatment. Common complaints of patients in this study included activity of daily living (ADL) changes, weight loss, and anorexia (Osato, Takano, Phillips, & Winne, 1993).

FTT presents a challenge to all nurses caring for older adults. Further research to better define the concept, and to create practice protocol for evidence-based care, is necessary. Creative interventions focusing on issues such as feeding strategies, which includes the offering of comfort foods and happy hours (Wood & Vogen, 1998), are essential. Nursing must continue to examine the complex relationships between malnutrition, depression, and functional decline in patients with FTT.

ELLEN FLAHERTY

See also:
CHRONIC ILLNESS
DEPRESSION AMONG OLDER ADULTS
NUTRITION
TERMINAL ILLNESS

GASTROESOPHAGEAL REFLUX DISEASE

Gastroesophageal reflux disease (GERD) is a spectrum of diseases. Symptoms of GERD include dyspepsia, heartburn, and regurgitation. Causes include gastric acid hypersecretion, impaired gastric motility, weakened pressure of the lower esophageal sphincter (LES), ineffective esophageal peristalsis, and loss of the integrity of the esophageal mucosa.

GERD is a common esophageal disorder among older adults and results in a lowered quality of life (Sallout, Mayoral, & Benjamin, 1999; Szarka & Locke (1999). Quality-of-life issues stem from esophageal complaints and other symptoms presented in the primary-care setting, including aspiration pneumonia, asthma, chest pain, chronic cough, halitosis, and hoarseness. Frequently new-onset asthma in older adults is associated with GERD (Mujic & Rao, 1999). Although it may occur without adverse consequences in the majority of cases (Kelley, 1997), GERD results in an overwhelming use of antacids, which often negate the effects of medications used to manage chronic diseases common to older adults (Meiner, 1997).

In untreated chronic cases, refluxed gastric juices may cause ulceration or erosion of the lower esophagus and can lead to changes in the cellular structure. This metaplasia is known as Barrett's esophagus and is a strong risk factor for adenocarcinoma. The successful treatment of GERD is essential to prevent Barrett's esophagus and the associated cancer risk (Shahin & Murray, 1999).

When lifestyle changes are not implemented, research findings have indicated limited effectiveness of other interventions used to manage GERD. Lifestyle changes are the cornerstone for effective reflux treatment, even with pharmacological interventions (Kelley, 1997; Spechler, 1992). Nursing research is needed to identify behavior modifications that are more likely to be sustained over time. Future nursing studies that may produce long-term lifestyle changes will need to include the following elements that are known to reduce GERD:

- Dietary modifications designed to avoid foods and fluids that lower LES pressure (e.g., tomatoes, peppermint, licorice, alcohol, and caffeine-containing foods and drinks such as coffee, tea, chocolate, and colas).
- Weight loss, when obesity is a factor.
- Elevating the head of the bed 4 to 6 inches with blocks (raising the entire angle of the bed).
- Eliminating all food and fluids for the 2 hours before bedtime.
- Smoking cessation.

Clinical manifestations of GERD are identified during the physical assessment in about 50% of patients with noncardiac chest pain; in about 75% of patients complaining of chronic hoarseness; and in 70%–80% of asthmatic patients (P. O. Katz, 1998; Scott & Gelhot, 1999). According to Claussen (1999), esophageal symptoms that do not respond to medications (e.g., omeprazole, 40 mg/day) call for prompt investigation. When heartburn is assumed to be GI-related, the potential for misidentification of GERD may lead to a delay in receiving treatment for angina pectoris or a myocardial infarction. When heartburn is assumed to be cardiac-related, the patient may limit all activities, thinking that the heartburn signals an imminent heart attack. Thus, additional research regarding symptom identification is needed to more rapidly differentiate GERD from other illnesses.

The effects of changing body position 1, 2, or more hours after eating also requires further study. When Koerselman et al. (1999) studied the use of oral anticholinergic drugs for GERD in upright and supine positions, findings indicated that the drugs' effectiveness depended on body position and whether the patient had fasted or eaten. The researchers recommended additional studies with medications and body position over time. This type of research is ideal for advanced-practice nurses in clinical and/or teaching institutions.

Studies have been done to observe the effect of low- and high-fat meals on LES motility and on GERD in healthy people (Pehl et al., 1999; Sifrim, Janssens, & Vantrappen, 1996). These studies found that ingestion of a low-fat meal (as opposed to a high-fat meal) did not affect the stimulation of GERD. However, the volume of the meal did make a difference. Nursing investigations directed toward the type and amount of food ingestion and GERD symptom management may provide material that can be disseminated to both clinicians and the general population.

GERD is a chronic problem among older adults. Few well-controlled trials have directly evaluated the overall efficacy of conservative treatment for patients with GERD. Nursing research may be undertaken to study ways of improving patients' willingness to make long-term lifestyle and dietary modifications. Studies that investigate symptomatic control may provide the foundation for improvement in the quality of life of older adults with GERD.

Advanced-practice nurses are currently able to effectively assess and manage 85%–90% of older adults with GERD. Only 10%–15% of patients with GERD need to be referred to a physician for invasive diagnostic procedures. This is necessary in refractory cases, or if surgery is being considered.

Transient LES relaxation is considered the most common cause of GERD. Drugs and foods that increase inappropriate LES relaxation must be identified. If medications that have a less relaxing effect on the LES are available, older adults with GERD should be encouraged to use them. Over-the-counter (OTC) drugs must be included in all medication histories and in the consideration of drug interactions. How many OTC drugs a patient uses, and how often, must be determined by a full medication review before considering medication adjustments. Several 1-day food diaries over a 2-week period, or at least one 3-day food diary, can usually produce a food history that can be used to detect foods that may relax the LES. This information can be obtained in a descriptive research study that could have widespread importance in the identification of drug-food and drug-drug interactions.

SUE E. MEINER

See also:
CHRONIC GASTROINTESTINAL SYMPTOMS

HIP FRACTURE

Fracturing a hip can be one of the most costly—and potentially deadly—events that an older person may experience. Due to the increasing number of people over the age of 65, it is estimated that total annual costs related to hip fracture in the United States will reach at least $31 billion by the year 2020 (Mossey, Knott, & Craik, 1990). Also, repair of hip fracture is becoming the most common surgical procedure for people over the age of 85, which attests to the increased incidence of hip fracture in higher age groups (Farmer, White, Brody, & Bailey, 1984; Kauffmann, Albright, & Wagner, 1987; Kenzora, McCarthy, Lowell, & Sledge, 1984; Levi, 1997). Many hip-fracture victims are frail, and have other chronic illnesses, such as dementia, that impede recovery.

Because advances in surgery now allow for early (if not immediate) ambulation, it should follow that recovery rates also improve. This is not the case. Mortality rates in the elderly population that experience hip fractures have held constant for the past three decades—about 20%–23% (Fitzgerald & Dittus, 1990; Fitzgerald, Moore, & Dittus, 1988; Kane et al., 1998; Kramer et al., 1997; Magaziner, Simonsick, Kashner, Hebel, & Kenzora, 1989; A. Myers et al., 1991). Many clients—reportedly as much as 50%—never regain their prefracture level of functional independence (Ceder et al., 1979; Hoenig, Sloane, & Kahn, 1998; Levi, 1997; Svennson, Stromberg, Ohlen, & Lindgren, 1996; Walheim, Barrios, Stark, Brostrom, & Olsson, 1990; Yarnold, 1999). It has become apparent that factors other than the actual physical recovery from the fracture itself (and subsequent surgery) have a profound effect on outcomes. This complex and devastating event constitutes a challenge for nurses. That is, how can we best facilitate better outcomes following hip fracture in people over the age of 65?

In the last three decades, studies of hip fracture clients have focused on the identification of factors that influence recovery or level of function measured by graded levels of activities of daily living (Katz, Ford, Heiple, & Newell, 1964). Based upon more recent research, this narrow definition of recovery has resulted in the identification of a number of other factors that affect recovery. These include demographic factors, general health status, type of fracture and surgical repair, psychosocial factors, confusion, depression, functional status, and environmental factors. This more comprehensive view has led to the framing of recovery in the context of a broad range of patient outcomes. It seems that it is the combination of several factors that is significant—rather than any one alone—when predicting hip-fracture outcomes.

When the data are adjusted for age and comorbidity, the type of fracture (and the type of repair) do not significantly affect in-hospital mortality or functional ability at 1-year postinjury (Dahl, 1980; Kramer, 1997; Levi, 1997; Svennson et al., 1996; Zuckerman, Fabian, Aharanoff, Kovel, & Frankel, 1993). Levels of recovery in Activities of Daily Living (ADL) and in walking ability are similar, regardless of the site of the fracture or the method of repair (Borquist, Ceder, & Thorngren, 1990; Ceder, Thorngren, & Wallden, 1980; Jette, Harris, Cleary, & Campion, 1987; Svennson et al., 1996; Walheim et al., 1990; Zuckerman et al., 1993).

The influence of general health status on recovery has been examined in terms of comorbidities, the number and type of which have been found to influence outcomes following hip fracture (Ogilvie-Harris, Botsford, & Worden Hawker, 1993; Svennson et al., 1996; Zuckerman et al., 1993). According to these researchers, the trauma caused by a hip fracture in an elderly person may affect the physiologic mechanisms that would normally compensate for changes among organ systems. These studies also demonstrate that older clients may need more intensive rehabilitation to hasten their recovery, and/or continuation of rehabilitation for longer periods of time in order to regain functional homeostasis.

Among the demographic factors studied, age is the most significant prognostic indicator for recovery in most studies; greater age correlates with poorer chances for recovery (Barnes, 1984; Ceder et al., 1980; Jette et al., 1987; Miller, C. W., 1978; Mossey, Mutran, Knott, & Craik, 1989; Svennson et al., 1996). However, Kauffman et al. (1987) reported outstanding rehabilitation outcomes in a study of 18 hip-fracture clients over the age of 90. They attributed their excellent survival rates (16/18) to early ambulation and to allowing for a longer recovery period. Mortality rates following hip fracture are greater in men than in women (Dahl, 1980; Levi, 1997; Yarnold, 1999), but Ceder et al. (1980) found no difference between sexes. To date, no studies have included ethnicity as a factor in determining outcomes for clients with hip fracture, although two studies have shown that African Americans are at a lower risk for hip fracture than are Caucasians (Farmer et al., 1984; Kelsey & Hoffman, 1987).

Psychosocial factors include emotional status, social functioning, living arrangements, and the ability to manage household responsibilities, such as those classified as Instrumental Activities of Daily Living (IADL). Depression among hip-fracture clients tends to increase the time required for rehabilitation (Berkman et al., 1986; Mossey et al., 1990; Stromberg, 1998). Other factors that are emerging as significant predictors of positive outcomes include the (prefracture) ability to visit friends or go shopping, to depend on others for support, to not be forced to live alone, to manage IADLs, and to maintain a positive emotional status (Ceder et al., 1980; Cobey et al., 1976; Levi, 1997; Stromberg, 1998). The ability to return home following hospitalization has also been associated with better recovery rates (Broos, Stappaerts, Lviten, & Gruwez, 1988; Ceder et al., 1980; Kauffman et al., 1987; Mossey et al., 1989; Naylor et al., 1999).

The use of Advanced Practice Nurses (APN) to improve the quality of care of a variety of clients has been reported (Aiken, 1990; Aiken et al., 1993; Brooten et al., 1986; Brooten et al., 1988; Brooten & Naylor, 1994; Burgess et al., 1987; Burl, Bonner, Rao, & Kahn, 1998; Kane et al., 1988, 1989c, 1991; Naylor, 1990; Naylor et al., 1994, 1999; Neidlinger, Scroggins, & Kennedy, 1987; Office of Technology Assessment [OTA], 1986; Safriet, 1992). These studies focused on outcomes of care provided after hospitalization, and included such outcomes as earlier hospital discharge, reduced rates of rehospitalization, and decreased posthospitalization complications. A recently completed study at the University of Minnesota, funded by the National Institute of Nursing Research (R01NRO-3490-01), demonstrated that improved outcomes were related to three commonly seen clinical problems in elderly nursing home residents when care was planned and coordinated by GAPNs (Ryden et al., 1999).

Research has demonstrated that the problems faced by older persons with hip fracture are complex and multifaceted. Their ability to recover is affected by many things besides rapid discharge from the hospital. There is persuasive evidence that GAPNs are the best solution to these problems. Because the scope of advanced practice nursing allows for caring beyond the boundaries of institutions, there is the potential for GAPNs to provide the missing link between care settings, and for them to fill the gaps experienced by clients and families. Some of these gaps have to do with a lack of information, and others have to do with the sense of being without resources once a patient is discharged. Based on their knowledge and expertise, GAPNs are able to design and implement a comprehensive plan of care that can address issues faced by individual clients and their families during the long process of recovery from hip fracture. The role of GAPNs is to improve outcomes for these older clients, and therefore to improve the quality of care that they receive.

KATHLEEN KRICHBAUM

See also:
ACTIVITIES OF DAILY LIVING
FALLS
FUNCTIONAL HEALTH
GERONTOLOGICAL NURSING: ADVANCED PRACTICE
MOBILITY

HYPERTENSION

Definition

Hypertension is the term applied to sustained and elevated levels of systolic and/or diastolic blood pressure. The exact level at which hypertension poses a health risk has been arbitrarily and continually redefined; however, the importance of hypertension is based on a rational association between sustained, elevated levels of arterial pressure and the probability of increased risk for morbidity and mortality from cardiovascular disease. The Joint National Committee on Detection, Evaluation and Treatment of High Blood Pressure (1993) defined hypertension as systolic blood pressure ≥140 mm Hg and/or diastolic blood pressure ≥90 mm Hg or taking antihypertensive medication. The committee reclassified hypertension into four stages and introduced the high normal category for use in medical diagnosis, evaluation, and treatment (see Table 1).

Sustained and elevated systolic blood pressure is now considered as crucial a measure as the diastolic level in evaluating the risks for cardiovascular disease. Elevated systolic blood pressure accompanied by normal diastolic levels, known as isolated systolic hypertension, is common in older populations. Primary hypertension, formerly known as essential hypertension, occurs in as many as 95% of all individuals with high blood pressure, as opposed to secondary hypertension, which is due to an identifiable and usually treatable cause (Kaplan, 1994).

Prevalence in the United States

Hypertension affects approximately 43 million Americans, almost one fourth of the U.S. adult population. In the 1988–91 National Health and

TABLE 1 Classification of Blood Pressure for Adults Age 18 Years and Older[a]

Category	Systolic (mm Hg)	Diastolic (mm Hg)
Normal[b]	<130	<85
High Normal	130–139	85–89
Hypertension[c]		
Stage 1 (mild)	140–159	90–99
Stage 2 (moderate)	160–179	100–109
Stage 3 (severe)	180–209	110–119
Stage 4 (very severe)	≥210	≥120

[a]Not taking antihypertensive drugs and not acutely ill. When systolic and diastolic pressures fall into different categories, the higher category should be selected to classify the individual's blood pressure status. For instance, 160/92 mm Hg should be classified as stage 2, and 180/ 120 mm Hg should be classified as stage 4. Isolated systolic hypertension (ISH) is defined as SBP ≥140 mm Hg and DBP <90 mm Hg and staged appropriately (e.g., 170/85 mm Hg is defined as stage 2 ISH).

[b]Optimal blood pressure with respect to cardiovascular risk is SBP <120 mm Hg and DBP <80 mm Hg. However, unusually low readings should be evaluated for clinical significance.

[c]Based on the average of two or more readings taken at each of two or more visits following an initial screening.

Note. In addition to classifying stages of hypertension based on average blood pressure levels, the clinician should specify presence or absence of target-organ disease and additional risk factors. For example, a patient with diabetes and a blood pressure of 142/94 mm Hg plus left ventricular hypertrophy should be classified as "stage 1 hypertension with target-organ disease (left ventricular hypertrophy) and with another major risk factor (diabetes)." This specificity is important for risk classification and management.

Nutrition Examination Survey (NHANES III), 32.4% of non-Hispanic Blacks, 23.3% of non-Hispanic Whites, and 22.6% of Mexican Americans had hypertension (Burt et al., 1995). Two thirds of hypertensive individuals were aware of their condition, and 53% reported being on drug therapy. In Mexican Americans, 35% of the hypertensive individuals were under treatment, but only 14% had controlled blood pressures; compared to 25% and 24% of the non-Hispanic Black and White populations, respectively, with controlled blood pressures. Given equal access to therapy, Black Americans, who are among the most affected population group, achieve similar blood pressure reductions. Almost 13 million people with normal blood pressures reported being told they were hypertensive on one or more occasions, and just over 50% of the 13 million reported self-compliance with lifestyle changes to maintain hypertension control.

Hypertension increases with age, is more common in Blacks, and is more prevalent among lower socioeconomic populations. Hypertension has a higher incidence in men throughout young adulthood to middle age. Thereafter, the incidence in women rises above that of men. The highest rates among women are found in non-Hispanic Black women and among men in non-Hispanic Black men. Among those with more severely elevated hypertension (DBP ≥115 mm Hg), Black men had four times higher incidence of complications than White men.

Detection and Measurement

Hypertension is not diagnosed by a single elevated reading but must be confirmed by multiple elevated blood pressure readings on several occasions. Standardized technique is strongly recommended to assure accurate and valid measurement (American Heart Association, 1993). Blood pressure is measured after 5 minutes of rest and without recent ingestion of alcohol, caffeine, or tobacco smoke, which can cause elevated readings. The blood pressure cuff must be the appropriate size for the patient and encircle the bare upper arm at heart level. The patient should be positioned with legs uncrossed, back supported, and feet resting flat on the floor. Systolic and diastolic readings should be measured by an accurately calibrated manometer. It is crucial that efforts be made to eliminate measurement errors, which result from observer bias, digit preference, and prior knowledge of patient blood pressure levels. At least two readings with a minimum of 2 minutes between measurements should be averaged.

Associated Factors

Hypertension seldom exists in isolation but most often occurs with other risk factors that potentiate the probability for cardiovascular disease. Factors commonly associated with hypertension that are nonmodifiable include low birthweight, older age, family history of high blood pressure, and history of diabetes mellitus, coronary heart disease, stroke, or end-stage renal disease. Modifiable confounders include smoking, alcohol consumption, high saturated dietary fats, excess dietary sodium, adiposity, and a sedentary lifestyle, as well as recreational and over-the-counter drugs. In addition, psychosocial and environmental factors create life stressors that may influence hypertension as well as care and management. Target-organ disease as a consequence of sustained, uncontrolled elevated blood pressure includes arteriosclerosis, heart failure, transient ischemic attacks (TIA), stroke, peripheral vascular disease, aneurysm, and end-stage renal disease.

Treatment

The ultimate goal for treatment is to prevent morbidity and mortality by the least intrusive means. The treatment regimen is determined by evaluating the severity of the blood pressure elevation, the presence of target-organ disease, and the effects of other coexisting risk factors. The inability to adhere to treatment recommendations is a major barrier in attaining and maintaining goal blood pressure levels in long-term management, evidencing the need for planned patient education programs. Traditional treatment strategies targeted to the general population lack cultural sensitivity, neglect active involvement of the patient in decision making, and fail to motivate and keep the patient in care. More individually oriented treatment methodologies that address the patients' concerns, including their social support system, employment status, health insurance, and barriers in daily life to meeting compliance goals, are required. Nursing can provide the training, education, and support to design planned health programs to increase the efficacy of interventions and improve overall compliance.

Lifestyle modification, formerly termed nonpharmacological therapy, includes interventions targeted toward healthier lifestyles and reducing the risks for cardiovascular complications at the family, community, and population levels. Lifestyle modifications for blood pressure control include reduction in weight, increased physical exercise, and dietary decreases in sodium, saturated fats, and alcohol consumption. Smoking, although not directly related to hypertension, is a major cardiovascular risk and should be avoided.

Pharmacological intervention is indicated in stages 1 and 2 hypertension only when blood pressure levels remain elevated for longer than 6 months despite lifestyle modifications (Joint National Committee, 1993). In stages 3 and 4 hypertension, it may be necessary to add a second or third agent if blood pressure levels remain uncontrolled. Hypertension management should include the simplest well-tolerated regimen and plans to gradually reduce dosages or the number of agents prescribed while vigorously incorporating lifestyle modifications into the treatment regimen.

The first preferred line of drugs used in initial therapy includes diuretics and beta blockers, followed by calcium antagonists, angiotensin converting enzyme (ACE) inhibitors, and alpha-1 receptor blockers. Factors such as side effects, effects of therapies on concomitant disease, and cost of therapy must be considered in selection of pharmacological treatment. As much as 80% of the total cost for hypertension treatment can be attributed to drug therapy. Newer classes of drugs are more costly than traditional and older pharmaceutical agents. Despite the costs involved, the reduction of blood pressure by using pharmacological treatment reduces the incidence of cardiovascular events and hospitalization.

Primary Prevention

Nonpharmacological therapy for treatment of hypertension is an evolving strategy in line with the objectives of Healthy People 2000 (U.S. Department of Health and Human Services, 1990). It represents a prevention area ideally suited for nursing practice and research. Public health prevention strategies focusing on lifestyle modification at the community and practice setting will help achieve an overall downward shift in the distribution of blood pressure levels in the general population. Interventions should target high dietary sodium, fats, alcohol, and low intake of potassium, as well as physical inactivity. Although these intervention strategies show promise in prevention of high blood pressure, societal barriers, such as the lack of satisfactory food substitutes, lack of access to care, and absence of economic resources, constrain compliance and achievement of intervention goals.

Gaps in Knowledge and Practice

Hypertension is a major independent risk factor for coronary artery disease and stroke, the first and third causes of mortality in the United States, yet its importance is not emphasized satisfactorily in research and practice. The individuals hardest to reach and at the highest risk are often not in care or are uninsured. Medical and behavioral intervention approaches lack cohesiveness and cultural relevance, therefore failing to achieve the strength of their impact as a combined intervention. Additional research is required to evaluate multidisciplinary strategies with a team approach to increase entry into care, remaining in care, and long-term compliance with prevention and treatment recommendations. Research also is needed to increase understanding of cost-benefit of interventions and the effects of self-monitoring and titration, including pharmacological vacations.

Nursing Practice and Research

Nurses can play leading roles in achieving improved health outcomes through lowering the rate and severity of hypertension and encouraging primary prevention. Nurses in all settings can provide case finding, referral, tracking and follow-up, and education and monitoring of patients with hypertension (Hill & Becker, 1995). Further important nursing interventions include developing more tailored patient-centered strategies to promote adherence by encouraging patient skill building and self-monitoring and using community outreach workers (Hill & Becker, 1995). Home visits and telephone contact strengthen understanding of the patient's environment and surrounding community, providing more insight into social, cultural, and psychosocial issues, including poverty, alcoholism, and substance abuse. Nursing research offers unlimited opportunities to improve hypertension prevention and care. Testing multidisciplinary approaches to patient-centered care allows for resource sharing, team building, and community partnerships to strengthen the supportive network among hospitals, local clinics, health agencies, and community providers. Finally, new discoveries in genetics and pharmacology promise exciting developments in the prevention of hypertension and cardiovascular disease.

MARTHA N. HILL
SUSAN DALE TANNENBAUM

See also:
ANGINA
CARDIOVASCULAR DISEASE
CEREBROVASCULAR DISORDERS
DIABETES MELLITUS
OBESITY AS A CARDIOVASCULAR RISK FACTOR

OBESITY AS CARDIOVASCULAR RISK FACTOR

Definition and Prevalence

For decades, cardiovascular disease (CVD) has been the leading cause of mortality and premature morbidity among midlife and older men and women, with obesity as the primary risk factor. Characterized by the storage of excess fat, obesity is defined as 20% or more over desirable weight, based on the midpoint of the range of weights for a medium frame from the 1983 Metropolitan Life Insurance height and weight tables. The body mass index (BMI) normalizes body weight for height so that relative degrees of obesity can be evaluated among individuals; it correlates highly with weight and is nearly independent of height. A BMI (weight in kilograms / height in meters)^2 of 27 or higher also defines obesity.

Based on four separate national surveys conducted since 1960 (National Health and Nutrition Examination Surveys), the prevalence of overweight in America increased 9%, from 24.3% in the 1960–1962 survey to 33.3% in the 1988–1991 survey. This occurred despite accelerated national emphasis on and awareness of healthy nutrition, as well as a marked increase in the availability of low-fat foods. Using the World Health Organization Expert

Commission obesity cutpoint as a BMI of 25, the National Center for Health Statistics estimated that the prevalence of obesity in America has soared to over 50%.

Empirical Evidence

Although there is little short-term relationship between obesity and morbidity or mortality, the long-term relationship is strong for both men and women. The Framingham Study included more than 5,000 men and women living in Framingham, Massachusetts, who were initially examined between 1948 and 1950 and reexamined at 2-year intervals thereafter. Even controlling for age, cholesterol level, systolic blood pressure, cigarette smoking, left ventricular hypertrophy, and glucose tolerance, higher BMI was significantly associated with the development of coronary heart disease (CHD) in these men and women, and in women it also was associated with an elevated risk of stroke. Moreover, weight gain was associated with increased blood pressure and increased serum levels of cholesterol and glucose. Weight gain after the young adult years increased the risk of CVD in both sexes. Data from the Nurses' Health study, established in 1976 with 121,770 female registered nurses and continuing to the present, corroborate and extend these findings (Manson et al., 1990). After adjusting for age and smoking, the risk of both nonfatal myocardial infarction and fatal coronary disease among women in the heaviest BMI category ($\geq$ 29) was more than three times higher than that in women with a BMI of 21 or less. Moreover, cardiac disease in women with a weight gain of more than 20 kg in the preceding 4 years was twice as high as in women whose weight was stable.

Even more important than adiposity per se is its distribution, with central obesity and its intermediary mechanisms shown to be related to CHD incidence (Larsson et al., 1984). In women as well as men, an upper body distribution of fat indexed as waist:hip ratio is an independent risk factor for ischemic heart disease, diabetes, stroke, and premature mortality. In middle-aged women, an upper body fat distribution was associated with significantly higher systolic blood pressure, total cholesterol, low-density lipoprotein cholesterol, triglycerides, and lower levels of high-density lipoprotein cholesterol, even after the data were statistically adjusted for BMI (Wing, Matthews, Kuller, Meilahn, & Plantinga, 1991). Nevertheless, the strong relationships between waist:hip ratio and degree of obesity make it difficult to ascertain whether obesity per se or the distribution of body fat is the major determinant affecting risk factors for CVD.

Analyzing data by both BMI and waist:hip ratio in women pre- and post–weight loss, Dennis and Goldberg (1993) reported that an upper body fat distribution in women worsens lipid risk factors for CVD posed by obesity, and weight loss is an effective intervention to improve lipid profiles in these women. Although weight loss reduced CVD risk factors regardless of BMI or waist:hip ratio, the magnitude of the increase in plasma high-density lipoprotein cholesterol and decrease in triglycerides in women with upper body fat distribution suggests that weight loss in these women has the greatest potential to reduce their risk factors for CVD.

A persistent argument is whether or not obesity is an independent risk factor for CVD. Although the uniform relationship between the degree of overweight and CVD holds in simple univariate analysis, obesity often fails to emerge as an independent risk factor in multivariate analysis. However, the failure of obesity to emerge in a regression equation that also includes its component risk factors may be more an issue of multicollinearity than of physiological processes.

Insulin has been identified as an important physiological mechanism underlying obesity as a CVD risk factor, for the insulin levels in both the fasted and postprandial state are elevated in obese individuals. Hyperinsulinemia secondary to insulin resistance impairs glucose tolerance, increases triglycerides and cholesterol, and lowers high-density lipoprotein cholesterol. Increased insulin secretion that ensues to compensate for insulin resistance and glucose intolerance increases production of hepatic very low density lipoprotein triglyceride; impairs the catabolism of triglyceride-rich lipoproteins by adipose tissue lipoprotein lipase; increases small, dense low-density lipoprotein particles; and reduces the synthesis of HDL_2 particles. Insulin resistance also raises blood pressure through its effects on sodium retention and peripheral vascular tone (Bierman, 1992).

Numerous studies (Dennis & Goldberg, 1993; Wing & Jeffery, 1995) regarding the beneficial impact of weight loss on CVD measure its metabolic risk factors (e.g., cholesterol, triglycerides, insulin sensitivity, blood pressure) rather than "hard" disease end points, presumably because the small sample sizes in these tightly controlled clinical trials are not likely to reach epidemiological proportions large enough to make statements about subsequent disease incidence in the population. Nevertheless, a consolidation of studies establishes causal links of obesity to CVD risk factors and then to CVD end points.

Nursing Research

Despite the overwhelming prevalence of obesity and its profound physiological, psychological, and sociological sequelae, consuming more than $50 billion annually, only a few nurse investigators have focused on this major health problem, and fewer have examined obesity as a cardiovascular risk factor. Using qualitative research methodology, Allan (1988, 1989) explored weight management practices among women, including how women interpret and use health information in weight management, their strategies for maintaining their weight, and the factors that influence the complex self-care activities for dealing with weight gain and values of thinness. Using triangulation methodology and a sensitivity to cultural diversity in weight management, Walcott-McQuigg (1995) examined the dynamics and relationships among stress and weight control in African American, European American, Mexican, Mexican American, and Puerto Rican women. Brink identified the characteristics of successful weight management and evolved a new definition of "success" from the construction of weight history based on changes in BMI as an adult.

Purfield and Morin studied the impact of weight gain during the pregnancy of previously normal-weight primigravidas on length of second-stage labor and mode of delivery. Although Morin noted that obesity was a significant predictor of pregnancy-induced hypertension, hypertension was conceptualized as an obstetric complication rather than a risk factor for CVD. The only nurse investigators who have studied obesity and its relationship to CVD risk are Hansen, Bodkin, and colleagues, who worked with nonhuman primates, and Dennis and colleagues, who examined obesity and metabolic risk factors for CVD in women. None of these nurse investigators, with one exception (Dennis & Goldberg, 1996), have as yet translated their findings into intervention studies that implement and evaluate strategies to help obese individuals reach their uniquely personal, weight-related health goals and reduce their risk for CVD.

Supported in part by 1 R01 NR03514 from the National Institute of Nursing Research, National Institutes of Health and the Geriatric Research Education and Clinical Center at the Maryland VA Health Care System, Baltimore.

Karen E. Dennis

See also:
ANGINA
CARDIOVASCULAR DISEASE
CEREBROVASCULAR DISEASE
DIABETES MELLITUS
NUTRITION
PERIPHERAL VASCULAR DISEASE

OSTEOARTHRITIS

Signs and Symptoms

Osteoarthritis, the most common of the rheumatic diseases, is characterized by progressive loss of articular cartilage and by reactive changes at the margins of the joints and in subchondral bone. Clinical features can include pain in the involved joint, which is typically worse with activity and relieved by rest; stiffness after periods of immobility; enlargement of the joint; instability; limitation of motion; and functional impairment. Depending on the absence or presence of an identifiable local or systemic etiological factor, osteoarthritis has been classified into idiopathic (primary) and secondary forms. Classification of the disease is based on various combinations of clinical, radiographic, and laboratory parameters (Schumacher, Kippel, & Koopman, 1993).

Epidemiology

The prevalence of osteoarthritis is strikingly correlated with age; it is uncommon in adults under 40, but it is the number-one chronic disease in late life, with more than 80% of those over the age of 75 being affected. Osteoarthritis is a major cause of disability in older adults, and knee osteoarthritis is more likely to result in disability than osteoarthritis of any other joint. However, the prevalence of osteoarthritis at all joint sites increases progressively with age, which is the most powerful risk factor for the disease. Women are about twice as likely as men to be affected, and African American women are twice as likely as Caucasian women to have knee osteoarthritis. The pattern of joint involvement also differs with sex: women have a greater number of joints involved and more frequent complaints of morning stiffness, joint swelling, and nocturnal pain. Factors that appear to be associated with osteoarthritis, based on cross-sectional and longitudinal studies, include obesity, bone density, trauma and repetitive stress, and genetic factors (Schumacher et al., 1993).

Impact of Osteoarthritis

The impact of osteoarthritis on function and costs of care are substantial. Patients with osteoarthritis are more likely to be limited in the amount and kind of major activities they can perform, have more restricted bed days, and are more likely to report disability. When disease prevalence figures were applied to estimates of health care utilization and disability for both rheumatoid arthritis and osteoarthritis, an aggregate economic impact some 30-fold greater was found for osteoarthritis than for rheumatoid arthritis (Kramer, Yellin, & Epstein, 1983). In addition to the functional disability and economic impact of osteoarthritis, older people with this disease experience an inordinate amount of suffering, depression, and diminished quality of life (Daltroy & Liang, 1993).

Treatment and Management

Treatment approaches to patients with osteoarthritis have been mainly pharmacological, usually combined with physical therapy and sometimes surgery. Although these interventions are useful, they often fail to control disease progression, and symptoms may be associated with high costs and many toxicities. In addition, they frequently fail to address important issues of patient concern, such as psychological stress, quality of life, and autonomy. Because of the chronicity of the disease, patients must learn to manage and cope with osteoarthritis on a day-to-day basis. The ability to succeed in this task differentiates those who are incapacitated from those who continue to lead full and active lives in the face of equal disease severity. For this reason, health education has a potentially important role.

One of the most common educational interventions used for chronic disease is self-management. Self-management has been described as the day-to-day tasks an individual must undertake to control or reduce the impact of disease on health status; it includes all the tasks for handling clinical aspects of the disease away from the hospital or physician's office. For persons with osteoarthritis this may include using medications, managing acute episodes and emergencies, maintaining adequate exercise and activity, using relaxation and stress-reducing techniques, seeking information, using community services, adapting to work, managing relations with significant others, and managing emotions and psychological responses to the illness. Studies of self-management programs for patients with osteoarthritis have shown that subjects gained an overall increase in knowledge, self-efficacy, management behaviors, functional ability, and overall health status. In addition, subjects showed an overall decrease in pain, depression, visits to physicians, and health care costs (Hawley, 1995).

Practice and Policy Implications for Nursing

The population is aging, and the number of aged is expected to increase from 33.2 million in 1994 (12% of the U.S. population) to 65 million (22%)

in 2030. By the year 2020, this group will account for approximately half of the nation's health care expenditures (Feldstein, 1994). This "graying of America" and its concomitant increase in the prevalence of osteoarthritis poses problems for an ever spiraling health care budget. Incurable by definition, management of osteoarthritis extends over time, creating continuous costs to both patient and provider. It is important that we examine innovative ways to deliver high-quality care for older adults with osteoarthritis in as efficacious and economical a manner as possible. Advanced practice nurses are in a unique position to help patients with osteoarthritis adjust to living with this chronic disease by educating them in the use of self-management skills. The use of advanced practice nurses in various settings has been shown not only to improve patient outcomes but also to decrease costs (Brooten, Naylor, York, et al., 1995). Randomized controlled clinical trials of self-management programs conducted by advanced practice nurses are needed to provide documentation of quality and cost-conscious health care delivery for older patients with osteoarthritis.

CAROL E. BLIXEN

See also:
ACTIVITIES OF DAILY LIVING
FUNCTIONAL HEALTH
MOBILITY
PAIN ASSESSMENT
PAIN MANAGEMENT

PAIN ASSESSMENT

Assessment of pain for older adults is a critical component of initial and ongoing evaluation of pain management. Health professionals who fail to ask about specific pain symptoms or effects place patients at risk for unidentified, misdiagnosed, and undertreated pain (Ferrell, 1993; Greipp, 1992). Standardized tools for assessing pain are not often used by nursing staff, although pain problems are recorded by nurses more often than by physicians, and the efficacy of pain treatments are assessed mainly by nursing staff (Bell, 1997; Gu & Belgrade, 1993; Sengstaken & King, 1993; Zalon, 1993). This entry critiques the literature regarding existing pain assessment instruments that have been identified as useful for elders and examines emerging research on tools recommended for assessing pain in cognitively impaired elders.

An important component of the assessment of pain requires the nurse to believe the patient's pain rating. Several studies have demonstrated that when compared with patients' ratings of pain, nurses' ratings routinely underestimate pain in older adults (Weiner, Ladd, Pieper, & Keefe, 1995). The most objective measure of patient pain is to use a scaled pain-assessment instrument.

The most commonly used pain assessment is a simple numeric rating scale (NRS) asked verbally: "On a scale of 1 to 10, with 1 being very little pain, and 10 being the worst pain you can imagine, how would you rank your pain?" This scale is problematic for some elders because of the need to abstract a "sensation" concept into a numeric concept. One-third of nursing home residents in general (not just cognitively impaired) were unable to use the 0–10 scale (Weiner et al., 1995) and less than half of cognitively impaired residents were able to respond to this scale (Ferrell, Ferrell, & Rivera, 1995). Recommended changes include collapsing the NRS to a five-point scale (0–4) to reduce confusion when rating moderate pain, and testing the scale with the word discomfort as well as pain (Fulmer, Mion, & Bottrel, 1996; Morrison et al., 1998).

The McGill pain questionnaire (MPQ), a widely used tool developed by Melzack (1975), includes a listing of 78 words which have been categorized into 20 groups, a body drawing, and a pain-intensity subscale which represent the sensory, affective, and evaluative dimensions of pain. The visual and hearing impairments of older subjects could interfere with comprehension and lengthen the time required for pain assessment using this tool. This may fatigue an already distressed patient (Herr & Mobily, 1991). Vocabulary-comprehension problems may also limit its usefulness in patients with lower educational levels or cognitive impairment. However, Melzack and his colleagues (1987) reported that cognitively intact, older postoperative patients with pain persisting for more than 4 days after surgery were likely to use more verbal descriptors of pain, rather than the fewer verbal descriptors used by younger patients, a finding supported by other pain researchers (Ferrell, Ferrell, & Osterweil, 1990). The Present Pain Intensity subscale (rating of "no pain," "mild," "discomforting," "distressing," "horrible," and "excruciating") of the MPQ has been used successfully with older adults, including those with cognitive impairment. The words may require higher educational levels. However, two-thirds (60-65%) of cognitively impaired elders in nursing home and hospital studies were able to rate their pain on this subscale (Ferrell, Ferrell, & Rivera, 1995; Mosier, Nusser-Gerlach, Manz, & Bergstrom, 1998; Raway, 1994; Weiner et al. 1995).

The Pain Experience Measure (Ferrell, Wisdom, & Wenzel, 1989) is an instrument that was developed to better characterize pain in cancer patients. The instrument helped to describe pain, to gain insight into etiology, and to describe management strategies used by patients. The instrument, later modified for use in a population of nursing home elders, was renamed the Pain Experience Interview (PEI). It was piloted using 20 frail elderly subjects with chronic pain at a veteran's facility and demonstrated an internal consistency of 0.85 (Cronbach's alpha) and a test-retest reliability of 87% (a comparison of assessments conducted 24 hours apart) (Ferrell, Ferrell, & Rivera, 1995). The semistructured interview consists of 31 questions, two-thirds of which are in a yes/no format for ease of use in the nursing home. A significant correlation (Pearson's $r = .67$, $p < .001$) between the pain frequency on the PEI and the Present Pain Intensity Scale has been reported (Ferrell, Ferrell, & Osterweil, 1990). Tests on hip-fracture patients revealed that, for the simple yes/no questions about pain on the PEI, cognitively impaired subjects did as well as intact subjects, with an 81% agreement between the initial test and the retest (Kappa = 0.601; $p < .001$) (Feldt, Ryden, & Miles, 1998).

The Visual Analogue Scale (VAS) is a simple 100-mm line with anchored words of "no pain" and "the worst pain possible." Elders are asked to place a mark on a line to indicate the degree of pain experienced. This tool has a failure rate of 7.1% for elders, a rate similar to failure rates of the general population (Herr & Mobily, 1993). Although highly correlated with other measures of pain intensity, retest reliability (within 5 mm of the previous mark) is poor (DeLoach, Higgins, Caplan, & Stiff, 1998; Herr & Mobily, 1993). A modified VAS with more anchored pain descriptors is recommended by the American Geriatrics Society Chronic Pain Management Guidelines (American Geriatrics Society Panel on Chronic Pain in Older Persons, 1998).

The pain intensity tool most preferred by the older subjects—and the one with the fewest failures—is the Verbal Descriptor Scale (VDS). The VDS is a variation of the Present Pain Intensity subscale developed by Melzack (1975). Pain-severity descriptions are, in simple language, "no pain," "slight pain," "extreme pain," and "pain as bad as it could be." The VDS was highly correlated ($r = .84$ to 1.00) with other measures of pain intensity (Herr & Mobily, 1993). This tool is understood by elders with lower education levels and has a low failure rate (2%). The VDS was successfully completed by 73% of cognitively impaired elders following hip-fracture surgery (Feldt, Ryden, & Miles, 1998). Both the PPI and VDS are limited by the single dimension of pain (intensity) that is measured.

The assessment of pain in cognitively impaired elders is complicated by the gradual global cognitive losses, including: short-term memory skills, impaired abstraction, impaired verbal skills (especially naming and word-finding problems), and eventually loss of verbalizations (Alzheimer's Disease Education and Referral Center, 1998). Nursing staff may discount complaints because of inconsistency or lack of reliability of patient report (Ferrell, Ferrell, & Rivera, 1995; Parmelee, Smith, & Katz, 1993; Weiner et al., 1995). Researchers suggest that clinicians attempt to use simple pain instruments for this population (Ferrell, Ferrell, & Rivera, 1995; Mosier et al., 1998) and also suggest that they attend to behavioral cues indicative of pain. Several scales are currently under development to measure these nonverbal indicators.

A scale for measuring discomfort in noncommunicative patients with advanced Alzheimer's type dementia has been developed (Hurley, Volicer, Hanrahan, Houde, & Volicer, 1992). Discomfort—defined by these researchers as a negative emotional and/or physical state subject to variation in magnitude in response to internal or environmental conditions—differs somewhat from the concept of pain (Simons & Malabar, 1995). The Discomfort in Dementia of the Alzheimer's type (DS-DAT) scale includes nine items, two positive and seven negative: noisy breathing, negative vocalization, content facial expression, sad facial expression, frightened facial expression, frown, relaxed body language, tense body language, and fidgeting. Observers scored each item on a continuous scale from absent (0) to extreme (100) based on the presence of the defining characteristics. Although initial testing showed good inter-rater reliability (.86 to .98) and tool reliability (Cronbach's alpha .86 to .89), the tool was used on a mostly male (90%), fairly small sample (N = 82) (Hurley et al., 1992). One of the items, noisy breathing, could be attributed to medical conditions, such as an upper-respiratory-tract infection or chronic obstructive pulmonary disease. Facial expressions of distress or discomfort may differ by gender and culture.

Researchers using the DS-DAT have identified difficulty with inter-rater reliability for specific items (relaxed body language, sad-facial expression, and frown), and have modified the tool to improve its reliability (Miller, Neelon, & Dalton et al., 1996). These researchers identified that the DS-DAT is not user-friendly for routine nursing care because of the in-depth training required to obtain accurate, reliable ratings. However, research assistants believed the DS-DAT is useful in reflecting relative changes in hospitalized patients' discomfort, and has been useful in detecting changes in comfort levels in nursing home populations (Miller, Neelon, Dalton et al., 1996; Kovach & Weissman, 1998).

Other scales for observer rating of pain behaviors in chronic-pain patients have been tested, although they were not designed for use with cognitively impaired elders. The University of Alabama Birmingham Pain Behavior Scale (UAB-PBS) (J. S. Richards, Nepomuceno, Riles, & Suer, 1982) is a tool designed for use in a hospital setting, and the Pain Behavior Checklist

(PBC) (Dirks, Wunder, Kinsman, McElhinny, & Jones, 1993) is a similar tool designed for use with chronic-pain patients in an outpatient or rehabilitation setting. The UAB-PBS 10-item scale includes observations of vocal complaints, grimacing, body language, and stationary restlessness. Similarly, the 16-item PBC includes grimacing, sighing, rigid posturing, bracing, and clutching or rubbing the pain site. The PBC was found to be highly correlated ($r = .68$, $p < 0.001$) with present pain ratings, and least and worst pain ratings of 395 pain patients (Dirks et al., 1993). The UAB-PBS tool was shown to have high inter-rater reliability (.94–.96) and a test-retest reliability coefficient of .89, indicating a high degree of stability for pain scores over 2 days (Richards et al., 1982). When the tool was compared to the McGill Pain questionnaire and a 0–10 analog scale, the UAB-PBS score did not significantly correlate, indicating that the relationship between observable manifestations of pain and self-report may not be a close one.

Both the UAB-PBS and the PBC tools include items which could lead to inaccurate scores for elders and dementia patients. For example, the UAB-PBS includes a category that requires the rater to identify the number of daytime minutes spent in bed due to pain, a difficult task for severely demented patients, who spend time in bed due to profound cognitive impairment rather than pain. These tools were developed for chronic-pain populations, and assume mobility. There is no explanation of how to rate nonambulatory elders on limping (PBC) or walking (UAB-PBS). Scores are higher (indicating greater pain) on both scales if they use support equipment such as canes or walkers, which may be used by elders for support or balance rather than in response to pain. In addition, the PBC includes items such as "hunched or unusual shoulder posture" (common in elders with osteoporosis); "number of stands/hr" and "has to walk" as measures of restlessness (would need redefining for nonambulatory elders); and "difficulty arising," "difficulty seating" (sometimes problematic for cognitively impaired elders due to simple perceptual changes with cognitive impairment).

Raway (1994) videotaped 22 hospitalized hip-fracture patients (11 of whom were cognitively impaired) to observe them for nonverbal pain behaviors. Pain-related facial expressions were coded using a facial coding system devised by Ekman and Friesen (1978). She reported coding problems due to poor camera placement to capture subject expression, blockage of the subject's face during transfers, and poor inter-rater reliability. Frequencies of "brow lowering" or "brow lowering with jaw drop" were similar to the items of "grimacing" found in the UAB and PBS tools. Other nonverbal pain behaviors noted on the videotapes included: bracing the leg while standing (95.6%), guarding the torso or whole body (86.4%), repositioning the foot or ankle on the affected side (68%), guarding the leg on the affected side (63.6%), and repositioning the leg on the affected side (50%). Only the guarding of the leg on the affected side occurred significantly less frequently in the confused group in her study. She noted three common nonlanguage vocalizations (sighing, grunting, and groaning/moaning) which were similar in the impaired and intact groups. However, four pain-related verbalizations were almost exclusively observed in the confused group (only one intact subject in her study had a pain-related verbalization) and included: words of protest ("no, no, no," "don't") observed in 46% of the subjects; exclamations, observed in 36% of the subjects; and profanity in 27% of the subjects. Correlations between observed pain behaviors and pain intensity were not reported.

Using the information from Raway's study and the UAB-PBS pain scale, Feldt (1996) developed a Checklist of Non-verbal Pain Indicators (CNPI). This scale with definitions includes 6 items: vocal complaints (expression of pain in moans, groans, grunts, cries, gasps, or sighs); facial grimaces/winces (furrowed brow, narrowed eyes, tightend lips, jaw drop, clenched teeth, or distorted expressions); bracing (clutching or grasping side rails, bed, tray, table, or affected area during movement); restlessness (constant or intermittent shifting of position, rocking, intermittent or constant hand motions, inability to keep still); rubbing (massaging affected area); and vocal complaints (words expressing discomfort or pain, "ouch," "that hurts"; cursing during movement, exclamations of protest "stop," "that's enough"). Inter-rater reliability for the CNPI showed 93% agreement on the dichotomous checklist items; Kappa statistic = 0.625 to 0.819 ($p = .019$ to .0057) for the behaviors observed. Initial testing on 87 hip-fracture patients revealed an alpha coefficient of .54 for observations using the scale while the patient was at rest, and an alpha coefficient of .64 for observations of patients during movement. The scale was modestly correlated with the VDS (CNPI at rest with VDS, Spearman correlation $r_s = .372$, $p = .001$; CNPI with movement with VDS, Spearman correlation $r_s = .428$, $p < .0001$).

Nursing home residents who had daily pain for at least 3 months were asked to identify behaviors that they engage in when they experience pain (Weiner, Peterson, & Keefe, 1999). These self-reported behaviors were compared with behaviors identified by nursing and family caregivers. Of the pain behaviors endorsed by at least half of each of the three groups (residents, nurses, and family caregivers), eight behaviors had a substantial test-retest agreement (kappa > 0.6). These included: using mechanical help (cane, walker, grabbing onto furniture); moving extremely slowly; taking (or asking for) medication; lying down; appearing upset or sad; sighing/moaning; having difficulty getting up after lying down or sitting; and asking someone to do something to help ease the pain. Interestingly, many behaviors identified by residents and caregivers are similar to those cited in the instruments recommended for use in cognitively impaired elders. These behaviors identify the effect of pain on function and the modification of function that is used by residents to manage pain.

Other measures are being developed, although their scoring and reliability have not yet been reported. These include the Observable Pain Behaviors Tool, an assessment instrument tested on 105 older hospitalized patients (Simons & Malabar, 1995) and the Behavior Checklist which identifies several behaviors indicative of pain in confused elders (Baker, Bowring, Brignell, & Kafford, 1996). The behaviors on these instruments are similar and include: moaning, outgoing, quiet, agitated, cheerful, withdrawn, mute, verbally abusive, cries easily, refuses food, aggressive, noisy breathing, friendly, rocking, disjointed verbalization, involved, eats well, describes pain, calling out, and picking. These behaviors are consistent with the behaviors identified by other pain researchers for this population (Bell, 1997; Parke, 1992; Herr & Mobily, 1991; Hurley et al., 1992; Marzinski, 1991; Ryden & Feldt, 1992; Sengstaken & King, 1993; D. K. Weiner et al., 1999).

An assessment of pain is essential to the evaluation of comfort- and pain-management strategies. Recommendations regarding appropriate pain-assessment instruments for elders have been established by pain guidelines (American Geriatrics Society Panel on Chronic Pain in Older Persons, 1998; Fulmer, Mion, & Bottrel, 1996). Future research on newer pain-assessment instruments should enhance our ability to provide better pain management for cognitively impaired elders.

KAREN S. FELDT

See also:
COMMUNICATION
PAIN MANAGEMENT
QUALITY OF LIFE

PAIN MANAGEMENT

Pain is "an unpleasant sensory and emotional experience associated with actual or potential damage or described in terms of such damage" (International Association for the Study of Pain, 1986, p. 249). This definition includes pain of pathophysiological and psychological origin. *Pain management* refers to the care and treatment of the pain. Pain is a common accompaniment of disease and illness and is the most common reason that people seek medical attention. It is the nursing diagnosis most frequently identified by nurses.

Pain generally is classified into two types: acute and chronic, with chronic further differentiated into pain associated with malignancy and pain not associated with malignancy. Acute pain subsides as healing takes place; it has a predictable end and is of brief duration, usually less than 6 months. Chronic pain most commonly is said to be that which lasts for longer than 6 months, although Bonica (1990) suggested that chronic pain is "pain that persists a month beyond the usual course of an acute disease or reasonable time for an injury to heal or that is associated with a chronic pathologic process that causes continuous pain or the pain recurs at intervals for months or years" (p. 19).

The undertreatment of pain has been well documented for at least the past 25 years (Marks & Sachar, 1973). Recent studies (Bookbinder, Coyle, & Thaler, in press; Miaskowski, Nichols, Brody, & Synold, 1994; Ward & Gordon, 1994) show that average present pain scores for hospitalized patients range from 3.6 to 4.3 (on a 0–10 scale), and worst pain in the past 24 hours scores range from 6.6 to 7.8. The undermanagement of pain has been particularly pronounced in children and in the elderly. Barriers to the effective treatment of pain include clinicians' lack of knowledge of pain management principles, clinician and patient attitudes toward pain and drugs, and overly restrictive laws and regulations regarding use of controlled substances.

The gate control theory published by Melzack and Wall (1965) provided a theoretical basis for showing how pain, transmitted peripherally to the brain, can be influenced by cognitive and affective as well as physiological factors. An understanding of the mind-body relationship exemplified in the experience of pain provides a basis for many of the strategies used to manage pain.

Nociception is the body's reaction to a noxious stimulus; pain describes the person's perception of that event. Tissue damage causes the release of pain-producing substances, such as serotonin, histamine, and bradykinin, which stimulate nerve endings called nociceptors. Nociception leads from the peripheral nervous system through the spinal cord to the central nervous system. Nerve fibers descending from the brain to the spinal cord can inhibit the perception of pain. Opiate receptors on the brain or spinal cord react both to opiates that are externally administered and to enkephalins and endorphins produced by one's own body to modulate pain.

Pain management includes pharmacological, cognitive-behavioral, physical, radiation, anesthetic, neurosurgical, and surgical techniques. Depending on the cause of the pain, one or more strategies may be used. Most pain can be managed by the use of analgesics administered orally or intravenously and by simple cognitive-behavioral techniques such as relaxation and distraction. More complex pain, such as that experienced by patients with reflex sympathetic distrophy or by cancer patients who have unrelieved pain from several origins, may require evaluation and treatment by a multispecialty pain management team. The successful management of pain depends on a careful assessment of the pain, including reassessment to determine the effectiveness of interventions used.

Pharmacological management of pain usually is by three types of drug: (a) aspirin, acetaminophen, and nonsteroidal anti-inflammatory drugs (NSAIDS); (b) opioids; and (c) adjuvant analgesics. Nonsteroidal anti-inflammatory drugs decrease the levels of inflammatory mediators generated at the site of tissue injury, thus blocking painful stimuli. They are useful in the management of mild pain and may be used in combination with opioids for moderate to severe pain. Opioids are morphinelike compounds that produce pain relief by binding to opiate receptors. They are used with moderate and severe pain and can be administered orally, subcutaneously, intramuscularly, intravenously, rectally, transdermally, epidurally, nasally, intraspinally, and intraventricularly. Patient-controlled analgesia (PCA) can be accomplished by mouth or by use of a special pump set to prescribed parameters to administer a drug intravenously, subcutaneously, or epidurally. Adjuvant drugs are used to increase the analgesic efficacy of opioids, to treat other symptoms that exacerbate pain, or to provide analgesia for specific types of pain (Jacox et al., 1994).

Physical modalities for pain management include use of heat and cold, counterstimulation such as transcutaneous electrical nerve stimulation (TENS), and acupuncture. Cognitive techniques are focused on perception and thought and are designed to influence interpretation of events and bodily sensations. Providing information about pain and its management and helping patients think differently about pain are examples of cognitive techniques. Behavioral techniques are directed at helping patients develop coping skills and modify their reactions to pain. Cognitive-behavioral techniques commonly used by nurses and other clinicians include relaxation, imagery, distraction, and reframing. Psychotherapy, structured support, and hypnosis also have been used successfully in pain management.

When the use of drugs, with or without physical and cognitive behavioral modalities, is not adequate to manage pain, other management techniques may be used. These depend on the cause of the pain and may be temporary or permanent. Radiation therapy is used to relieve metastatic pain and symptoms from local extension of primary disease. Nerve blocks include the injection of a local anesthetic into a spinal space and peripheral nerve destruction. Surgical procedures are used to remove sources of pain, such as debulking a tumor that is pressing on abdominal organs or removing bone spurs that are compressing nerves. Neuroablation techniques include peripheral neurectomy, dorsal rhizotomy, cordotomy, commissural myelotomy, and hypophysectomy.

It is difficult to know how frequently each of the above management strategies is used. Estimates of their frequency in the management of cancer pain are as follows: oral, transdermal and rectal drugs, 75% to 85% of patients; intravenous and subcutaneous drugs, 5% to 20%; epidural and intrathecal, 2% to 6%; and nerve blocks, palliative surgery, and ablative surgery, 1% to 5% (Jacox et al., 1994).

During the past 10 years, various agencies and organizations have published guidelines for the management of pain. These have included the American Pain Society's (1995) principles of analgesic use in acute and cancer pain and the Agency for Health Care Policy and Research guidelines for the management of acute pain, cancer pain, and low back problems (Bigos et al., 1994; Carr et al., 1992; Jacox et al., 1994). In addition to these, the American Pain Society Quality of Care Committee (1995) published guidelines for using quality-improvement mechanisms in institutions to improve the management of acute and cancer pain. There is greater consensus regarding how to manage acute and cancer pain than for chronic nonmalignant pain.

ADA JACOX

See also:
COMMUNICATION
MEDICATIONS IN THE ELDERLY
PAIN ASSESSMENT
QUALITY OF LIFE

PERIPHERAL VASCULAR DISEASE

Peripheral Vascular Disease (PVD) is a term used to describe a group of conditions resulting from the interference of blood or lymph flow to or from the extremities. The conditions included in PVD are: peripheral-arterial disorders (PAD); lower extremity arterial disease (LEAD); carotid artery disease; aneurysms; venous disorders; venous stasis ulcers; varicose veins; deep vein thrombosis; lymphatic disorders; lymphedema vasomotor disorders (Raynaud's phenomenon and Buerger's disease), and congenital disorders (arterial-venous malformation). It is estimated that peripheral vascular disease affects 30% of the adult population, and two-thirds of all cases are asymptomatic (Federman, Trent, Froelich, Demirovic, & Kirsner,

1998). Conditions such as deep-vein thrombosis (DVT) and its potentially fatal *sequela* of pulmonary emboli (PE) may occur in healthy people, but is more prevalent in the immobilized population and in the elderly population (Fahey, 1999). Age is not a risk factor for varicose veins, lymphedcma, or vasomotor problems. This review focuses on the normal changes of the aging vasculature, as well as the three most common PVDs seen in older adults. Risk factors and treatments for PVD follow, as well as suggestions for future research and practice.

Peripheral Arterial Disorders (PAD)

The most commonly occurring PVD among older adults is PAD, resulting from artherosclerosis and its systemic manifestations. The prevalence of PAD increases sharply with age. Estimates in the geriatric population range from 10% of the population aged 60 and above (AHA, 1996) to over 20% in people over the age of 75 (Vogt, Wolfson, & Kullerler, 1992). A study of elderly Japanese American men reflects this dramatic increase of risk with age. In this study, the prevalence of PAD among 71–74 year-old men was 8%, but rose to 27.4% in those aged 85–93 (Curb et al., 1996).

Because PAD is largely asymptomatic, patients often present with advanced vascular disease. The symptoms of PAD range from intermittent claudication (IC) or ischemic muscle pain precipitated by activity and relieved by rest, to ulceration and gangrene. Epidemiological studies indicate that up to 5% of men—and 2.5% of women aged 60 and above—have symptoms of IC (AHA, 1996). Although the differing prevalence (based on sex) diminishes with advancing age, males continue to exhibit more severe forms of PAD than do females (Criqui & Denenberg, 1998). Because restrictions on walking are often rationalized and attributed to other causes, older adults do not always seek medical attention for IC. Meijer and colleagues (1998) report that the actual prevalence of IC may be underestimated. Individuals with symptomatic PAD are 2–4 times as likely to have coronary-artery disease (CAD) (Federman et al., 1998). Not only is PAD a strong predictor of CAD mortality, but the risk of increased CAD—and associated mortality—increases with the severity of PAD (Criqui & Denenberg, 1998).

Inexpensive and noninvasive measures such as ankle-brachial pressure index (ABI) and noninvasive carotid duplex scans (CDS) are currently used to assess and monitor the progression of PAD. ABI is a reflection of systemic artherosclerotic disease. Low ABI (< 0.9) requires further assessment. Vogt, Cauley, Newman, Kuller, and Hulley (1993) found that a decrease in ABI was a strong predictor of mortality in older men and women. The literature suggests the use of ABI during routine physical examinations of elderly persons who exhibit other risk factors for PAD.

Aneurysms

Aneurysmal problems commonly result from the combination of hypertension (HTN) and artheriosclerotic disease, and are largely asymptomatic. Age is a risk factor for aneurysmal disease, the only cure for which is surgical treatment. It is estimated that 6% of men over 65 years of age have detectable aneurysms. Another study places the prevalence at 14% for men with a history of cigarette smoking and PVD (Roland & Radnich, 1996). The most common form of aneurysmal disease is abdominal aortic aneurysms (AAA) above the infrarenal arteries. There is a high degree of mortality associated with the rupture of aneurysms greater than 6 cm. Studies suggest that age alone should not influence the decision for elective aneurysm repair (Harris et al., 1986).

Carotid Artery Stenosis (CAS)

CAS affects older men and women equally (Gudwin & Padussis, 1994), and is positively correlated with HTN. The disease was found in 25% of hypertensive elderly participants, as compared to 7% of normotensive elders (Bots, Hofman, de Bruyn, de Jong, & Grobbee, 1993; Lewis, Padayachee, Ariyanayagam, & Gosling, 1988; Sutton-Tyrrell, Alcorn, Wolfson, Kelsey, & Kuller, 1993; Tells et al., 1994). Characteristic symptoms of CAS, such as dizziness or other transient neurologic symptoms, are often attributed to "forgetfulness" and natural aging. Therefore it is imperative that diagnostic measures be taken to prevent further morbidity and mortality. Due to the high prevalence of asymptomatic CAS among patients with PAD, CDS is warranted in the elder population (Ascher, DePippo, Salles-Cunha, Marchese, & Yorkovich, 1999). A 1997 study indicates that pulse pressure is another effective predictor of CAS in older adults (Franklin, Sutton-Tyrrell, Belle, Weber, & Kuller, 1997).

Risk Factors for PVD

Individuals with both systolic HTN and evidence of PAD are at high risk for cardiovascular events. The Systolic Hypertension in the Elderly Program (SHEP) followed participants identified as having PAD for cardiovascular events. The mortality rate for those identified as having no atherosclerotic disease was 4.8%, for those having subclinical atherosclerosis was 16.7%, and for those with clinical artherosclerosis was 23%. Fatal and nonfatal cardiovascular events for the three groups were 10.9%, 29.8%, and 58.3%, respectively (Sutton-Tyrrell, Alcorn, Herzog, Kelsey, & Kuller, 1995). Smoking and PVD are strongly related. Therefore, smoking cessation is the most important intervention needed to prevent the development of the disease. It has been found that smoking is a stronger risk factor for PAD than CAD (Price et al., 1999).

Each year more than 56,000 lower extremity amputations (LEA) resulting from PVD are attributed to Diabetes Mellitus (DM) (Schoonmaker, 1998). Elders account for more than half of these amputees. Increased glucose levels associated with DM may cause microvascular changes and a thickening of the vascular smooth muscle, resulting in the development of PAD. It is estimated that 90% of LEA in the Western world are the consequence of the combination of PAD and DM (Schoonmaker, 1998).

Treatment

First-line interventions for PVD target modifiable risk factors such as smoking and HTN. Nursing is ideally suited to provide education and desimate guidelines regarding these risk factors. Home-care nurses can assess and screen for risk factors and early signs of PVD, such as foot-related problems (van Rijswik, 1998). Many relatively common foot disorders can become very serious in the elderly. Delays in referrals to vascular surgeons for severe PAD can increase the likelihood of limb loss (Zeltsman & Kerstein, 1998).

Although amputation is the most extreme treatment of PAD, other treatment modalities include angioplasty and revasculariztion. Studies show that elders tolerate procedures such as percutaneous transluminal angioplasty (PTA) well and with very effective results (Krikorian, Kramer, & Vacek, 1996). As the cost of postamputation rehabilitation is extensive, revascularization is a more cost-effective means of treating severe arterial-occlusive disease In working with individuals who have a diagnosis of PVD, nurses are confronted with a population who have several complex associated conditions such as DM and HTN. Whether the patient is hospitalized for an ulcer or revascularization, the nurse will have a limited amount of time to assess and provide education about the disease process. Follow-up care for this population is critical. There is little nursing research literature regarding the elder-PVD population. Further research is needed on the prevention, evaluation, and treatment of this disease.

DINA SHAH

See also:
  ANGINA
  CARDIOVASCULAR DISEASE
  CEREBROVASCULAR DISEASE
  HYPERTENSION
  PRESSURE ULCERS

PRESSURE ULCERS

Pressure ulcers are defined as any skin lesion caused by unrelieved pressure, resulting in damage of underlying tissue. Pressure ulcers usually occur over bony prominences and are graded from Stage 1 (nonblanchable erythema) to Stage 4 (full-thickness skin loss with tissue necrosis and destruction extending to muscle, bone, or supporting structures) (Panel for Prediction and Prevention of Pressure Ulcers, 1992). Pressure ulcers are a persistent, not a new clinical problem. It is difficult to estimate the incidence and prevalence of pressure ulcers, but one recent survey of 143 hospitals indicated that 11% of the patients had ulcers (Meehan, 1994). This problem is higher among critical care patients and elderly nursing home residents. The cost of treatment and the cost in human suffering, delayed rehabilitation, and an increased use of health care resources are difficult to determine, but one recent estimate suggested that \$1.3–\$6.8 billion may be spent on pressure ulcer treatment of hospitalized patients alone.

The goal of good patient care is to prevent pressure ulcers. This goal was supported by the Agency for Health Care Policy and Research (AHCPR) with the assistance of a multidisciplinary panel that created clinical practice guidelines (Panel for Prediction and Prevention, 1992) based on a comprehensive review and synthesis of scientific evidence and the judgment of clinical experts. In general, preventive measures recommended in this document include assessing risk of all bedfast or chairfast individuals on admission to a health care setting, reducing the amount and duration of pressure to which the tissue is exposed; keeping tissues clean, supple, and free from undue exposure to moisture or to dryness; and providing for adequate dietary intake.

Predicting pressure ulcer risk has been a goal of nurses for several decades. Early work by Phyllis Verhonick at Walter Reed Army Hospital and Doreen Norton in Great Britain focused on understanding the etiology of pressure ulcers with a view to predicting risk. This work in the late 1950s and early 1960s drew attention to the problem. The Norton Scale (Norton, McLaren, & Exton-Smith, 1962/1975), reported in 1962 and 1964, was the first tool tested for predictive validity. Attempts were continued in the early 1970s by Davina Gosnell (1973) and in the 1980s and 1990s by Barbara Braden and Nancy Bergstrom (Bergstrom, Braden, Laguzza, & Holman, 1987). The Braden Scale for Predicting Pressure Sore Risk© was introduced in 1987 and has been studied extensively since that time, proving effective in predicting who will develop pressure ulcers.

The Braden and Norton scales were recommended for use on all bedfast and chairfast individuals in the guidelines. The Braden Scale, now more commonly in use, is composed of six subscales (Mobility, Activity, Sensory

Perception, Nutrition, Moisture, Friction, and Shear) that address major conceptual risk factors. The total of these scores indicates the level of risk. This tool has very good sensitivity and specificity; that is, it accurately identifies who is at risk and who is not at risk. Individuals known to be at risk receive care based on the specific factors placing them at risk.

The hallmark of an effective pressure ulcer prevention program is teamwork. It is important for a multidisciplinary team to put a systematic prevention plan in place. Staff education and participation is essential. Planning mechanisms that focus on the processes of care and mechanisms for ensuring that risk is assessed and preventive practices are delivered have been most effective. Susan Horn and colleagues (Horn, Ashton, & Tracy, 1994) from Intermountain Health System have demonstrated that computer-assisted decision support based on risk assessment and accompanied by risk reduction as recommended by the AHCPR guidelines can reduce pressure ulcer incidence among even the most severely ill. Cost savings have been documented to accompany this improved patient outcome.

When pressure ulcers develop, it is important to create a comprehensive plan of care and a mechanism for systematic delivery of care. A management program, suggested by the AHCPR guideline and based on best evidence synthesis (Bergstrom, Bennett, & Carlson, 1994), suggests including the following factors: assessment of wounds, selection of support surfaces to reduce the amount and duration of exposure to pressure, incontinence management, and selection of dressings, wound cleansing agents, moisture barriers, and skin cleansing agents. Treatment plans must be written, communicated, and carried out regularly. Wounds should be evaluated at each dressing change and at periodic intervals to ensure that healing is occurring and the wound is not worsening. Signs of beginning healing are usually evident in 2 weeks for large ulcers. It is also important to monitor the patient for signs of complications, such as local and systemic infection and osteomyelitis.

A wound assessment guide developed by Barbara Bates-Jensen (1990) is useful for quantifying the size and depth of the wound and other wound characteristics. Another wound assessment schema is also under development by the National Pressure Ulcers Advisory Panel. Wound assessment serves as the basis for planning care and monitoring progress.

Pressure reduction, using specialty beds, has been shown to provide an environment for wound healing. Reducing exposure to pressure is central to the healing of pressure ulcers. Some support surfaces are more effective than others in achieving this objective, but even those that provide for lower interface pressures often have high interface pressures over the heels. It is important to provide for pressure relief by keeping the heels off the mattress surface, keeping in mind the fact that the support surface alone is not sufficient to heal wounds.

Wound care includes debridement, cleansing, and appropriate dressing. Pressure ulcers must first be debrided to reduce the bioburden and promote healing. This can be accomplished in a number of ways, depending on the condition of the wound and the condition of the patient. At each dressing change, the wound should be cleansed, using products that are not cytotoxic (usually normal saline) and mild pressure. Products such as betadine and other skin cleansers should be avoided. Dressings that provide for a moist (not wet) wound environment should be used. The moist environment can be achieved with gauze moistened with normal saline or with occlusive dressings. Occlusive dressings are more expensive but do not need the frequent changing required to keep saline gauze moist.

Skin surrounding the wound should be kept dry and supple. Wound contamination and damage to surrounding tissue are important issues for incontinent individuals. Skin cleansing, toileting, special collection devices, and moisture barriers for the skin are all important. Adequate nutrition is a key factor in wound healing. Provision of calories and protein sufficient to meet the individual's requirements should be ensured.

Perhaps the most useful concept to emerge from the pressure ulcer treatment guideline is the expectation that wounds make progress toward healing in 2 weeks. Clear expectations of healing, a comprehensive plan of care, and continuous monitoring of the effectiveness of the treatment plan can promote healing and prevent pressure ulcers from becoming chronic wounds.

NANCY BERGSTROM

See also:
PERIPHERAL VASCULAR DISEASE

PROSTATE CANCER

The prostate, a walnut-size gland that sits at the base of the bladder and encircles the urethra, produces the whitish fluid ejaculated during orgasm. In fertile men, this fluid contains sperm. The prostate gland enlarges as men age, but the mechanism of this enlargement is not fully understood. The cellular proliferation may be either benign (as in benign prostatic hyperplasia) or malignant. Benign prostatic hyperplasia (BPH) and prostate cancer are androgen-dependent for growth. However, the location of growth differs. Benign prostatic hyperplasia typically occurs in the central, or transitional, zone of the prostate, while cancer is found in the peripheral zone (Pienta & Esper, 1993).

Prostate cancer is identified as either histologic or clinical. Autopsy studies indicate that histologic, or latent, cancer is evident in 15% to 30% of men over the age of 50 years and that the prevalence increases to 60% to 70% in men over the age of 80 years (Picnta & Esper, 1993). Latent prostate cancer found at autopsy is typically small, well differentiated, and confined to the gland itself (Ohori, Wheeler, Dunn, Stamey, & Scardino, 1994). Results of several epidemiological studies indicate that the incidence of histologic prostate cancer is constant across different groups of men, suggesting that environmental factors play a role in the development of clinically evident prostate cancer after initiating events occur (L. Baker et al., 1996). Some researchers believe histologic prostate cancer eventually leads to clinically evident cancer (Pienta, Goodson, & Esper, 1996), while others suggest that histologic prostate cancer has no impact on survival (L. Baker et al., 1996). It is not known why the incidence of prostate cancer increases more with age than all other major cancers (Pienta et al., 1996). With expectations of a continued rise in the incidence of both latent and clinically detectable prostate cancers among "baby boomers," prostate cancer will continue to be a disease of the elderly. Therefore, basic research is needed to better understand the biologic potential of latent cancers, the function of aging in prostate cancer, and the relationship between latent and clinically evident prostate cancer.

One in five men will develop clinical prostate cancer during their lifetimes (Pienta et al., 1996). The Gleason score grades clinically evident cancer. This score—using a scale of 1 to 10—is based on the degree of differentiation of cellular tissue and the relationship of that tissue to the surrounding stroma (L. Baker et al., 1996). Men aged 55 to 74 years with a Gleason score of 2 to 4 (low-grade to highly differentiated tumor) at diagnosis face a minimal risk of death from prostate cancer within the next 15 years, whereas those with a Gleason score of 7 to 10 (high-grade or poorly differentiated tumor) face a high risk of death from prostate cancer when treated conservatively (Albertsen, Hanley, Gleason, & Barry, 1998). A complex predictive model for grouping men according to the clinical stage of the tumor uses clinical stage of tumor, presurgical Gleason score, presurgical PSA level, and postsurgical tumor stage (Garnick & Fair, 1998). It is important to determine the spread of the disease, as well. Local metastasis most often occurs to the pelvic lymph nodes, seminal vesicles, urinary bladder, and pelvic side walls, while distant spread is to bone, lungs, liver, or adrenals (L. Baker et al., 1996).

Although prostate cancer is highly prevalent, incidence varies among racial groups. African American men have a 35% greater incidence rate and a 223% greater mortality rate than do Caucasians (Pienta et al., 1996). While common in North America and northwestern Europe, prostate cancer is rare in Asia, Africa, and South America (American Cancer Society, 1999).

In the United States, prostate cancer is the most prevalent cancer in men, with 179,300 new cases diagnosed in 1999 (Landis, Murray, Bolden, & Wingo, 1999). Incidence rates in the United States and other developed countries have been influenced by intensive screening efforts, the use of prostate-specific antigen (PSA), and the diagnosis of asymptomatic, latent cancers (Parkin, Pisani, & Ferlay, 1999). In fact, the incidence of prostate cancer in the U.S. doubled in the ten-year period from 1984 to 1994 (Landis et al., 1999). While prostate cancer is not a prominent cause of death in men worldwide, in the U.S. it is the second leading cause of cancer-related deaths among men. This is attributed to the fact that those men diagnosed in their forties and fifties tend to have more aggressive disease (Garnick & Fair, 1998), and also to the large numbers of African American males who often go undiagnosed until the late stages of the disease.

Risk factors for prostate cancer include modifiable factors, such as dietary fat intake, and unalterable factors, such as age, race, genetic predisposition, and positive family history (Pienta & Esper, 1993; L. Baker et al., 1996). Social factors—such as access to care, willingness to seek treatment, and literacy—may also play a role in risk (C. Bennett et al., 1998; Haas & Sakr, 1997). Other factors that have been linked to an increased risk of prostate cancer include vasectomy, zinc and cadmium exposure, and sexually transmitted diseases (Haas & Sakr, 1997).

Traditionally, the gold standard method of detecting prostate cancer has been the digital rectal examination (DRE). During the DRE, the prostate gland is palpated for size and detectable lumps. A major disadvantage of the DRE is that microscopic cancers are often missed until they grow large enough for detection. Therefore, the development of a less invasive method that provides earlier detection was desirable. In the past decade, the use of PSA to detect and monitor prostate cancer increased dramatically. Both normal and malignant cells secrete PSA, but the level of PSA is often elevated in the presence of cancer cells.

Controversy, however, surrounds the use of PSA as a general screening tool. A major problem with using the PSA as a general screening method is its lack of specificity (Litwin & deKernion, 1994; Mettlin et al., 1994; Olsson & Goluboff, 1994; Woolf, 1994). Lange (1994) noted that there is a 95% accuracy rate in predicting significant cancer, but only a 66% accuracy rate in predicting insignificant cancer. Therefore, it is certain whether routine PSA testing should be recommended due to its lack of specificity, the potentially unnecessary interventions initiated by screening, the resultant significant complications, and the increased cost (Agency for Health Care Policy and Research [AHCPR], 1999; Handley & Stuart, 1994). Cantor,

Spann, Volk, Cardenas, and Warren (1995) concluded that when quality-of-life preferences of men are considered, annual screening of asymptomatic men is not recommended. Conversely, others believe that screening is absolutely necessary to decrease the large numbers of prostate cancer deaths reported annually. In addition to this debate, the precise age at which to start annual prostate cancer screening begs an answer (von Eschenbach, Ho, Murphy, Cunningham, & Lins, 1997).

Although prostate cancer is the most prevalent cancer among men in the United States, we still have a poor understanding of which prostate cancers will smolder on, producing few or no symptoms without intervention, and which will claim a life despite intervention (A. Porter et al., 1996). As a result, disease management is highly controversial within the medical community. The fact is that no one treatment has proved capable of providing a cure for prostate cancer. This is complicated by several variables including the man's age, the timeliness of the diagnosis, and the fact that prostate cancer essentially behaves as four different entities, ranging from early localized nonmetastatic disease to advanced metastatic disease.

The treatment of choice for localized prostate cancer is radical prostatectomy (Garnick & Fair, 1998). Other treatments for prostate cancer include external-beam radiation; brachytherapy, hormonal therapies, hormone ablation, cryotherapy, and conservative management, or "watchful waiting," often used in men over the age of 65. There is also a growing interest in complementary and alternative therapies, such as vitamin and mineral supplementation and special diets, either in tandem with or instead of the traditional Western treatments mentioned above (Nam et al., 1999). The reader is directed to the National Prostate Cancer Practice Guidelines for in-depth discussion of treatment options (L. Baker et al., 1996).

Prostate cancer treatment is not necessarily consequence-free and ironically many men are left with posttreatment effects that often remain long after the fear of cancer has dissipated. Three important side effects of prostate cancer treatment that can have a major impact on a man's quality of life are impotence, urinary incontinence, and diarrhea (Marshall, 1994; US TOO, 1999; Moore, 1999). In addition to the negative impact on quality of life that these sequelae may cause, psychosocial morbidity (i.e., uncertainty and fear of cancer) has been described in relation to the "watchful waiting" treatment.

The known variations in the incidence of mortality from prostate cancer among ethnic groups offer compelling evidence of the need for culturally sensitive screening tools, and determination of patient preference for treatment options. Nursing plays a major role in symptom management, providing patient education, management of the common side effects of treatment—impotence, urinary incontinence, and diarrhea. These conditions have profound effects on men's work, social, and interpersonal activities. The focus of nursing research has been screening and early detection, symptom management, behavioral and psychosocial aspects of care, and quality of life. Because nursing incorporates a broad perspective of healthcare, environmental factors that appear to play a role in the development of prostate cancer should be the focus of nursing action and research in an effort to reduce risk. Nurse researchers need to advocate for adequate funding of both basic and clinical prostate cancer research. Special initiatives must be directed at high-risk men, especially those of African American descent and those with positive family histories. Nurse researchers need to be part of interdisciplinary teams that are intent on discovering accurate predictive models of screening, diagnosis and prognosis, and efficacious interventions that preserve not only life, but its quality, for affected men and their loved ones.

MARY H. PALMER
LORRIE L. POWEL

See also:
CANCER CARE: CHEMOTHERAPY
CANCER SURVIVORSHIP
SEXUALITY RESEARCH

TERMINAL ILLNESS

A terminal illness is defined as one in which a patient's remaining life is judged to be limited. The last phase of such an illness is the phase that eventuates in death. Usually, conventional therapies have been unsuccessful in effecting a cure, and care is directed toward the palliation of symptoms. Terminal illness implies that there has been an onset and a termination with various phases in between. It also suggests a history of chronicity. Thus, a death resulting from an acute insult to the body's functioning in which death ensues within hours or days thereafter would not be construed as having been the outcome of a terminal illness.

Florence Wald engaged in pioneering work in this area. Wald was dean of the School of Nursing in 1963 when Dame Cicely Saunders first came to Yale's School of Medicine to explore care of the dying in the United States. A series of visits by Dr. Saunders, the founder of St. Christopher's Hospice in London, culminated in a study of the care of the dying in New Haven by Wald and her colleagues, which resulted in the development of what is now the Connecticut Hospice (Wald, 1994).

The research undertaken by Wald investigated the adequacy and efficacy of the care of the dying. Other investigators have continued to explore this topic by contrasting settings for care as well as the comparative effectiveness of different approaches to symptom control. Although there continues to be a major concern with pain control, other troublesome symptoms such as anorexia, pressure ulcers, delirium, and dyspnea also have been studied. Much of this research has taken place in the setting of cancer care.

The experience of dying and the fact of death as a field of scholarly inquiry was stimulated by the work of Herman Feifel with the publication of his book *The Meaning of Death* in 1959. Feifel's endeavors and those of Robert Fulton in sociology, Elizabeth Kubler Ross in psychiatry, Robert Kastenbaum in psychology, Jean Quint Benoliel in nursing, and a small coterie of colleagues resulted in a renewed interest in the field and subsequently an increase in research. A number of the initial studies in the field of terminal illness concerned the attitudes of providers toward caring for the dying. This is not entirely surprising given the fact that nurses' attitudes in general were a subject for investigation at the time.

In one of the first studies conducted by a nurse researcher in terminal illness, Jan Folta (1965) found that staff nurses showed higher levels of anxiety about caring for dying patients than did nurses in other positions. This continues to be a subject of interest to researchers and clinicians, but the emphasis has shifted to questions of the prevention of burnout and more recently spirituality. There also has been a recent surge of studies about the knowledge and attitudes of health care providers toward the care of those infected with the human immunodeficiency virus (HIV).

The study of terminal illness in the hospital has been an important part of the life work of Anselm Strauss. His emphasis was on the staff and the manner in which they handled dying patients. Strauss, with his colleague Barney Glaser, found that health care providers have to answer questions regarding certainty and the time of death for every terminally ill person (Glaser & Strauss, 1965, 1968). Another important contribution has been the work on trajectory, which schematically depicts the path and shape of a chronic illness with its disease-specific perturbations, culminating in a terminal phase (Corbin & Strauss, 1991). By way of contrast, Benita Martocchio (1980) introduced a categorical approach to defining the health-illness course of patients, with such distinctions as well, acutely ill, chronically ill, high risk of dying, dying, and dead.

Another early researcher in the field of terminal illness, Jeanne Quint Benoliel (1994) joined Glaser and Strauss as an associate after her prior studies on women who had mastectomies. She contributed to their work (cited above), which she described as being concerned with the influence of cultural values and social context characteristics on (1) what patients were or were not told about their situation, (2) different patterns of dying associated with different diseases, and (3) the education of student nurses for work involving death and dying patients. (Benoliel, 1994, p. 6; see also Quint, 1967)

Benoliel and her students continued their interest in death education for student nurses and also developed a transition service that would allow terminally ill persons to die at home. The transition service provided the clinical base for further research.

Ida Martinson also was concerned with allowing individuals to die at home, but the subjects for her investigation were children. The impact of children dying at home on the children themselves, their parents, and in more recent studies, on their siblings has opened the door for the home care of dying children (Martinson et al., 1978).

The focus of research on the adult terminally ill has broadened to include studies of their family caregivers and the support required by these individuals. A number of studies have explored the congruence of expectations and perceptions between the terminally ill and either the professional or the family caregiver, as well as the needs of the terminally ill and their satisfaction with care and quality of life.

Research on the terminally ill person with acquired immunodeficiency syndrome (AIDS) has examined the needs of those dying from this disease, their partners, and family members. Although there have been papers on multiple loss, the literature on living and dying as a result of AIDS has not sufficiently exposed the experience of terminal illness in the context of an epidemic, as contrasted with dying of a disease without the public attention given to HIV/AIDS. Further research also is needed on the dying family, that is, the family where two or more generations are infected or where all of the siblings are infected.

Other areas requiring investigation include the impact of managed care on the care of the terminally ill; the manner in which care of the terminally ill will be affected by the presence or absence of health care provider–assisted suicide; and the nature of terminal illness care in an aging society. If the research on symptom control leads to the desired improvements in care, then future researchers will find that the terminally ill are able to live and die well.

Inge B. Corless

See also:
HOSPICE
SUICIDE

URINARY INCONTINENCE

Definition

Urinary incontinence was defined by the International Continence Society Committee on Standardisation of Terminology in 1973 as "involuntary loss of urine which is objectively demonstrable and a social or hygienic problem" (ICS, 1990). The committee defined four specific types of incontinence: (a) genuine stress, (b) urge as described by the patient, (c) reflex, and (d) overflow incontinence, as evidenced by urodynamic demonstration of urine loss.

In 1992 an Agency for Health Care Policy and Research (AHCPR) expert panel defined incontinence as "involuntary loss of urine which is sufficient to be a problem" (Diokno, McCormick, Colling, et al., 1992, p. 1). The expert panel deleted the words "objectively demonstrable and a social or hygienic problem." It was the judgment of the panel that the literature would not support science-based evidence that changes in outcomes of urinary incontinence were "objectively demonstrable." For several days the AHCPR panel deliberated what outcomes could be measured in incontinence. If involuntary loss of urine is the problem, then it was determined the outcome was dryness or no voluntary loss of urine. Dryness was measured in episodes or accidents per day, per week, or per month. To measure dryness, a toileting diary was recommended as the tool to collect measurable outcomes of dryness.

Four Types of Incontinence

The four types of incontinence result from four different pathophysiological mechanisms. Therefore, the correct nursing diagnosis is important because the treatment must be specific to the diagnosis to achieve an appropriate outcome.

The symptom of urge incontinence is the involuntary loss of urine associated with a strong desire to void (urgency). Urge incontinence is usually, but not always, associated with urodynamic findings of involuntary detrusor contractions, referred to as detrusor instability (DI). When this symptom is associated with a neurological lesion, it is called detrusor hyperreflexia (DH), which is seen in patients with stroke. In patients with multiple sclerosis and suprasacral spinal cord lesions, DH is accompanied by detrusor sphincter dyssynergia (DSD), inappropriate contraction of the external sphincter with detrusor contraction. In older adults this symptom is associated with detrusor hyperactivity with impaired bladder contractility (DHIC).

The symptom of stress incontinence is seen in patients who involuntarily lose urine during coughing, sneezing, laughing, or other physical activities that increase intraabdominal pressure. Stress urinary incontinence is defined as urine loss that occurs with an increase in intraabdominal pressure, in the absence of a detrusor contraction or an overdistended bladder. The most common cause of stress incontinence in women is a floppy uterus or urethral hypermobility. It is also common in men after prostatectomy.

Reflex incontinence occurs without any warning or sensory awareness, often in patients with paraplegia. It is also called unconscious incontinence.

Overflow incontinence is involuntary loss of urine associated with overdistention of the bladder. This type of incontinence causes constant dribbling. Overflow may be caused by an underactive or acontractile detrusor. The bladder may be underactive or acontractile secondary to use of drugs, to neurological conditions such as diabetic neuropathy or low spinal cord injury, or to radical pelvic surgery that interrupts the motor innervation of the detrusor muscle.

Nursing research has contributed to the definition of functional incontinence, which is urine loss caused by factors outside the lower urinary tract, such as a physical or cognitive impairment. A patient who is immobile and cannot toilet in time is functionally incontinent.

Prevalence and Costs

Urinary incontinence affects approximately 13 million Americans, with the highest prevalence in the elderly in both community and institutional settings (National Kidney and Urologic Diseases Advisory Board, 1994). Urinary incontinence is estimated to cost $11.2 billion annually in community-dwelling persons and $5.2 billion in nursing homes (based on 1994 dollars) (Fantl et al., 1996).

Risk Factors

Nursing research has provided identification of important risk factors in adult urinary incontinence. The risk factors validated by nurses are low fluid intake, environmental barriers, estrogen depletion, and pelvic muscle weakness (Fantl et al., 1996). These are in addition to other risk factors, including immobility, impaired cognition, medications, morbid obesity, diuretics, smoking, fecal impaction, delirium, high-impact physical activities, diabetes, stroke, childhood nocturnal enuresis, race, and pregnancy, vaginal delivery, or episiotomy.

Nursing Assessment and Diagnosis

The diagnosis of incontinence is based on a structured history, physical exam, urinalysis, and postvoid residual volume measurement. Recommended questions for the history include frequency of episodes, duration of the problem, volume of accidents, precipitating factors and questions related to risk factors. The physical exam should include tests for neurological abnormalities, abdominal examination, rectal examination, genital and pelvic examinations, and direct observation of urine loss using a cough stress test.

Treatment

There are three basic treatments of incontinence: medications and behavioral and surgical interventions. The most significant contributions of nursing science have been in the behavioral interventions. Nurse researchers have conducted research on toileting assistance, bladder retraining, and pelvic muscle rehabilitation.

Toileting assistance includes scheduled toileting, habit training, and prompted voiding. Studies have been conducted in outpatient populations and in nursing home residents. Nursing staff have achieved significant reductions in urinary incontinence during a 4–9-week intervention—about 80% improvement. Four clinical trials in nursing homes, three controlled and one uncontrolled, demonstrated that prompted voiding reduced incontinence by 0.8–1.8 episodes per patient per day (Fantl et al., 1996).

Bladder training is a procedure that includes education, scheduled voiding with systematic delay, and positive reinforcement. A controlled, randomized clinical trial of 131 women with sphincteric incompetence and unstable detrusor function showed that of the 60 women in the treatment group, 12% became dry, and 75% had a 50% reduction in incontinent episodes (Fantl et al., 1996).

Pelvic muscle rehabilitation (Kegel exercises) may be done alone or augmented with bladder biofeedback therapy or vaginal weight training. This type of intervention is most beneficial in patients with stress urinary incontinence. In a study of 65 women aged 35 to 75, a 62% reduction in incontinence episodes was documented. In another uncontrolled study, 20 women aged 35 to 65 were reported to have a 95% reduction in urinary incontinence episodes. In a nurse-directed project, when pelvic muscle exercise was compared with phenylpropanolamine hydrochloride treatment, patients experienced a 77% reduction with exercise and 84% with drugs (Fantl et al., 1996).

When pelvic muscle exercise is augmented by bladder inhibition with biofeedback therapy, a range of 54%–87% improvement has been demonstrated. Biofeedback that uses feedback from pelvic muscle contraction and abdominal and detrusor activity shows the greatest improvement, with a 75.9%–82% improvement rate across six studies involving 166 subjects. Overall, the literature indicates that pelvic muscle exercise and other behavioral strategies, with or without biofeedback, can cure or reduce incontinent episodes.

Pelvic muscle exercise also can be augmented with vaginal weight training. Women insert cone-shape weights (20–100 g) into the vagina. They try to retain the cone by contracting the pelvic muscle for up to 15 minutes. Research from 103 premenopausal women indicated a subjective cure or improved status of 68%–80% after 4–6 weeks of treatment.

Pelvic floor electrical stimulation is another intervention used by nurses and supported by nursing research. Pelvic muscle electrical stimulation produces a contraction of the levator ani and external urethral and anal sphincters, accompanied by a reflex inhibition of the detrusor. Two randomized controlled trials have been conducted. Using electrical stimulation, 86% of patients improved or were cured, compared to 33% in the control group. Behavioral therapies are very effective and carry no risks.

Pharmacological and Surgical Treatments, and Other Management Options

Several medications have been tested in clinical trials for specific types of urinary incontinence. As with most drugs, there is a risk of side effects, and persons taking more than one drug should be observed for adverse drug interactions. Various procedures have been described in AHCPR clinical practice guidelines (Fantl et al., 1996) to treat incontinence surgically. The objectives of surgical treatments depend on the underlying anatomical and physiological etiology; the purpose is to circumvent the underlying pathophysiology that is causing urine loss. As with any surgery, there are possible complications and risks.

Other measures and supportive devices can be used to manage rather than treat or cure incontinence. Nursing has contributed to the development and evaluation of several measures, including intermittent catheterization, indwelling urethral catheterization, suprapubic catheters, external collection systems, penile compression devices, pelvic organ support devices, and absorbent pads or garments.

Psychological Impact of Incontinence

Nursing research has identified the quality-of-life and psychological impact of incontinence on the adult and the nursing staff or other caregiver

(Palmer, 1996). Incontinent adults often remove themselves from social situations where the risk of an accident would be embarrassing. Family members caring for the incontinent patient often find the care burdensome or tiring, and they become resentful. Health care providers are consumed by the labor-intensive care required by the incontinent patient. They may avoid the person, complain about the burden of care, or even blame the patient for accidents. Standardized questionnaires have been developed by nurse researchers to determine the psychological impact of incontinence.

KATHLEEN A. MCCORMICK

See also:
ACTIVITIES OF DAILY LIVING
FUNCTIONAL HEALTH
HYDRATION
PRESSURE ULCERS

Part VI

COGNITIVE AND NEURO-BEHAVIORAL ISSUES IN AGING

INTRODUCTION

Particularly over the last decade, views have significantly changed regarding cognitive functioning and aging. Rather than as a normal consequence of aging, cognitive decline is now primarily seen as a disease process. As the general population ages, the number of cognitively impaired (CI) individuals will rise exponentially over the next 30 years. Currently approximately 4 million individuals with Alzheimer's disease and other cognitive impairments live in the United States, with this number increasing by several hundred thousand in the next 5 years, and by more than a million in the next 15 years (Administration on Aging, 1999). Costs to care for persons with Alzheimer's disease have been estimated at $80 to $90 billion per year in the United States (Rice, Fox, & Max, 1993).

Cognitive decline can be the primary manifestation of a disease, such as dementia of the Alzheimer's type, or can occur as a secondary problem of another disease, such as cognitive changes of Parkinson's disease. No matter what the cause, cognitive impairment in the elderly is associated with significant decline in ability to function in the community, and the end of community tenure with placement in long-term care (Osterweil, Martin, & Syndulko, 1995).

Nursing researchers, in conjunction with researchers of many fields, are making great strides in understanding how to treat patients with cognitive impairment and how to maintain normal cognition as one ages. Each chapter in this section will detail the current research in a particular area of cognitive problems in the aging population. A wide variety of currently funded nursing research is being conducted in the area of cognitive impairment. Nurse researchers are currently funded to study many problems of the aging person and their caregivers, such as sleep, agitation of dementia, memory loss, and quality of life.

Because the research in cognitive changes is currently so active in many biomedical fields, a general overview of topics currently being investigated in addition to nursing research is of interest. Current research can be divided into three categories: the cause of cognitive impairment, the assessment to determine the presence of CI, and treatments for CI.

A wide variety of mechanisms are being investigated to determine what pathologic changes are associated with cognitive decline and the cause of that pathology. Pathologic changes may include the formation of plaques and neurofibrillary tangles, reduction in neurotransmitters, such as acetylcholine, changes in the mass of brain tissue in critical regions, production of neurotoxic proteins (Grammas, Moore, & Weigel, 1999), and changes resulting from an excess of oxygen free radicals (Venters et al., 1997). Some of these changes may be initiated or caused by genetic abnormalities, such as APO-E$_4$ allele homogeneity. As understanding of the pathology of cognitive decline improves, treatments can be devised to reverse and hopefully prevent cognitive impairment.

A number of factors may delay the onset of CI, including estrogen, use of nonsteroidal antiinflammatory drugs, and long-term use of Vitamin E. Other factors, such as high blood pressure, previous history of head injury, low levels of vitamin B$_{12}$, and hypothyroidism, are associated with an increased incidence of CI.

As more treatments for cognitive impairment become available, early assessment to identify cognitive impairment becomes more critical. A book published in 1997 provides a comprehensive compilation of measures used to assess cognitive status in elderly individuals (Teresi, Lawton, Holmes, & Ory, 1997). Brain scanning techniques are currently being validated for their sensitivity and specificity in diagnosing dementia premorbid. Additionally, researchers conducting the Nun Study are providing a detailed account of longitudinal measures of cognitive function throughout an individual's adult life, and neuropathologic changes found on autopsy (Snowdon et al., 1997). Using a novel approach, researchers found that high levels of a neural thread found in the urine may be diagnostic of Alzheimer's disease.

Drug treatments for cognitive impairment in the elderly currently include traditional and alternative medicine options. Several researchers have demonstrated the value of using donepezil to improve cognitive function in dementia (A. Burns et al., 1999; McLendon & Doraiswamy, 1999). High doses of vitamin E have also become standard treatment (van Reekum, Simard, & Farcnik, 1999). There is less evidence that vitamin C, ginkgo biloba, and other herbal extracts have a positive effect on cognitive function. Limited research has shown that dietary factors, such as strawberries and spinach, may effect cognition (Joseph et al., 1998).

Behavioral therapies hold significant promise for the treatment of agitation and behavioral problems manifested in cognitive impairment. Many therapeutic activities have been devised and tested by nurse researchers, including mental stimulation, reminiscence, physical activity, and improvement of sleep. Other allied health fields are making significant contributions to interventions research (Buettner & Greenstein, 1997).

As the incidence of CI rises with the aging of the baby boomer generation, more research is being conducted. Obtaining access to this information can be done through the a variety of organizations and web sites. A sampling of useful internet sites include: *www.alz.org* (Alzheimer's Association); *www.alzheimers.org* (National Institute of Health and Aging); *www.alzheimers.com* (public information site); and *www.mednwh.unimelb.edu.au* (National Ageing Research Institute, Australia).

MEREDITH ROWE

ALZHEIMER'S DISEASE

Alzheimer's disease (AD) is the most common form of the dementias, a group of illnesses that affect the brain, eventually resulting in death. Alzheimer's disease is a progressive neurological disorder that proceeds in stages over months or years and gradually destroys reason, memory, judgment, language, and functional ability, according to the Agency for Health Care Policy and Research Practice Guidelines (Costa, Williams, Somerfield, et al., 1996). Although cognitive impairment is a major symptom, changes in mood and personality often occur. In the early stages of the illness, AD is sometimes confused with delirium (an acute reversible mental confusion) or psychiatric depression; both conditions occur in older adults. Depression may be an early part of AD, when the individual is aware of a decline from previous level of competence and is having multiple memory problems.

Alzheimer's disease is characterized by an accumulation of cortical neuritic plaques and neurofibrillary tangles in excess of those found in normal aged persons (Berg, 1994) and can be diagnosed accurately only by brain biopsy or autopsy. Thus, most cases are diagnosed as probable AD. Computerized tomography is sometime used to show changes in the size and shape of the brain, which may indicate probable AD but is not a definite measure. Because of insufficient knowledge about the illness, criteria for probable AD have been developed only recently. These criteria are found in the *Diagnostic and Statistical Manual of Mental Disorders* (DSM-IIIR).

Approximately 4 million people are diagnosed with dementia of the Alzheimer's type, formerly thought to be a presenile disease. Its prevalence increases as individuals reach old age. It is estimated that 20% of those 80 and over can be expected to develop AD (Dungee-Anderson & Beckett, 1992). The diagnosis of early AD is based on mental status exams and changes in behavior rather than by laboratory instruments. Alzheimer's disease continues to baffle the health professions although much light has been shed on the illness since it was discovered in 1920 by the German physician Alois Alzheimer. In early assessment of the illness, differentiation must be made between AD and delirium and between AD and depression so that proper counseling can be established. Medications that may cause symptoms of cognitive impairment also need assessment.

Delirium is an acute reversible organic brain syndrome and a treatable medical condition. It is a disease that affects the memory and is common in older people with acute and chronic illnesses. Depression is a psychological reaction, an altered mood state usually activated by a serious loss of self-esteem and negative self-image. Depression occurring in older adults is frequently related to rapid and constant losses among elderly persons.

Dementia, on the other hand, is a chronic irreversible brain syndrome that results from the death of brain cells. Each of the three conditions may present as the other, or they may coexist.

Quality-of-Life Issues

Quality-of-life issues have been raised for persons with AD because of the progressive decline that occurs in several stages. Reissberg (1984) has identified nine different stages of the disease process. Thus, early identification of AD is extremely critical for planning quality care. Once the diagnosis of probable AD has been established, the question arises as to what type of care is needed. The AD patient may require minimal care in the early stages, but the need for care escalates as the individual experiences increased cognitive impairment. As the disease progresses, the quality of life changes, independent self-functions decrease, and the individual becomes totally dependent on caregivers. Loss of control of body functions and the inability to carry out the activities of daily living require continuous attention from caregivers, who are often family members.

Unfortunately, the direct care of the AD patient affects the quality of life of the caregiver and of family members who are forced to provide informal caregiving services. The term "sandwich generation" has been used to describe the plight of middle-aged women who are sometimes caregivers to parents with AD at the same time that they are caregivers to their children. These caregivers often need help to determine how best to care for their relatives with AD and how not to neglect their own health. Studies have shown that there is increased morbidity and mortality among caregivers of persons with AD (George & Gwyther, 1986).

The care of persons with AD has a major impact on nursing practice. Special care needs of dementia patients require appropriate nursing interventions at different stages of decline and for individual variation in symptomatology. The task is often difficult when the major goal is to maintain as much quality of life as possible for the patient. There is no known cure for AD, and therefore it is a major challenge for health care professionals. The emotional component that accompanies the illness affects formal caregivers as well as persons with AD and their families. The degenerative nature of the disease, together with the cognitive and functional impairment, requires an increasing amount of caregiving time. Determining the distinctions between stages of dementia is necessary for planning nursing interventions. Nursing care for the AD patient begins with accurate assessment, diagnosis of the stages, expected outcomes, care planning and implementation, and evaluation of effective interventions.

Nursing practice with patients who have AD is a field that is ripe for nurse researchers. Nursing care is the single mode of treatment for the disease even though a few drugs for improving memory are on the market. There is a particular need to develop specific models of care for this complex illness. Watson's (1988) nursing model of human care is one example of a framework that provides a conceptual basis for provision of nursing care to AD patients and their families. The nursing activity is intentional and based on a knowledge of the changing needs of the person with AD. The nurse is a key part of the human transaction and is equally important in the relationship with the family caregiver. Watson's model is based on a humanistic view of the individual.

Because of the severe mental impairment and functional decline manifested by the disease, nursing research is sorely needed to deliver competent nursing care to the AD patient. Patients need help with bathing, feeding, toileting, dressing, mobility, and communications, and the caregiver needs social support as well as help to plan care and to utilize community services. One problem is the tendency of AD patients to develop behavior problems (Wykle & Morris, 1994). In research studies of caregivers, behavior problems are listed most often as major stress inducers for the caregiver. Acting out behavior is sometimes related to excitement, inability to remember faces, and strange environments. Behavior problems such as wandering or actions brought about by delusions, disorientation, and communication problems, vary in these individuals depending on the disease course.

Part of the nursing assessment should include a psychiatric evaluation simply because AD patients often have high levels of anxiety and depression. The nursing practice theory of progressively lower stimuli therapy (PLST), developed by Buckwalter (1989), is designed to provide a nonstimulating environment that will cause less catastrophic behavior reactions. Recently, there has been a trend toward designing special care units for AD patients who are placed in a nursing home or hospital. These special care settings take into consideration the individual needs of the client as well as the type of staffing pattern necessary to provide quality care and maintain a safe environment. There is also a trend toward using alternative methods of intervention, such as massage therapy and horticulture therapy. Nevertheless, there is still much that is unknown about AD, its manifestations, and effective nursing interventions. This disease that profoundly affects older adults and their quality of life is a high priority for nursing outcome research.

May L. Wykle
Gwi-Ryung Son

See also:

ALZHEIMER'S DISASE: SPECIAL CARE UNITS IN LONG-TERM CARE

CAREGIVER
COGNITIVE DISORDERS
COGNITIVE IMPAIRMENT
DEPRESSION AMONG OLDER ADULTS
NEUROBEHAVIORAL DISTURBANCES OF THE OLDER ADULT:
  DELERIUM AND DEMENTIA

CEREBROVASCULAR DISORDERS

The term *cerebrovascular status* was first attached to nursing research regarding patients with critical neurological conditions in 1984 by L. Claire Parsons at the University of Virginia (Parsons & Wilson, 1984). It appropriately captures the underlying dynamics and craniocerebral mechanisms that threaten neuronal integrity in patients with a variety of acute intracranial disorders.

Cerebrovascular status broadly encompasses the relationships among the components of the intracranial system: blood, brain, and cerebrospinal fluid. In such conditions as acute head injury and hemorrhagic stroke, trauma to brain tissues sets in motion a cascade of events that may create local ischemia as well as compensatory vasodilation of large areas of the brain to maintain adequate overall cerebral perfusion. If intracranial pressure begins to rise due to the increase in blood volume or if brain hemorrhage acts as a mass, cerebrospinal fluid may be moved into the spinal sac to attempt to keep cerebrospinal fluid and tissue pressure from rising. Ordinarily, changes in systemic blood pressure do not change local cerebral perfusion pressure because of a phenomenon called autoregulation. However, in the injured brain, autoregulation may fail and allow cerebral perfusion pressure to rise and fall with systemic blood pressure. Conversely, in acute conditions such as ischemic stroke, major arterial vessels of the brain may receive too little blood, creating ischemia distal to that artery and setting in motion the same injury cascade as with direct brain trauma.

Clinical nursing research with people who have either acute or chronic effects of cerebrovascular disorders has involved (a) protection from effects of secondary insults such as hypoxia, reduced perfusion pressure, and environmental triggers to these events and (b) restoration and rehabilitation following the primary effects of brain injury and stroke. Reviews of nursing research regarding patients with neurological disorders have shown that essentially no nursing research was done until the mid-1960s and that the body of literature has grown only since the 1980s (DiIorio, 1990). The majority of this research focused on critically ill patients with acute cerebrovascular problems. A smaller body of research has involved issues related to restoration and rehabilitation of people with chronic effects of cerebrovascular damage. That body of research also has grown since the 1980s but not nearly to the extent of the acute care– and trauma-focused research.

Despite the growing number of research studies in the area, relatively few nurse investigators have sustained programs of research in either acute or chronic areas of cerebrovascular problems. The only sustained programs in cerebrovascular responses of patients with increased intracranial pressure (ICP) to nursing interventions have been the groups of Dr. Pamela Mitchell, University of Washington; Drs. Ellen Rudy and Mary Kerr, University of Pittsburgh; and Dr. Claire Parsons and Lee Crosby, University of Arizona (see, e.g., Crosby & Parsons, 1992; Kerr, Rudy, Brucia, & Stone, 1993; Mitchell, Kirkness, Burr, March, & Newell, in press). Margo Hugo (1992) of South Africa is the only investigator who has published a series of studies in the area of nursing interventions and ICP outside the United States.

In contrast, long-term care programs in restoration and rehabilitation of people with cerebrovascular problems have been mostly in Scandinavia, in the work of Elisabeth Hamrin and Astrid Norberg with patients recovering from stroke and those with neurodegenerative diseases. Deborah Webb of Baylor built a program of systems of care to enhance recovery of stroke patients. Dr. Margaret Kelly-Hayes is a nurse investigator who has been active in the longitudinal Framingham study regarding epidemiology of stroke.

The largest body of studies has examined the effects of various bedside nursing care activities on ICP and cerebral perfusion pressure, indirect indices of the adequacy of perfusion to brain tissues. Extension, flexion, and rotation of the neck is the only activity that uniformly increased ICP and often decreased cerebral perfusion pressure. Other activities studied, such as being suctioned, being repositioned, having the head of the bed elevated, and being subjected to painful procedures and assessments showed highly individualized patient responses. Current research is attempting to identify better predictors regarding which patients are apt to respond adversely to these common nursing care activities. These patients are said to have the nursing diagnosis of decreased adaptive capacity, intracranial. They may be identified by abnormal intracranial waveform (elevated P_2 waveform), increased amplitude of waveforms, or large and sustained increase in intracranial pressure to stimuli. Level of ICP does not appear to be a good predictor (Mitchell, Kirkness, Burr, et al., in press).

The studies regarding recovery and rehabilitation from acute stroke are sufficiently scattered in focus to preclude a summary of findings. Studies continue in Scandinavia and the United States to determine the effect of interdisciplinary stroke care teams on functional outcomes and costs

(Webb, Fayad, Wilbur, Thomas, & Brass, 1995). Thus far the evidence is mixed, with the positive effects on functional outcomes often confounded by bias in selection of experimental and control groups. The issues of specific therapy versus natural recovery in ameliorating such impacts as altered communication, mobility, and the like are still unresolved despite decades of research in a variety of disciplines.

The advent of thrombolytic therapy to reverse stroke in progress has reenergized public and professional interest in stroke prevention and early treatment. One hopes to see an active nursing research agenda in such areas as community interventions for stroke prevention as well as interventions designed to reduce secondary brain injury in both cerebrovascular trauma and completed stroke.

PAMELA H. MITCHELL

See also:
APHASIA
COGNITIVE DISORDERS
COGNITIVE IMPAIRMENT
CRITICAL CARE NURSING

COGNITIVE DISORDERS

Cognition has been defined as the activity of knowing: the acquisition, organization, and use of knowledge. All of our mental abilities—perceiving, remembering, and reasoning—are organized into a complex system with the overall function of cognition. Other descriptions refer to the mental processes of comprehension, memory, judgment, and reasoning, as opposed to emotional processes (McDougall, 1990). These definitions provide variability in terminology and represent the paradigms or theories that guide research. Therefore, cognition is defined as the supraordinate construct that includes all mental operations, such as attention span, concentration, and memory. The literature is vast in this area because work occurring simultaneously in gerontology, neuroscience, nursing, psychiatry, and rehabilitation does not always cross over or interrelate.

The theories of adult cognition, such as genetic-epistemological (represented by Piaget), information processing (represented by the computer), psychoanalytic (represented by Freudian analysis), postformal (represented by dialectics), and psychometric (represented by intelligence testing), denote different disciplines and methods of research that are not always appropriate for application to clinical research and practice (Rybash,

Hoyer, & Roodin, 1986). There is substantial knowledge development on 14 nursing diagnoses formulated for cognition, based on the work of the North American Nursing Diagnosis Association. They include altered thought processes, sensory/perceptual alterations, potential for injury, self-care deficit, knowledge deficit, altered growth and development, altered sexuality patterns, altered parenting, altered role performance, impaired adjustment, self-esteem disturbance, social isolation, ineffective family coping, and altered family process.

The generic terms *confusion* and *disorientation* are global and insensitive for determining the specific cognitive processes diminished or compromised. A content analysis of cognitive impairment research was implemented, and the following 11 screening instruments were found to be of most use in clinical practice: the Dementia Assessment Inventory (DAT), Brief Cognitive Rating Scale (BCRS), Blessed Dementia Scale (BDS), Cognitive Capacity Screening Examination (CCSE), Cognitive Levels Scale (CLS), Function Reason Orientation Memory Arithmetic Judgment Emotion (FROMAJE), Global Deterioration Scale (GDS), Mini-Mental State Exam (MMSE), Mental Status Examination (MSE), Clinical Dementia Rating (CDR), and the Short Portable Mental Status Questionnaire (SPMSQ) (McDougall, 1990).

Screening instruments are best suited to measure the presence, absence, and severity of impairment. Older adults in various settings should be routinely screened for cognitive function and mental status by clinicians and health care providers. Recommendations from research and practice are specific. Because cognitive impairment often goes undetected in nonpsychiatric settings, routine screening of older medical patients is recommended. Selection of a screening instrument must be discriminating and based on a clearly understood purpose, that is, cognitive function, mental status, or combinations of those categories.

Screening instruments were designed to measure the presence, absence, and severity of cognitive impairment. Typically, adults with less than an eighth-grade education may be incorrectly identified as cognitively impaired. Screening instruments were never designed to be the sole measure of cognitive function or mental status. Data from 1983 show that a reduction in length of stay by 1 day through accurate assessment of cognitive function would save between $1 and $2 billion each year (Levkoff, Besdine, & Wetle, 1986). The common types of cognitive disorders will be defined for heuristic purposes.

Cognitive impairment is a term describing a disturbance in cognitive functioning. Cognitive functioning is a broad construct that includes a number of categories: attention span, concentration, intelligence, judgment, learning ability, memory, orientation, perception, problem solving, psychomotor ability, reaction time, and social intactness. The assessment of cognitive functioning need not include all of these dimensions, but typical screening instruments such as the MMSE include many of them and give the clinician and researcher a gross indication of whether cognitive impairment is present. Assessment of cognitive function and a complete mental status examination are essential components in the diagnosis of delirium, dementia, and pseudodementia (McDougall, 1995).

Alzheimer's disease is a progressive disorder marked by dementia and the accumulation of cortical neuritic plaques and neurofibrillary tangles in excess of those found in normal aging. The only accurate method of diagnosing Alzheimer's disease is to perform a brain biopsy or autopsy (National Institute of Neurological and Communicative Disorders and Stroke [NINCDS]–Alzheimer's Disease and Related Disorders Association [ADRDA], 1985). Without either of these two methods, the diagnosis is "possible" Alzheimer's disease. Criteria for the clinical diagnosis of Alzheimer's disease were developed only in 1984 (McKhann, Drachman, Folstein, et al., 1984), and they are not fully operational because of insufficient knowledge about the disease. The criteria are compatible with the current *Diagnostic and Statistical Manual of Mental Disorders* and the *International Classification of Diseases.*

The criteria for the diagnosis of probable, possible, and definite Alzheimer's disease are presented by McKhann and colleagues (1984). Probable Alzheimer's disease can be clinically diagnosed if there is a typical insidious onset of dementia with progression and if there are no other systemic or brain diseases that could account for the progressive memory loss and other cognitive deficits. Excludable disorders include drug intoxication, manic-depressive disorder, multiinfarct dementia, and Parkinson's disease. Examples of other disorders that may cause dementia include thyroid disease, vitamin B_{12} deficiency, luetic brain disease and other chronic infections of the nervous system, subdural hematoma, occult hydrocephalus, Huntington's disease, Creutzfeldt-Jakob disease, and brain tumors. There are numerous other disorders causing or simulating dementia that have not been mentioned (see Office of Technology Assessment, 1987).

The diagnosis of dementia cannot be made if delirium is present. Although the official nomenclature for the syndrome is delirium, it has been given many other names: acute confusional state, acute brain syndrome, confusion, metabolic encephalopathy, and toxic psychosis. Delirium is a transient mental disorder with a relatively rapid onset, a course that typically fluctuates, and a brief duration. The essential features of delirium are (1) reduced ability to maintain attention to external stimuli and to appropriately shift attention to new external stimuli and (2) disorganized thinking, as manifested by rambling, irrelevant, or incoherent speech. There is sensory misperception, a disordered stream of thought, and difficulty in shifting, focusing, and sustaining attention to both external and internal stimuli. Irrelevant stimuli can easily distract the delirious individual. Also common are perceptual disturbances that result in misinterpretations, illusions, and hallucinations. In addition, disturbances of sleep-wakefulness and psychomotor activity are present. Nurse investigators have contributed to understanding the phenomena of concern to gerontology nurses caring for patients with cognitive disorders.

Sundown syndrome is a common behavioral problem manifested in patients with cognitive impairments and resembles delirium. Nurses often describe it as the agitation, restlessness, confusion, and wandering behavior of older adults when the sun goes down. Risk factors that have been identified for sundown syndrome in the elderly include physiological factors, such as dehydration, mental impairment, frequent night awakening for nursing care, dementia, and urine odor, and psychosocial factors, such as being in a room less than 1 month, recent admission to facility, and higher evening levels of confusion (Evans, 1987).

This term *confusion* is used by nursing to describe general affect and behaviors of patients; however, it is not specific and appears to have a great deal in common with delirium. The issue seems to be whether the terminology belongs to another discipline (Foreman, 1993). Assessment of behavior and discrimination of terms are important for planning appropriate nursing care of patients with cognitive disorders.

Graham McDougall

See also:
ALZHEIMER'S DISEASE
COGNITIVE IMPAIRMENT

COGNITIVE IMPAIRMENT

Although most older adults live without cognitive difficulties, an estimated 15% of those over 65 have cognitive impairment. Most at risk are the oldest, those over 85, currently the fastest-growing segment of the population (Abrams, Beers, Berkow, & Fletcher, 1995). As more aged live longer, the number of older adults with cognitive impairments who seek healthcare is expected to rise dramatically. These increasing numbers pose a significant public health problem with major implications for morbidity and mortality, quality of life, and healthcare costs for older adults and their families.

Cognitive impairment, or confusion, can result from a number of causes. Dementia and delirium are the most common. Dementia is a degenerative disease of the brain that causes cognitive, functional, and affective losses that are progressive, severe, and irreversible (Reisberg, Ferris, & deLeon, 1982). Alzheimer's disease (AD) is the most common type of dementia. Prevalence rates vary widely—from 11% in people over 65 years old to an estimated 47% in people over 85, which is the population most at risk for AD (D. A. Evans et al., 1990). AD has an insidious onset and is difficult to diagnose in its early stages, often resulting in underrecognition and underreporting of the disease.

AD primarily involves the cerebral cortex of the brain, the region responsible for reason, language, judgment, and personality. Cognitive symptoms include impairments in orientation, memory, language, and judgment; visuospatial changes; and impairment of executive function, such as planning, organizing, and abstracting. Because of cognitive losses, behavioral symptoms appear, such as wandering, disruptive verbalizations, aggression, or apathy. Adverse affect (mood) and functional symptoms are also results of AD. Affective symptoms include irritability, labile mood, or apathy. Function gradually deteriorates in the later stages of AD until the impaired person requires extensive assistance in all aspects of self-care, including decision making. AD and vascular dementia (dementia from cardiovascular causes) are the most common types of dementia. Other types—including Parkinson's dementia, Huntington's chorea, and Pick's disease—account for approximately 15% of dementias.

Delirium, an acute confusional state, is the second most common cause of cognitive impairment in older adults. In contrast to the insidious onset of dementia, delirium occurs suddenly (within hours or days) and heralds an underlying biophysical disorder. The cardinal symptom of delirium is a reduced level of consciousness, manifested by an inability to focus, sustain, or shift attention. Perceptual disturbances (illusions, delusions, hallucinations) and mood disturbances (labile mood, irritability, depression, or euphoria) typically occur. The incidence (new onset during hospitalization) of delirium ranges from 4% to 53.2%. Hospital staff often fail to recognize delirium, or misdiagnose it as dementia or depression. Delirium is potentially reversible if the underlying etiology is recognized and treated. Since prognosis depends on rapid detection, evaluation, and treatment, a nurse's expertise in assessment and treatment is critical (Milisen, Foreman, Godderis, Abraham, & Broos, 1998).

Neuropsychiatric disorders may also impair cognition, mood, or function in the elderly. Unipolar depression is the most common mood disorder in the elderly. Depression is also often unrecognized or misdiagnosed in the elderly. Symptoms of depression may include poor cognitive performance, sleep disturbances, and lack of interest in activities—symptoms that often occur in people with dementia. Population studies of older adults have reported prevalence rates for depression of 1.4–4.1%. Among people with irreversible dementias, such as AD or vascular dementia, estimates rise sharply, to 20%–25% (Meyers & Bruce, 1998). Suicide is the most serious consequence of depression, and older white males have the highest suicide rate of any age group in the United States. Less common psychiatric illnesses, such as delusional disorder, bipolar disorder, anxiety disorders, and schizophrenia—may coexist in elderly clients, often remaining unrecognized or undertreated.

Psychotic symptoms (delusions and hallucinations) may be mistaken for dementia. Medical conditions or medications may obscure psychotic symptoms. Several conditions predispose the elderly to psychotic symptoms; these conditions include comorbid physical illnesses, social isolation, sensory deficits, cognitive changes, polypharmacy, and substance abuse. Illusions (misperceptions about reality), delusions, and hallucinations are common in both dementia and delirium. Institutionalized elderly have the highest prevalence of psychiatric disorders; it is estimated that as many as 80%–90% have at least one psychiatric diagnosis. Like physical illnesses, psychiatric illnesses may present in an atypical fashion in the elderly. Careful evaluation of recent and past symptoms, including psychiatric symptoms, is critical in establishing the causes of cognitive or mood impairments.

The frequency of multiple comorbidities, as well as the complex interplay of cognition, mood, behavior, and function, makes assessment of cognitive impairment in older adults an ongoing challenge. Comprehensive assessment begins with a thorough history and physical examination to establish all of the possible causes for impairments. Researchers have developed several screening tools to assess cognition, but each of the tools assesses only specific cognitive domains, such as memory or visuospatial changes (clock drawing test). The Mini-Mental State Examination (MMSE) (Folstein, Folstein, & McHugh, 1975) is the tool most widely used to assess for delirium and dementia in geriatric populations. The MMSE is an excellent screening tool to evaluate changes in cognition over time, but several disadvantages persist. Five to twenty minutes are typically required to administer the tests. Pain, fatigue, sensory deficits, poor language skills, and altered consciousness make testing difficult and render the findings hard to interpret. Short cognitive-screening tests are not diagnostic tools, the results are tentative, and they must be compared to the broader findings of the comprehensive history and physical examination.

Mood disorders and other neuropsychiatric disorders in the elderly often impair cognitive function, so a careful evaluation of mood is important. Screening tools have been developed for depression and anxiety, but any suspicion or overt symptoms of a mood disorder need to be further evaluated or referred to a mental-health practitioner. Evaluation of function and behavior are vital components of any assessment of cognition. Evaluation of function includes assessment of instrumental activities of living (shopping, managing finances, cooking) and activities of daily living (continence, eating, bathing). Standardized measures of function (Katz, Ford, Moskowitz, Jackson, & Jaffee, 1963) and behavior (Cohen-Mansfield, 1999) are most commonly used in evaluation of institutionalized elderly, or in the ongoing evaluation of people with memory impairments in the community. A careful history from a caregiver of the impaired person's functioning abilities and behavioral symptoms typically suffices for diagnostic and treatment purposes. In the case of AD, a diagnosis based on a comprehensive history and physical has been found to be 85%–90% accurate when compared to autopsy findings.

Biomedical researchers are currently exploring the neurobiological mechanisms of the brain to understand the causes of neurocognitive disorders. Many neurotransmitters are depleted in the brains of people with AD. Acetylcholine, critical for memory, is among these depleted neurotransmitters. Acetylcholinesterase inhibitors, a new class of drugs for cognition, are postulated to work by prolonging the breakdown of acetylcholine at the synapse, thus delaying the onset of cognitive symptoms. Other neurotransmitters found to be deficient are serotonin, somatostatin, and norepinephrine, the deficiency of which is believed to contribute to the sensory disturbances, aggressive behavior, and neuron death seen with dementia. Genetic research has discovered evidence of a link between AD and genes on three chromosomes—14, 19, and 21. Scientists have also identified beta amyloid plaques in the brain. These neurofibrillary tangles, containing a protein fragment called beta amyloid, are believed to be responsible for the brain damage in AD. Research exploring the role of antioxidants, calcium, anti-inflammatory drugs, and estrogens is ongoing. Researchers hope to discover the causes of and cure for dementia and other neurocognitive disorders (National Institute on Aging, 1999).

While biomedical researchers continue to search for more effective treatments and possible cures, extensive research is being done to minimize the adverse consequences of the behavioral and functional symptoms of cognitive impairment. Behavioral disturbances contribute significantly to morbidity, institutionalization, and mortality of impaired adults. Functional and behavioral symptoms are frequently reported to be the most troublesome for families and nursing staff to manage. Researchers are attempting to identify the factors that cause or worsen disturbing behavioral symptoms, such as aggression or disruptive vocalizations (Cohen-Mansfield & Werner, 1998a; Sloane et al., 1997). Many factors make it difficult to study behavioral symptoms. Researchers do not agree about what constitutes a problem behavior symptom or how to define it. People who assess behaviors—family, staff, and researchers—may give different ratings for the same behavior. The time of assessment is important—some behavioral symptoms are worse in the evening (sundowning). Without reliable and accurate measurement, it remains difficult to track treatment interventions and monitor the effects of pharmacologic and behavioral interventions.

The treatment of behavioral symptoms of confusional states remains predominantly pharmacologic. Antipsychotics, such as Haldol, are the most commonly used pharmacologic agents. Benzodiazepines are also commonly used, but their association with falls and sedation in the elderly limits their usefulness to the short term. Newer antipsychotic medications (e.g., Risperdal) have fewer side effects, including fewer extrapyramidal symptoms, but use of these drugs in older adults with multiple comorbidities and polypharmacy continues to pose significant clinical challenges. Non-pharmacologic behavioral interventions are becoming more common. Although there is little empirical evidence to determine which strategies have produced the most favorable outcomes, many researchers and clinicians are optimistic based on early findings. Forbes (1998), in an extensive review of the literature of behavioral management strategies, found that attention-focusing programs, functional skills training, music, and pet therapy were among the most successful strategies reported. Overall, these strategies improved social interaction, self-care abilities, day/night disturbances, and wandering in confused older adults.

In advanced stages of dementia, persons with AD need extensive assistance with self-care. However, aggression or delusions often cause resistance to care. Most studies of maintaining or improving self-care abilities in AD patients have been small or have been practice-based. In a study of 90 cognitively impaired nursing home residents, nursing staff used behavioral strategies to improve independent dressing self-care. Significant improvements in dressing ability, without clinically significant increases in staff time, resulted (Beck et al., 1997).

Another extensive area of research is exploring the caregiving of persons with cognitive impairments. Most older adults with cognitive impairments live in the community, and an estimated 80%–90% of their care is provided by family. Caregiving research has been overwhelmingly quantitative, and has been concerned primarily with the difficulties that families experience in caregiving. Many caregivers report negative outcomes to themselves as a result of caregiving, including poorer physical health and psychological morbidities, especially depression. Some caregivers have reported positive outcomes for themselves as a result of caregiving, including finding purpose in life (a sense of meaning), renewed affection, and self-acceptance (Farran,

Keane-Hagerty, Salloway, Kupferer, & Wilken, 1991; Kramer, 1997; Quayhagen & Quayhagen, 1996). Researchers are investigating ways to alleviate the distress of at-risk caregivers, thereby improving the well-being of both the family caregiver and the impaired older adult (Chang, 1999; Mittleman et al., 1995).

Researchers continue to work in diverse areas that promise to improve care of confused older adults. These diverse areas include: pain management, recognition and management of delirium, dementia special-care units, elder abuse, nutrition, ethics, advance directives, holistic therapies (therapeutic touch, massage), interdisciplinary team training, physical restraint reduction, and environmental design. Advances in these areas offer tremendous hope in improving the quality of life for older persons with cognitive impairments and their families.

The future holds many challenges for nurses who care for older adults. Older adults are extremely diverse and complex compared to younger persons. Older adults are more likely to have biophysical conditions, and they are more likely to have a marked dissimilarity in the presentation of their physical and psychiatric disorders. Today, more that ever, nurses need to increase their gerontological expertise. Knowledge about cognition and its relationship to the well-being of individuals and their families is rapidly expanding. As the challenge of properly using that knowledge emerges, nurses need to be ready to meet it head-on.

MARY SHELKEY

See also:
  ALZHEIMER'S DISEASE
  COGNITIVE DISORDERS

COGNITIVE INTERVENTIONS

Cognitive interventions are designed to change some aspect of cognitive function, such as attention, concentration, or memory. An intervention may be defined as a programmatic attempt at altering the course of life-span development. Interventions may be classified as concrete technologies involving such parameters as the goal: enrichment, prevention, or alleviation; the target behavior: cognition, social interactions, or attitudes; the setting: family, classroom, community, or hospital; and the mechanism: training-practice, psychotherapy, or health delivery (Baltes & Danish, 1980). These interventions may be applied to many patient or client populations such as the elderly in long-term care and young head-injured individuals in rehabilitation settings. (See Psychosocial Interventions.)

The body of research literature or data-based publications is stronger in the specialty of gerontology. The burgeoning elderly population of the United States, some 31.6 million people as estimated by the 1989 census, represents one of the biggest challenges facing the nation today in health care. Adults 55 years of age and older complain of memory problems frequently. General or specific incidents of forgetting are often used by older adults to interpret the effectiveness of their memory ability and awareness. The treatment for negative self-evaluation of memory in normal, healthy elderly persons takes two forms. The most frequent intervention is simply to tell the individual, "Don't worry, there is nothing wrong with you." This advice is rarely heeded, and the person continues to seek help or silently remains concerned.

The second approach is for the older adult to attend memory training programs. Memory training programs designed for older adults operate on two basic assumptions: (a) older adults with less than optimal performance will benefit from intense exposure to memory aids, and (b) participation in training will increase the use of these memory aids. The aim of memory training is to teach older adults to use internal memory strategies such as elaboration and rehearsal and external strategies such as calendars and lists to enhance their remembering.

A review of 39 published studies of memory training with older adults documented that the elderly may improve their memory performance on episodic memory tasks (Verhaeghen, Marcoen, & Goossens, 1992). The training was most effective when carried out in groups, when subjects were younger, when sessions were relatively short (less than 90 minutes), and when pretraining was provided in imagery or relaxation techniques. These conclusions are valid only for memory performance on classical episodic memory tasks; however, nothing can be inferred about the impact of memory training on everyday memory performance or on metamemory (memory awareness). More research is needed in this area, and older adults should be encouraged to continue learning. Specific examples of cognitive interventions designed to improve cognitive function are presented as prototypes.

Memory Interventions

In the community, Dellefield and McDougall (1996) designed a study to test the effects of a 2-week, four-session group intervention with healthy older adults to increase memory self-efficacy and memory performance. A total of 145 community-dwelling older adults with an average age of 71 years participated in the study, which was based on Bandura's self-efficacy theory. The intervention significantly increased both memory self-efficacy and memory performance in the treatment group. In addition, the treatment group's perception of control in memory-demanding situations was strengthened, and their perception of negative changes in memory over time was diminished. The control group experienced a significant decline in memory self-efficacy over time. Memory performance was not significantly related to memory self-efficacy. Those individuals with depression had significantly lower memory self-efficacy scores than did those without depression; however, there was no difference in memory performance between depressed and nondepressed subjects. From the posttest to the follow-up period, depressed subjects receiving the intervention showed a significant decrease in memory self-efficacy, whereas nondepressed subjects showed no change.

Interventions for Cognitive Impairment

The International Classification of Impairments, Disabilities, and Handicaps (ICIDH) uses the three conceptual levels of impairment, disability, and handicap to facilitate the collection and use of data (Brown, 1993). Handicap is defined by the World Health Organization (WHO) as a disadvantage that limits or prevents fulfillment of a role that is normal and depends on age, gender, and social and cultural factors. Both the nature and extent of handicap are important to assess within the framework of the Americans With Disabilities Act and the WHO model of disablement. Although rehabilitation professionals have developed numerous objective measures of cognitive disability, they have not produced subjective measures of handicap. The framework of handicap is useful to guide these interventions.

An increasing proportion of the elderly in the Unites States will live or reside in nursing homes during their life span. The nation's nursing home population grew by 24.2% in the 10-year period from 1980 to 1990 as reported in a recent 1990 Census Bureau report. Of the 500,000 to 600,000 individuals who suffer from strokes annually, most are older adults, with 90% over age 55 and 80% over age 65. Many of these individuals will most likely spend time in nursing homes.

Rosswurm (1991) developed an attention-focusing program to stimulate perceptual and cognitive processing, improve functional performance, and increase participation in group activities in three skilled nursing facilities. The findings showed that there were significant improvements in perceptual processing of information and in the social interactions of the persons in the attention-focusing group. Abraham, Neundorfer, and Currie (1992) implemented a study to test the effects of three cognitive-behavioral group interventions on cognition and depression in nursing home residents. Based on Beck's model of cognitive therapy, the 24-week interventions failed to reduce depression, hopelessness, or increase life satisfaction scores in the residents; however, they improved overall cognitive function. In another study of nursing home residents with severe cognitive impairment and behavior disturbances, Goddaer and Abraham (1994) used relaxing music with a slow tempo and an unpredictable rhythm to reduce agitation. The music had a therapeutic effect on the negative behaviors and significantly reduced agitation as well as exhibition of physical and verbal agitated behaviors.

Nursing has developed a body of knowledge related to the design, implementation, and testing of psychosocial and psychoeducational interventions that is broader in perspective than cognitive interventions (see Psychosocial Interventions).

GRAHAM McDOUGALL

See also:
CEREBROVASCULAR DISORDERS
COGNITIVE DISORDERS
COGNITIVE IMPAIRMENT
FUNCTIONAL HEALTH
GERONTOLOGIC CARE
MUSIC THERAPY

DEMENTIA CARE

Implications for Research

The nursing care of persons with dementia, historically a process of trial and error (Hall & Buckwalter, 1987), has recently become the basis for the development of *middle-range theories* in nursing. These theories focus on a limited number of variables, are more amenable to empirical testing, and are positioned between grand theories and microtheories embodied in care procedures (Fitzpatrick & Whall, 1996). Utilizing the criteria of publication and dissemination within nursing, the following middle-range theories were selected for review: need-driven, dementia-compromised behavior (Algas et al., 1996), progressively lowered stress threshold (PLST)

(Hall & Buckwalter, 1987), individualized care for frail elders (Happ, Williams, Strumpf, & Berger, 1996), and decision-making process for level of assistance with activities of daily living (Beck, Heacock, Rapp, & Mercer, 1993). In addition, several other theories are cited but not reviewed due to space limitations.

Need-Driven, Dementia-Compromised Behavior

The need-driven, dementia-compromised behavior approach views the person with dementia as experiencing an unmet need or goal that results in need-driven behaviors such as aggression, wandering, or disturbing vocalizations. These behaviors reflect the interaction of salient background and proximal factors found either within the person or in his or her immediate environment or both. Background variables include neurological, cognitive, health status, and psychosocial factors. Proximal factors include personal characteristics and the physical and social environment. Need-driven, dementia-compromised behavior is evaluated on dimensions of frequency and duration. Nursing's role is to identify those at risk and to intervene with strategies under various sets of environmental circumstances. The theory has been applied to the study of aggression by Whall and to the study of wandering by Algase. Research efforts are focused on the identification of variables common to and different from each of the disturbing behaviors and the application of linear modeling to further build the theory.

Progressively Lowered Stress Threshold

Hall and Buckwalter's (1987) framework views the person with dementia as experiencing baseline anxious and dysfunctional states throughout the course of the disease. Anxious behavior occurs during stress, and if stress continues, dysfunctional states such as panic occur. Six principles guide nursing care: (a) maximize the level of safe function by supporting all areas of loss in a prosthetic manner, (b) provide unconditional positive regard, (c) use behaviors indicating anxiety to determine limits of stimuli and activity, (d) teach caregivers to "listen" and evaluate verbal and nonverbal responses, (e) modify environment to support losses and enhance safety, and (f) provide education, support, care, and problem solving for caregivers. Evaluation research at 13 long-term care facilities has utilized such designs as pre- and posttests and longitudinal experimental approaches. Research has also identified behavioral characteristics and interventions for four types of wandering and has led to the classification of factors influencing dysfunctional behavior.

Individualized Care for Frail Elders

The individualized care for frail elders approach (Happ, Williams, Strumpf, & Berger, 1996) embodies an interdisciplinary approach to care. It emphasizes four critical attributes: (a) knowing the person (life story and patterns of response), (b) the relationship (staff continuity and reciprocity), (c) choice (decision making and risk taking), and (d) resident participation (daily planning). Evans's (1996) cross-cultural observations in four European countries supported these propositions and delineated three factors that contributed to individualized care: congruent societal and health care values, commonalties of patient needs in all settings, and primacy of caring through knowing the person. Rowles and Dallas (1996) found that family involvement in nursing home decision making served to individualize care and provided a continuing link to the residents' personal history and preferences. Several studies supported cost-effectiveness linked to lowered medication costs and staff turnover. Further research concerning resident outcomes and refinements in definitions, goals, and critical attributes is indicated.

Decision-Making Process for Level of Assistance With Activities of Daily Living

This algorithmic framework (Beck, Heacock, Rapp, & Mercer, 1993) emphasizes that each elder has an individual pattern of cognitive deficits that must be assessed to improve the quality of life and interactions; these include attention deficits, language impairment, sequencing problems, and impaired judgment. Seven levels of assistance are defined: stimulus control, verbal prompt, modeling/gesturing, physical prompt, physical guidance, occasional physical guidance, and complete physical guidance. The decision-making process of prescribing strategies is displayed in a flowchart algorithm that results in selection of the most appropriate level of assistance. The process is based on research to improve dressing behaviors in nursing home residents with cognitive impairment.

A number of nurse scientists have explicated some of the bases for middle-range theory work and have produced instruments to assess demented subjects. Most notable are Tappen and Barry's (1995) Dementia Mood Picture Test, Hurley's Discomfort Scale (Hurley, Volicer, Hanrahan,

Houde, & Volicer, 1992), Ryden's Aggression Scale (Ryden, Bossenmaier, & McLachlen, 1991), and Burgener's Modified Interaction Behavior Measure (Burgener, Jirovec, Murrell, & Barton, 1992). Utilizing decision trees to clarify nursing strategies for disturbing behaviors is an important new approach (Richie, 1996).

The latter decades of this century have been characterized by the designing and examination of middle-range theories and models of dementia care. The nursing approaches described above have been at the forefront of this exploration and provide effective and humane approaches for behavioral disturbance in dementia. As these efforts are supported by multiple programs of research, they hold great promise for more effective dementia care in the decades ahead.

KATHLEEN BYRNE COLLING
ANN L. WHALL

See also:
ALZHEIMER'S DISEASE
COGNITIVE DISORDERS
FAMILY CAREGIVING TO FRAIL ELDERS
FUNCTIONAL HEALTH

MINI-MENTAL STATE EXAMINATION

The Mini-Mental State Examination (MMSE) (Folstein, Folstein, & McHugh, 1975) is a measure frequently used to assess cognitive status. It is almost invariably used by nurse researchers who study ways to improve care for the vulnerable group of people who suffer from dementia of the Alzheimer type (DAT).

The MMSE (Folstein et al., 1975) was developed to be a brief, easy-to-administer clinical evaluation tool, with acceptable reported psychometric properties, to quantitatively assess cognitive status. The MMSE was devised for the serial testing of the cognitive mental state of patients on a neurogeriatric ward. The MMSE consists of nine items that test a range of cognitive skills: orientation; memory; attention; the ability to name objects; the ability to follow verbal and written commands; the ability to write a sentence spontaneously, and the ability to copy two intersecting pentagons.

To enhance cooperation and avoid unpleasant reactions, administration procedures instruct the tester to make the patient comfortable, establish rapport, praise success, and avoid pressing items that the patient finds difficult. The tester scores verbal answers to questions (date, location, immediate recall of three unrelated objects, performing serial sevens, or spelling the word *world* backward, delayed recall of the three objects, names of two common objects, and repetition of a phrase); and assesses the patients' ability to follow a three-stage verbal command, to read and obey a command, to write a spontaneous sentence, and to copy a design. Items are scored and summed and provide a scale total score with a range of 30 (all correct responses) to 0 (no correct responses). Norms exist for determining cognitive capacity, but these need to be interpreted in the context of age and education (Crum, Anthony, Bassett, & Folstein, 1993).

Initial measurement reliability, using two samples and several raters, was adequate for interrater agreement and retest stability (Folstein et al., 1975). Convergent and discriminant validity, as well as sensitivity and specificity, were supported by (a) hypothesized similarities/differences between scores from normal, demented, and depressed subjects with and without cognitive symptoms; (b) clinicians' ratings; and (c) response to treatments. During the last quarter century the MMSE has become almost a gold standard. It has been used to describe subjects for research projects; to provide an estimate of the cognitive capacity of questionably impaired patients (to make treatment and research decisions); and to assess the need for, and/ or the efficacy of cognition-enhancing medications.

The reliability and validity of the MMSE in reported studies, regardless of settings, subjects, and raters, illustrates the stability of the initially reported psychometrics. The MMSE has been translated into several languages, and modifications have been made for versions that are culturally and linguistically appropriate, e.g., see Folstein (1998).

Our research team has used the MMSE in all our studies conducted since 1990 with persons who have DAT and found measurement properties of interrater reliability to be adequate by rater agreement (Volicer, Hurley, Lathi, & Kowall, 1994) and internal consistency by acceptable Cronbach alpha (Camberg et al., 1999; Hurley, Volicer, & Volicer, 1996; Hurley, Volicer, Hanrahan, Houde, & Volicer, 1992; Hurley, Volicer, Mahoney, & Volicer, 1993; Hurley et al., 1999; Mahoney et al., 1999). Our experience is that research assistants can easily learn to administer the MMSE, are accurate and consistent in its administration to patients following training, and do not upset patients when using it. Because the MMSE is used in so many studies, it is almost incumbent on researchers to include the MMSE to characterize subjects so that consumers of research have a benchmark of cognitive capacity for comparing results across studies.

The above statement is one reason why our team uses the MMSE despite the fact that our research program focuses on persons with late-stage dementia who bottom out on the MMSE because their advanced disease precludes answering questions (aphasia), performing commands (apraxia), and identifying objects (agnosia) and thus score 0. This floor effect of the MMSE does not allow further comparisons for late-stage patients, regardless of clinically evident cognitive differences. We report MMSEs by score, e.g., mean scores of 0 to 2 (out of a possible 30) indicated severe cognitive capacity (Hurley et al., 1992, p. 372); by means and standard deviations by groups, e.g., 0.68 ± 1.4 (Mahoney et al., 1999, p. 30); and by percentage of zero score (scores were 0 in 92% of patients on MMSE) (Volicer et al., 1994, p. M224).

The strengths and limitations of the MMSE, as with all clinical assessment instruments, need to be considered when planning one's study and when interpreting the results of others' research. As is intended by its developers, the MMSE is a brief scale that is accurate, and easy to administer by a variety of persons, in many settings, to patients with different levels of cognitive impairment. This lack of complexity in administration leads to high levels of rater reliability—a very important feature. The MMSE can be scored without a calculator, and the total can be entered into the patient's record (or data set) as a standardized measure of a range of cognitive functions.

Many researchers have grappled with the issue of how to describe the cognitive capacity of patients who bottom out on the MMSE. Albert and Cohen (1992) identified ways to test cognitive capacity that are not captured by the MMSE: for example, to distinguish between a person who writes his/her name instead of a sentence and a person who can write nothing at all; or a person who responds to the handshake gesture and shakes hands with the tester. Our group found that this Test for Severe Impairment (Albert & Cohen, 1992) further characterized patients with severe DAT, but our late-stage patients scored a zero on this test as well (Volicer et al., 1994). Thus, we developed a measure of disease severity for late-stage patients, the BANS-S, that combines ratings of cognitive and functional deficits with the occurrence of pathological symptoms (Volicer et al., 1994).

The MMSE is only a brief screening test. MMSE scores were never intended to be a proxy for DAT disease severity, a criterion to justify third-party payment for cognition-enhancing medication, or a guideline for determining capacity to provide informed consent. Perhaps because the MMSE is so widely accepted and employed, some users unintentionally extrapolate meanings never intended and extend the MMSE's use beyond the stated purpose.

For research with subjects who have an MMSE-testable level of cognitive capacity and can respond to questions, the MMSE is a very useful measure, but it should be used as designed. Since the MMSE neither provides an early diagnostic marker for Alzheimer's disease nor characterizes disease severity of the large group of people suffering from late-stage disease, other instruments should be used for those purposes.

For the former, a scale such as the Alzheimer Disease Assessment Scale, Cognitive subscale (ADAS-Cog) (Rosen, Mohs, & Davis, 1984) is suggested. The ADAS-Cog is a screening test that takes 30 minutes to administer, is only minimally influenced by age and education, and is useful for both early detection and staging. For the latter, since cognitive ability and testing ability are so diminished in late-stage disease, examination of disease severity by the BANS-S, a seven-item scale, completed by a caregiver familiar with the patient, is recommended.

DAT is a complex problem that affects cognitive and other capacities. To adequately describe people with DAT for nursing research, we recommend using the MMSE, as well as other assessment instruments, to characterize subjects in research projects.

ANN C. HURLEY
LADISLAV VOLICER
ELLEN MAHONEY

See also:
 ALZHEIMER'S DISEASE
 COGNITIVE DISORDERS
 COGNITIVE IMPAIRMENT

NEUROBEHAVIORAL DISTURBANCES

Impairments in cognitive functioning from disturbances in the brain's physiology can easily occur in older adults. Disturbances in processing information and in behaving in socially adaptable ways can result from neurological changes in the brain and the mind's attempts to compensate for these changes. The most frequent causes of neurobehavioral disturbances in older adults are organic brain disorders, the most common are delirium and dementia. The most challenging behavioral disturbances to caregivers are agitation and aggression.

Delirium, or acute mental confusion, is transient, often abrupt and fluctuating, and typically reversible. Key symptoms include anxiety, incoherent or disoriented thinking and perceiving, reduced ability to sustain and shift attention, and agitated behavior. Precipitants are related to physical illness (e.g., cardiovascular disease), infection, hormone disorders, or nutritional deficiencies. Most frequent precipitants are metabolic disturbances, fluid and electrolyte imbalances, drug and alcohol toxicity, and unfamiliar and excessive sensory-environmental stimuli. Delirium may be life-threatening and is a medical emergency (Early Alzheimer's Disease Guideline Panel, 1996).

Dementia is a neurological brain syndrome that affects cognitive and functional abilities. Dementia is usually chronic and progressive; some dementias are reversible. Key symptoms include impairments in memory, language, judgment, and visual-spatial motor skills. Personality changes include lack of initiative, paranoia, and aggressiveness. Aggressive behavior is considered the most serious behavioral disturbance associated with dementia. Alzheimer's disease, the most prevalent form of irreversible dementia, proceeds in stages insidiously over months or years and results in functional dependence and death, usually from secondary causes. Genetic factors may be more important in the etiology of Alzheimer's disease than previously thought. Common to both delirium and dementia is depletion of older adults' already limited cognitive reserves, making adaptation to even minor changes in either health status or social environments challenging.

Nursing research historically has focused on identifying risk factors, developing assessment tools, and evaluating nursing interventions by using anecdotal or case study evidence. With increased sophistication in designing intervention studies, nurses are conducting research on the care of persons with delirium (for a review, see Cronin-Stubbs, 1996), dementia (for a review, see Maas & Buckwalter, 1991), and behavioral disturbances (for a review, see Taft & Cronin-Stubbs, 1995).

Early identification and prompt treatment of the causes of delirium prevent irreversible dementia and death, with nursing interventions targeted to reversing physiological disturbances and preventing sensory deprivation (Neelon & Champagne, 1992). Limited evidence suggests efficacy for reality orientation, perioperative management of hypoxia and orthostatic hypotension, postoperative pain management, and curtailment of excessive or meaningless stimuli (Cronin-Stubbs, 1996). Rehabilitation models and cognitive-behavioral principles have guided development of interventions for dementia, including cognitive retraining and skills training in activities of daily living (for a review, see Beck, Cronin-Stubbs, Buckwalter, & Rapp, in press). The Progressively Lowered Stress Threshold model targets minimizing stressful stimuli as a way of bolstering functional reserves in persons with dementia (Hall, Gerdner, Zwycart-Stauffacher, & Buckwalter, 1995).

Caregiver research to date has focused on global psychosocial and educational interventions delivered for brief periods of time (8–10 weeks) and targeted to reducing caregiver distress (for a review, see Light, Niederehe, & Lebowitz, 1994). Multifaceted programs that include long-term effects on caregivers' health status and institutionalization rates are beginning to be tested, with particular attention to the facets of the program that pertain to specific levels of service intensity (Knight, Lutzky, & Macofsky-Urban, 1993).

Agitation and aggression in persons with delirium and dementia have been studied cross-sectionally with correlational-descriptive designs (Taft & Cronin-Stubbs, 1995). Longitudinal studies are needed to map the natural history of behavioral symptoms, and experimental and quasi-experimental studies are needed to identify alternatives to chemical and physical restraints for persons with agitation and aggression. Low doses of haloperidol for treating neurobehavioral disturbances have demonstrated efficacy in recent clinical trials. Nutritional interventions are being tested for curbing aggressive episodes. Special care units that integrate behavioral, nutritional, and environmental interventions are beginning to demonstrate treatment efficacy.

One issue in the conduct of intervention studies of neurobehavioral disturbances is the match between the definition of the syndrome and the items included on the instruments to measure them. Studies of delirium and dementia and their behavioral sequelae have used assessment measures of varying degrees of psychometric rigor. Most mental status exams, for example, are measures of general cognitive function and do not distinguish types of cognitive impairment. Another issue in the conduct of these studies is the design and implementation of the interventions. Intensity, frequency, and duration of the intervention delivery requires standardization, and assessments must be made to determine if the intervention that was intended matches the intervention that was delivered.

Even when outcomes of the intervention study suggest efficacy, the mechanisms or the active ingredients of the intervention are not known. In testing multifaceted intervention packages, for example, the relative efficacy of each component must be matched to specific outcomes if results are to be replicated and cost-effective generalizations to diverse patient care situations are to be made.

Future research directions include establishing the efficacy of interventions for eventual generalization to diverse settings. However, research has not advanced to the development and testing of standardized protocols in randomized clinical trials. Nor has efficacy of interventions been determined in subgroups of older adults (young-old vs. old-old, men vs. women, Blacks vs. Whites). Commonly used methods to control behavioral disturbances are known to either intensify target behaviors (physical restraints) or further impair cognition and active involvement in treatment programs (neuroleptic medications).

Future directions also include the continued development of interventions that promote rehabilitation and recovery. Combinations of pharmacological, behavioral, and environmental approaches warrant testing, and algorithms for individualizing and dosing interventions are needed. Methods for educating caregivers about managing behaviors associated with delirium and dementia also are needed. Nurses are challenged to develop, systematically evaluate, and use nonrestrictive strategies for responding to the behaviors associated with cognitive impairment experienced by older adults in all settings.

DIANE CRONIN-STUBBS

See also:
ALZHEIMER'S DISEASE
ALZHEIMER'S DISEASE: SPECIAL CARE UNITS IN LONG-TERM CARE
CAREGIVER
COGNITIVE DISORDERS
COGNITIVE IMPAIRMENT
DEMENTIA CARE

PARKINSON'S DISEASE

Parkinson's Disease (PD) is a progressive neurological disorder affecting the area of the brain that is responsible for control and regulation of movement. The prevalence increases with age, and has been associated with an increased risk of mortality (Janko & Shannon, 1996). In the majority of clients, the cause of the disease is unknown. The disease most frequently occurs in the fifth or sixth decade of life, and occurs in approximately 1% of the total United States population over the age of 60. It is the second most common neurological disorder among older adults. Furthermore, the percentage of older adults with the disease is likely to rise along with the life expectancy of the population (Masterman & Cummings, 1998).

The pathophysiology of the disease results from the loss of the neurotransmittor, dopamine, in the substantia nigra and corpus striatum of the brain. Dopamine has an important inhibitive function in the central control of movement. Although dopamine exists in high concentrations in normal conditions, it is depleted in the substantia nigra and corpus striatum in PD sufferers (Birtwhistle & Baldwin, 1998). Beyond the loss of control of movement common to PD, Delieu and Keady (1997) report that the loss of dopamine may have detrimental effects on other parts of the central nervous system resulting in dementia.

The major manifestations of PD are impaired movement, muscular rigidity, tremor, muscle weakness, and loss of postural reflexes. Early signs of the disease include stiffening of the extremities and a cogwheel rigidity in the performance of movements. Other characteristics of the disease include loss of normal arm swing, facial expression, and postural reflexes. Difficulty in pivoting and loss of balance may lead to frequent falls. Several studies have been conducted in an attempt to explore the symptoms experienced by sufferers of PD.

A study by Abudi, Bar-Tal, Ziv, and Fish (1997) explored the frequency and severity of symptoms of 39 PD subjects, in an attempt to validate the symptoms stated in the literature with patients' self-report of symptoms bothering them. The results showed consistency between the present literature and patient self-report of dyskinesia/tremor, walking, freezing gait, and changing position. Dressing self, getting in/out of bed, morning stiffness, and deficit in cognitive sequencing were less bothersome to subjects than had been suggested by researchers. Subjects reported a high severity of mental and psychosocial symptoms followed by problems in completing activities of daily living.

A study of 101 PD patients was designed to explore the severity of symptomatology of the disease. Motor, cognitive, and psychological-problems scales were formed and correlated with demographic, disease-related, and psychosocial variables. The demographic variables were not significantly correlated with the three scales. However, PD staging was significantly related to scores on the motor scale. Measures of functional ability were significantly correlated with all three scales. The researchers report that the patient may view PD symptoms more broadly than clinicians and researchers (Brod, Mendelsohn, & Roberts, 1998).

Depression—a common symptom of PD—is the subject of much research. In a study of 132 community-dwelling patients and their caregivers, depressive symptoms were examined as a possible predictor of caregiver depression. Depression, disease severity, and cognitive function were assessed in the patients, and depression was measured in the caregivers. The results revealed that 64% of the PD patients and 34% of the caregivers were depressed. Increased depression correlated with increased severity and longer duration of the disease, as well as impaired cognitive function. Depression of the caregiver was accurately predicted by the level of depression in the patient. The results of the study confirm the high level of depression in PD and the relationship between depression, cognitive function, and the severity and length of the disease (Meara, Mitchelmore, & Hobson, 1999).

The prevalence of sleep disturbances in patients with PD and their spouses was examined in a sample of 153 PD patients and their spouses and 103 healthy controls. The predictive ability of demographic, psychological, and disease variables was examined on the standardized sleep ratings of the three groups. The data revealed that sleep disturbances occurred frequently in 25% of male and 41% of female PD subjects. Frequent sleep disturbance was reported by 27% of male and 48% of female spouses. Depression best predicted sleep disturbances of both patient and spouse (Smith, Ellgring, & Oertel, 1997).

Chronic sorrow as a symptom of PD was studied by Lindgren (1996) as the result of "the grief experienced from continual loss during the trajectory of an illness or disability." Six PD sufferers and their spouse caregivers (n = 4) were surveyed for the presence and severity of sorrow related to the disease. Four of the six PD patients and two of the four caregivers confirmed the presence of chronic sorrow using a standardized instrument. Strategies used to cope with the sorrow included problem-solving and emotion-focused coping. The sample reported that the losses and restrictions placed on them by the disease often triggered the sorrow. Both physicians and close family were reported as sources of support among the sample.

The loss of control common to the experience of PD was the subject of a study involving PD subjects and their caregivers. The effects of perceived control over symptoms (PCS) and perceived control over disease progression (PCDP) of both patient and caregiver were examined regarding patient and caregiver well-being and caregiver burden. The data showed that PCS was significantly related to patient well-being, caregiver well-being, and caregiver burden. No relationships were found between PCDP and the outcome variables. The researchers underscore the need for symptom management and the inclusion of the caregiver in patient care (Wallhagen & Brod, 1997).

The physical deterioration and chronicity of PD often result in the dependence of the patient on a caregiver. Several studies have been conducted to examine the burdens placed on the caregiver by the PD sufferer. One study of 30 spousal caregivers and elderly PD patients, by Berry and Murphy (1995), explored the correlation between the stage of PD and physical and social functioning, and caring spouse's physical, social psychological, and economic well-being. The results revealed a correlation between the stage of PD and the patient's functional ability, and between the patient's functional and social ability and the number of hours of care received. Caregivers' health was related to the declining health of PD patients. Caregivers' age, number of years of marriage, and educational level were also related to their social, psychological, and financial well-being. Once again the researchers underscored the need for caregiver involvement in nursing care.

Another study by Whetten-Goldstein, Sloan, Kulas, Cutson, and Schenkman (1997) was conducted to explore the burden of PD on family and society. A sample of 109 PD subjects were interviewed, using standardized measures of income, health status, health-related costs, and household activities. The data revealed that the healthcare burden on society was approximately $6000 per year, consisting mostly of compensation for the lost earnings of those less than 65 years old. The loss of income joined informal caregiving as the greatest burdens reported by caregivers. The researchers suggested a more holistic approach to the care of PD patients to include these caregiver burdens.

Treatment for PD includes both pharmacological and nonpharmacological interventions. However, as the disease progresses, drug therapy is inevitable. Stevenson (1997) explored the pharmacological strategies frequently used to correct the imbalance of dopamine in the CNS. Medications frequently used include: antimuscarinic drugs to counteract the excessive effects of acetylcholine, and levodopa, dopamine agonists, as well as selegiline and amantadine to supplement or improve the effects of dopamine. Often these treatments cease their effectiveness after a period of time, and have many residual side effects.

In a study of 42 PD patients, hope and health-promoting lifestyle were examined in order to expand the basis from which nursing interventions may evolve. Subjects completed standardized questionnaires. Significant relationships were found between hope, total health-promoting lifestyle, spiritual growth, and interpersonal relations subscales. The researchers reported that, on the whole, subjects viewed themselves as hopeful and were engaged in a health-promoting lifestyle (Fowler, 1997).

Surgical treatments for PD are among the newly developed treatments for the disease. Medial pallidotomy, a procedure in which the pallidum of the brain is lesioned to lessen the symptoms of PD, was originally developed in the 1950s. Gilbert, Counsell, and Snively (1996) report that modern technology has allowed a resurgence of the procedure with PD sufferers. In a study of 27 late-stage PD patients who underwent the procedure, improvement was seen in drug-induced dyskinesia, akinesia, rigidity, and tremors (Duff & Sime, 1997).

Parkinson's Disease is a chronic neurological disorder resulting in impaired physical mobility. Much research has focused on describing and validating the physical symptoms of the disease. Physical symptoms such as dyskinesias, tremors, walking difficulties, freezing gait, and difficulty with changing position and functional impairments are supported by the literature. In addition, depression, sleep disturbances, and chronic sorrow were evidenced among PD patients. Further research is needed to explore the complex physical and emotional symptoms of PD.

The burden of PD on caregivers has been the subject of several research studies. However, they remain descriptive in nature. Intervention studies are needed to provide nurses with the information they need to help relieve their burden as caregivers. The interventions used to manage PD include drug therapy, hope, health-promoting lifestyle, and surgical pallidotomy. Further research on the implementation and effectiveness of these treatments is essential to provide care to PD patients.

MEREDITH WALLACE

See also:
ACTIVITIES OF DAILY LIVING
COPING
FALLS
FUNCTIONAL HEALTH

REFERENCES

AACN (1999). http://www.nursingworld.org/

Aaronson, L., Carlon-Wolf, W., & Schoener, S. (1991). Pressures that fall on rising: Ways to control postural hypotension. *Geriatric Nursing, 12,* 67.

AARP (1999a). Financial planning: A must for midlife and older women, 3 p. Available: http://www.aarp.org/finance99/older.html [June 28, 1999].

AARP (1999b). Baby Boomers envision their retirement: An AARP segmentation analysis, 7p. Available: http://research.aarp.org/econ/boomer_seg_1.html [June 23, 1999].

Aarsland, D., Cummings, J. L., Yenner, G., & Miller, B. (1996). Relationship of aggressive behavior to other neuropsychiatric symptoms in patients with Alzheimer's disease. *American Journal of Psychiatry, 153,* 243–247.

Aber, C. S. (1992). Spousal death, a threat to a women's health: Paid work as a "resistance resource." *Image: Journal of Nursing Scholarship, 24,* 95–99.

Abidin, R. R. (1990). *Parenting Stress Index* (3rd ed.). Charlottesville, VA: Pediatric Psychology Press.

Abraham, I. L., Bottrell, M. M., Dash, K. R., Fulmer, T. T., Mezey, M. D., O'Donnell, L., & Vince-Whitman, C. (1999). Profiling care and benchmarking best practice in care of hospitalized elderly: The geriatric institutional assessment profile. *Nursing Clinics of North America, 31,* 239–255.

Abraham, I. L., Neundorfer, M. M., & Currie, L. J. (1992). Effects of group interventions on cognition and depression in nursing home residents. *Nursing Research, 41,* 196–202.

Abrams, W. B., Beers, M. H., Berkow, R., & Fletcher, A. J. (Eds.). (1995). *The Merck Manual of Geriatrics.* New Jersey: Merck Research Laboratories.

Abudi, S., Bar-Tal, Y., Ziv, L., & Fish, M. (1997). Parkinson's disease symptoms—patient's perceptions. *Journal of Advanced Nursing, 25,* 54–59.

Acello, B. (1998). Protecting the patient who wanders. *Nursing 98, 28*(6), 18–21.

Achenbaum, W. A. (1995). *Crossing frontiers: Gerontology emerges as a science.* Cambridge: Cambridge University Press.

Acton, G., Mayhew, P., Hopkins, B., & Yauk, S. (1999). Communicating with individuals with dementia the impaired person's perspective. *Journal of Gerontological Nursing, 25*(2), 6–13.

Adams, F. (1988). Fluid intake: How much do elders drink? *Geriatric Nursing, 9,* 218–221.

Adams, W. (1996). Alcohol use in retirement communities. *Journal of the American Geriatrics Society, 44,* 1082–1085.

Adams, W. L., Barry, K., & Fleming, M. F. (1996). Screening for problem drinking in older primary care patients. *Journal of the American Medical Association, 276,* 1964–1967.

Adams, W. L., Yuan, Z., Barboriak, J. J., & Rimm, A. A. (1993). Alcohol related hospitalizations of elderly people: Prevalence and geographic variation in the United States. *Journal of the American Medical Association, 270,* 1222–1225.

Ades, P. A., & Grunvald, M. H. (1990). Cardiopulmonary exercise testing before and after conditioning in older coronary patients. *American Heart Journal, 120,* 585–589.

Ades, P. A., Waldmann, M. L., McCann, W. J., & Weaver, S. O. (1992). Predictors of CR participation in older coronary patients. *Archives of Internal Medicine, 152,* 1033–1035.

Ades, P. A., Waldmann, M. L., Polk, D. M., & Coflesky, J. T. (1992). Referral patterns and exercise response in the rehabilitation of female coronary patients aged > 62 years. *American Journal of Cardiology, 69,* 1422–1425.

Adkins, C. B., & Fields, J. (1992). Health care values of homeless women and their children. *Family Community Health, 15*(3), 20–29.

Administration on Aging (1998a). *Profile of older Americans: 1998,* 12 p. Available: http://www.aoa.gov/aoa/stats/profile/default.htm [June 23, 1999].

Administration on Aging (1998b). Health and health care. *Profile of Older Americans: 1998* (On-line), 14 p. Available: http://www.aoa.gov/aoa/stats/profile/default.htm [August 24, 1999].

Administration on Aging. (1999). Projections of the 65+ population of states: 1995 to 2025.

Agency for Health Care Policy and Research. (1996). *Smoking cessation* (Publication No. 96-0692). Rockville, MD: Author.

Agency for Health Care Policy and Research. (1999). Prostate studies focus on barriers to early diagnosis, candidates for conservative treatment, and urinary tract symptoms. *AHCPR Research Activities, 224,* 8–9.

Ahern, D. K., Gorkin, L., Anderson, J. L., Tierney, C., Hallstrom, A., Ewart, C., Capone, R. J., Schron, E., Kornfeld, D., Herd, J. A., Richardson, D. W., & Follick, M. J., for the CAPS investigators. (1990). Biobehavioral variables and mortality or cardiac arrest in the Cardiac Arrthymia Pilot Study (CAPS). *American Journal of Cardiology, 66*(1), 59–62.

Aiken, L. (1990). *Educational innovations in gerontology: Teaching nursing homes and gerontological nurse practitioners.* Washington, DC: Association for Gerontology in Higher Education.

Aiken, L. H., Lake, E. T., Semaan, S., Lehman, H. P., O'Hare, P. A., Cole, C. S., Dunbar, D., & Frank, I. (1993). Nurse practitioner managed care for persons with HIV infection. *Journal of Nursing Scholarship, 25*(3), 172–177.

Aiken, L. H., Sloane, D. M., Lake, E. T., Sochalski, J., & Weber, A. L. (1999). Organization and outcomes of inpatient AIDS care. *Medical Care, 37,* 760–772.

Ainlay, S., Singleton, R., & Swingert, V. (1992). Aging and religious participation: Reconsidering the effects of health. *Journal for the Scientific Study of Religion, 31,* 175–188.

Albert, M. S., & Cohen, C. (1992). The test for severe impairment: An instrument for the assessment of patients with severe cognitive dysfunction. *Journal of the American Geriatrics Society, 40,* 449–453.

Albertsen, P., Hanley, J., Gleason, D., & Barry, M. (1998). Competing risk analysis of men aged 55 to 74 years at diagnosis managed conservatively for clinically localized prostate cancer. *Journal of the American Medical Association, 280,* 975–980.

Alessi, C. A., Stuck, A. E., Aronow, H. U., Yuhas, K. E., Bula, C. J., Madison, R., Gold, M., Segal-Gidan, F., Fanello, F., Rubinstein, L. Z., & Beck. J. C. (1997). The process of care in preventive in-home comprehensive geriatric assessment. *Journal of the American Geriatric Society, 45,* 1044–1050.

Alford, D. (1991). Tips on promoting food and fluid intake in the elderly. *Journal of Gerontological Nursing, 17*(11), 44–46.

Algase, D. L. (1992a). A century of progress: Today's strategies for responding to wandering behavior. *Journal of Gerontological Nursing, 18*(11), 28–34.

Algase, D. L. (1992b). Cognitive discriminants of wandering among nursing home residents. *Nursing Research, 41,* 78–81.

Algase, D., Beck, C., Kolanowski, A., Whall, A., Berent, S., Richards, K., & Beattie, E. (1996). Need-driven dementia-compromised behavior: An alternative view of disruptive behavior. *American Journal of Alzheimer's Disease, 11*(6), 10–19.

Algase, D. L., Kupferschmid, B., Beel-Bates, C. A., & Beattie, E. R. A. (1997). Estimates of stability of daily wandering behavior among cognitively impaired long-term care residents. *Nursing Research, 46,* 172–178.

Allan, J. D. (1988). Knowing what to weigh: Women's self-care activities related to weight. *Advances in Nursing Science, 11*(1), 47–60.

Allan, J. D. (1989). Women who successfully manage their weight. *Western Journal of Nursing Research, 11,* 657–675.

Allen, K. R., & Chin-Sang, V. A. (1990). A lifetime of work: The context and meanings of leisure for aging black women. *Gerontologist, 30*(6), 734–740.

Allen, K., & Blascovich, J. (1996). The value of service dogs for people with severe ambulatory disabilities: A randomized trial. *Journal of the American Medical Association, 275,* 1001–1006.

Alliance for Aging Research. (1998). When Medicine Hurts Instead of Helps: Preventing Medication Problems in Older Persons. Washington, DC: Alliance for Aging Research Publication.

Alston, M. H., & Robinson, B. H. (1992). Nurses' attitudes toward suicide. *Omega: Journal of Death and Dying, 25,* 205–215.

Alston, M. H., Small, E. B., & Whiteside, M. D. (1992). Loneliness in Black elderly. *Journal of National Black Nurses Association, 5,* 37–44.

Alzheimer's Association (1992). *Guidelines for Dignity: Goals of Specialized Alzheimer/Dementia Care in Residential Settings (1st Edition).* Chicago, IL: Author.

Alzheimer's Association (1996). *Facts about Alzheimer's Disease.* Chicago IL: Author.

Alzheimer's Association (1997). Future outlook on Alzheimer's improving. *Journal of Psychosocial Nursing, 35*(9), 9.

Alzheimer's Association supports first large-scale clinical trial on prevention of Alzheimer's disease, March 15, 1999, http://www.alz.org/news1/rtlargescale.htm.

Alzheimer's Disease Education and Referral (ADEAR) Center (1998). *Progress report on Alzheimer's disease.* Silver Spring, MD: Author.

Amella, E. J. (1996). Choking and aspiration. In C. Wanich-Bradway (Ed.), *Geriatric emergencies* (pp. 154–170). New York: Springer Publishing.

Amella, E. J. (1998). Assessment and management of eating and feeding difficulties for older people: a NICHE protocol. *Geriatric Nursing, 19,* 269–274.

Amella, E. J. (1999). Dysphagia: Differential diagnosis in long-term care. *Lippincott's Primary Care Practice, 3,* 135–149.

American Academy of Nursing. (1995). *Promoting cultural competence in and through nursing education.* Washington, DC: Author.

American Association of Colleges of Nursing. (1994). Position Statement: *Certification and Regulation of Advanced Practice Nurses.* American Association of Colleges of Nursing: Washington, D.C.

American Cancer Society. (1999a). *Cancer Facts & Figures.* Atlanta, GA. Author.

American Cancer Society. (1999b). Colon and Rectum Cancer: Prevention and Risk Factors. *Prevention* [On-Line]. Available: http://www3.cancer.org/.

American Cancer Society. (1999c). The importance of nutrition in cancer prevention. Prevention and Early Detection [On-Line]. Available: htt://www2.cancer,-org/.

American College of Sports Medicine, *American College of Sports Medicine's Guidelines for Exercise Testing and Prescription,* 5th Edition. (1995). Baltimore, MD: Williams & Wilkins.

American Geriatrics Society Panel on Chronic Pain in Older Persons. (1998). The management of chronic pain in older persons. *Journal of the American Geriatrics Society, 46,* 635–651.

American Heart Association. (1993). Human blood pressure determination by sphygmomanometry. *Circulation, 88,* 2462–2465.

American Heart Association. (1994a). *Caring for a Person with Aphasia.* Dallas, TX: Author.

American Heart Association. (1994b). *How Stroke Affects Behavior.* Dallas, TX: Author.

American Heart Association. (1995). Preventing heart attack and death in patients with coronary disease. *Circulation, 95,* 2329–31.

American Heart Association. (1996). *Diagnosis and Treatment of Chronic Arterial Insufficiency of the lower extremities: A critical review.* Dallas, TX: Author.

American Heart Association. (1997). Guide to primary prevention of cardiovascular diseases. *Circulation, 95,* 2329–2331.

American Heart Association. (1997). *Heart and stroke statistical update.* Dallas, TX: Author.

American Heart Association. (1998). *Heart and stroke facts and statistics.* Dallas, TX: Author.

American Nurses Association. (1982). *A challenge for change: The role of gerontological nursing.* Kansas City, MO: Author.

American Nurses Association. (1985). *Code for nurses.* Washington, DC: Author.

American Nurses Association (1992). *Position Statement: Registered Nurse Utilization of Unlicensed Assistive Personnel.* Washington, DC: Author.

American Nurses Association. (1992b). *Nursing and the American Nurses Association.* Washington, DC: Author.

American Nurses Association. (1993). *Nursing facts ANA.* Washington, DC: Author.

American Nurses Association (1995). *Nursing: A social policy statement.* Washington, DC: Author.

American Nurses Association. (1997). Position Statement: *Continuing Nursing Education.* American Nurses Association: Washington, DC: Author.

American Nurses Association. (1997). *End of life care: Ethical dimensions.* A Continuing Education Monograph for Nurses. Research Triangle Park, NC: Glaxco Wellcome Health Care Education.

American Nurses Credentialing Center. (Spring, 1998). *Credentialing News, 1*(2).

American Nurses Credentialing Center. (September, 1998). *Credentialing News, 1*(3).

American Nurses Credentialing Center. (October 3, 1998). *Credentialing News, 1*(3).

American Nurses Credentialing Center. (December, 1998). *Credentialing News, 1*(4).

American Pain Society, Quality of Care Committee. (1995). Quality improvement guidelines for the treatment of acute pain and cancer pain. *Journal of the American Medical Association, 274,* 1874–1880.

American Psychiatric Association (1987). *Diagnostic and statistical manual revised 3rd ed.* Washington, DC: Author.

American Psychiatric Association. (1994). *Diagnostic and statistical manual of mental disorders* (4th ed. rev.). Washington, DC: Fiest, M. B. (ed.).

American Thoracic Society: Medical Section of the American Lung Association. (1991). Lung function testing: Selection of reference values and interpretive strategies. *American Review of Respiratory Diseases, 144,* 1202–1218.

Anderson, C., & Weber, J. (1993). Preretirement planning and perceptions of satisfaction among retirees. *Educational Gerontology, 19,* 397–406.

Anderson, I. (1997). The Malmo mammography screening trial: Update on results and a harm-benefit analyses. In *NIH Consensus Development Conference: Breast cancer screening for women ages 10 49: Program and abstracts* (pp. 51–53). Bethesda, MD: National Institutes of Health.

Anderson, K. L., & Dimond, M. F. (1995). The experience of bereavement in older adults. *Journal of Advanced Nursing, 22,* 308–315.

Anderson, M. A., Wendler, M. C., & Congdon, J. C. (1998). Entering the world of dementia: CAN interventions for nursing home residents. *Journal of Gerontological Nursing, 24*(11), 31–37.

Andreucci, V. E., Russo, D., Cianciaruso, B., & Andreucci, M. (1996). Some sodium, potassium and water changes in the elderly and their treatment. *Nephrology Dialysis Transplant, 11*(Suppl. 9), 9–17.

Anonymous. (1997). What you need to know about certification and accreditation. *Texas Nursing, 71*(3), 4–5.

Ansell, D., Lacey, L., Whitman, S., Chen, E., & Phillips, C. (1994). A nurse-delivered intervention to reduce barriers to breast and cervical cancer screening in Chicago inner cities. *Public Health Reports, 1,* 104–111.

Applegate, W. B., Graves, S., Collins, S., Zwaag, R. V., & Akins, D. (1984). Acute myocardial infarction in elderly patients. *Southern Medical Journal, 77,* 1127–1129.

Aradine, C. R., & Hansen, M. R. (1970). Interdisciplinary teamwork in family health care. *Nursing Clinics of North America, 5,* 211–222.

Aravanis, S. C., Adelman, R. D., Breckman, R., Fulmer, T., Holder, E., Lachs, M., O'Brien, J. G., & Sanders, A. B. (1992). *Diagnostic and treatment guidelines on elder abuse and neglect.* Chicago: American Medical Association.

Archbold, P. G., & Stewart, B. J. (1996). The nature of the family caregiving role and nursing interventions for caregiving families. In E. A. Swanson & T. Tripp-Reimer (Eds.), *Advances in gerontological nursing* (Vol. 1, pp. 133–157). New York: Springer Publishing.

Armer, J. M. (1993). Elderly relocation to a congregate setting: Factors influencing adjustment. *Issues in Mental Health Nursing, 14,* 157–172.

Armstrong-Esther, C., & Browne, K. (1986). The influence of elderly patients' mental impairment on nurse-patient interaction. *Journal of Advanced Nursing, 11,* 379–387.

Armstrong-Esther, C., Browne, K., & McAfee, J. (1994). Elderly patients: Still clean and sitting quietly. *Journal of Advanced Nursing, 19,* 264–271.

Armstrong-Esther, C. A., Browne, K. D., Armstrong-Esther, D. C., & Sander, L. (1996). The institutionalized elderly: Dry to the bone! *International Journal of Nursing Studies, 33,* 619–628.

Aronow, W. S. (1987). Prevalence of presenting symptoms of recognized acute myocardial infarction and of unrecognized healed myocardial infarction in elderly patients. *American Journal of Cardiology, 60,* 1182.

Aronow, W. S., Starlin, L., Etienne, F., D'Alba, P., Edwards, M., Lee, N. H., & Parungao, R. F. (1986). Risk factors for coronary artery disease in persons older than 62 years in a long-term health care facility. *American Journal of Cardiology, 57,* 518–22.

Ascher, E., DePippo, P., Salles-Cunha, S., Marchese, J., & Yorkovich, W. (1999). Carotid screening with duplex ultrasound in elderly asymptomatic patients referred to a vascular surgeon: Is it worthwhile? *Annals Vascular Surgery, 13,* 164–8.

Assisted Living Federation of America (1997). *The assisted living industry, 1996.* Fairfax, VA: Author.

Atchison, J. H. (1998). Perceived job satisfaction factors among nurse assistants employed in midwest nursing homes. *Geriatric Nursing, 19,* 135–8.

Atchley, R. (1977). *Social forces in later life.* Belmont, CA: Wadsworth.

Atchley, R. C. (1991). *Social forces and aging: An introduction to social gerontology* (6th ed.). Belmont: Wadsworth.

Atkinson, R. (1990). Aging and alcohol use disorders: Diagnostic issues in the elderly. *International Psychogeriatrics, 2,* 55–72.

Atkinson, R. M., Turner, J. A., & Tolson, R. L. (1998). Treatment of older adult problem drinkers: Lessons learned from "the class of 45." *Journal of Mental Health and Aging, 4*(2), 197–214.

Ayus, J. C., & Arieff, A. I. (1996). Abnormalities of water metabolism in the elderly. *Semin Nephrology, 16*(4), 277–288.

Baker A., Bowring L., Brignell A., & Kafford D. (1996). Chronic pain management in cognitively impaired patients: A preliminary research project. *Perspectives, 20,* 4–8.

Baker, L., Hanks, G., Gershenson, D., Kantoff, P., Lange, P., Logothestis, C., Sandler, H., & Walsh, P. (1996). NCCN Prostate Cancer Practice Guidelines. *Oncology, 10*(11) (Suppl. #), 265–288.

Baldwin, B. (1990). Family caregiving: trends and forecast. *Geriatric Nursing, 10,* 172–175.

Baltes, M. M., & Horgas, A. L. (1997). Long-term care institutions and the maintenance of competence: A dialectic between compensation and overcompensation. In S. L. Willis, K. W. Schaie, & M. Hayward (Eds), *Societal mechanisms for maintaining competence in old age* (pp. 142–164). New York: Springer Publishing Co.

Baltes, P. B., & Danish, S. J. (1980). Intervention in life-span development and aging. In R. R. Turner & H. W. Reese (Eds.), *Life-span developmental psychology* (pp. 49–78). New York: Academic Press.

Bandriet, L. M. (1993). *Changing nurse aide behavior to decrease learned helplessness in nursing home elders.* Unpublished doctoral dissertation, University of Utah.

Barba, B. E. (1995). The positive influence of animals: Animal-assisted therapy in acute care. *Clinical Nurse Specialist, 9,* 199–202.

Barnes, B. (1984). Ambulation outcomes after hip fracture. *Physical Therapy, 64,* 317–321.

Barnes, P. (1992). Poorly perceived asthma. *Thorax, 47,* 408–409.

Barusch, A. S. (1994). *Older women in poverty: Private lives and public policies.* New York: Springer Publishing.

Barzilay, J. I., & Kronmal, R. A. (1998). Coronary heart disease in diabetic and nondiabetic patients with lower extremity arterial disease. *American Heart Journal, 135,* 1055–1062.

Bates-Jensen, B. (1990). New pressure ulcer status tool. *Decubitus, 3*(3), 14–15.

Bauer, T., & Barron, C. R. (1995). Nursing interventions for spiritual care: Preferences of the community-based elderly. *Journal of Holistic Nursing, 13,* 268–279.

Baumgarten, M., Becker, R., & Gauthier, S. (1990). Validity and reliability of the Dementia Behavior Disturbance scale. *Journal of the American Geriatrics Society, 38,* 221–226.

Baun, M. M., Bergstrom, N., Langston, N. F., & Thoma, L. (1984). Physiological effects of human/companion animal bonding. *Nursing Research, 33,* 126–130.

Bayer, A. J., Chadha, J. S., Farag, R. R., & Pathy, M. S. (1986). Changing presentations of myocardial infarction with increasing old age. *Journal of the American Geriatrics Society, 34,* 263–266.

Bearn, J., & Wessely, S. (1994). Neurobiological aspects of the chronic fatigue syndrome. *European Journal of Clinical Investigation, 24,* 79–90.

Beck, A. T. (1978). *Cognitive therapy and emotional disorders.* New York: International Universities Press.

Beck, C., Heacock, P., Mercer, S. O., Walls, R. C., Rapp, C. G., & Vogelpohl, T. S. (1997). Improving dressing behavior in cognitively impaired nursing home residents. *Nursing Research, 46,* 126–132.

Beck, C., Heacock, P., Rapp, C. G., & Mercer, S. O. (1993). Assisting cognitively impaired elders with activities of daily living. *The American Journal of Alzheimer's Care and Related Disorders & Research, 8*(6), 11–20.

Beck, C., Ortigara, A., Mercer S., & Shue, V. (1999). Enabling and empowering certified nursing assistants for quality dementia care. *International Journal of Geriatric Psychiatry, 14,* 197–212.

Beck, C., Rossby, L., & Baldwin, B. (1991). Correlates of disruptive behavior in cognitively impaired elderly nursing home residents. *Archives of Psychiatric Nursing, 5*(5), 281–291.

Bell, M. L. (1997). Postoperative pain management for the cognitively impaired older adult. *Seminars in Peri-operative Nursing, 6,* 37–41.

Benfield, R., & Williams, M. D. (1999). Health and Illness. In K. Berger & M. Williams (Eds.), *Fundamentals of Nursing Vol. 1* (2nd ed). Stamford, CT: Appleton & Lange.

Benjamin, B. A. (1995). *Relationship between literacy skills and actual and estimated job performance of the nurse's aide.* Columbia University Teachers College. 1995 EdD.

Benner, P. (1985). Quality of life: A phenomenological perspective on explanation, prediction, and understanding in nursing science. *Advances in Nursing Science, 8*(1), 1–14.

Bennett, C., Ferriera, M., Davis, T., Kaplan, J., Weinberger, M., Kuzel, T., Seday, M., & Sartor, O. (1998). Relation between literacy, race, and stage of presentation among low-income patients with prostate cancer. *Journal of Clinical Oncology, 16,* 3101–3104.

Bennett, D., & Dancer, J. (1997). Communication screening in older adults with vision loss. *Perceptual and Motor Skills, 84,* 1097–1098.

Benoliel, J. Q. (1983). Nursing research on death, dying, and terminal illness: Development, present state, and prospects. In H. H. Werley & J. J. Fitzpatrick (Eds.), *Annual Review of Nursing Research: Vol 2.* (pp. 101–130).

Benoliel, J. Q. (1983). Nursing research on death dying and terminal illness: Development, present state, and prospects. In H. Hurley & J. Fitzpatrick (Eds.), *Annual review of nursing research* (Vol. 1, pp. 105–123). New York: Springer Publishing.

Benoliel, J. Q. (1994). Death and dying as a field of inquiry. In I. B. Corless, B. B. Germino, & M. Pittman (Eds.), *Dying, death and bereavement: Theoretical perspectives and other ways of knowing* (pp. 3–14). Boston: Jones & Bartlett.

Benton, A., & Anderson, S. W. (1998). Aphasia: Historical perspectives. In M. T. Sarno (Ed.), *Acquired aphasia* (3rd ed.) (pp. 1–20). San Diego: Academic Press.

Berenson, R. A. (1984). *Intensive care units: Clinical outcomes, costs, and decision making* (OTA-HCS-28). Washington, DC: U.S. Government Printing Office.

Berg, L. (1994). Alzheimer's disease. In J. C. Morris (Ed.), *Handbook of dementing illnesses* (pp. 229–242). New York: Marcel Dekker.

Bergstrom, N., Bennett, M. A., & Carlson, C. E. (1994). *Treating pressure ulcers.* Clinical practice guideline No. 15 (AHCPR Publication No. 94-0047). Rockville, MD: U.S. Department of Health and Human Services, Agency for Health Care Policy and Research.

Bergstrom, N., Braden, B., Laguzza, A., & Holman, V. (1987). The Braden Scale for Predicting Pressure Sore Risk. *Nursing Research, 36,* 205–210.

Berkman, L., Berkman, C. S., Kasl, S., Freeman, D. H., Leo, L., Ostfeld, A. M., Cornori-Huntley, J., & Brody, J. A. (1986). Depressive symptoms in relation to physical health and functioning in the elderly. *American Journal of Epidemiology, 124,* 372–388.

Berkman, L. F., Leo-Summers, L., & Horowitz, R. (1992). Emotional support and survival after myocardial infarction: A prospective population based study of the elderly. *Annals of Internal Medicine, 117,* 1003–1009.

Berkman, L. F., & Syme, S. L. (1979). Social networks, host resistance, and mortality: A nine-year follow-up study of Alameda County residents. *American Journal of Epidemiology, 109,* 186–204.

Bernard, M. (1998). Backs to the future? Reflections on women, aging and nursing. *Journal of Advanced Nursing, 27,* 633–640.

Berrio, M., & Levesque, M. (1996). Advance directives: Most patients don't have one—do yours? *American Journal of Nursing, 96*(8), 25–29.

Berry, D. L., & Catanzaro, M. (1992). Persons with cancer and their return to the workplace. *Cancer Nursing, 13,* 40–46.

Berry, R. A., & Murphy, J. F. (1995). Well-being of caregivers of spouses with Parkinson's disease. *Clinical Nursing Research, 4,* 373–386.

Biegel, D. E., Sales, E., & Schulz, R. (1991). *Family caregiving in chronic illness: Alzheimer's disease, cancer, heart disease, mental illness, and stroke.* Newbury Park, CA: Sage.

Bierman, E. (1992). Atherogenesis in diabetes. *Arteriosclerosis and Thrombosis, 12,* 647–656.

Bigos, S., Bowyer, O., Braen, G., Brown, K., Deyo, R., Haldeman, S., Hart, J. L., Johnson, E. W., Keller, R., Kido, D., Liang, M. H., Nelson, R. M., Nordin, M., Owens, B. D., Schwartz, R., Stewart, D. H., Jr., Susman, J., Triano, J. J., Tripp, L. C., Turk, D. C., Watts, C., & Weinstein, J. N. (1994). *Acute low back problems in adults* (Clinical Practice Guideline No. 14). Rockville, MD: U.S. Department of Health and Human Services, Agency for Health Care Policy and Research, Public Health Service.

Birtwhistle, J., & Baldwin, D. (1998). Adult/elderly care nursing. Role of dopamine in schizophrenia and Parkinson's disease. *British Journal of Nursing, 7,* 832, 834, 836.

Bissonnette, A., & Hijjazi, K. M. (1994). Elder homelessness: A community perspective. *Nursing Clinics of North America, 29,* 409–416.

Bjurstam, N., Bjorneld, L., & Duffy W. S. (1997). The Gothenburg breast screening trial: Results from 11 years follow up. In *NIH Consensus Development Conference: Breast cancer screening for women ages 40–49: Program and abstracts* (pp. 63–64). Bethesda, MD: National Institutes of Health.

Blair, K. (1990). Aging: Physiological aspects and clinical implications. *Nurse Practitioner, 2,* 14–28.

Blair, K. A., & White, N. (1998). Are older women offered adequate health care? *Journal of Gerontological Nursing, 24*(1), 39–44.

Blesch, K., Paice, J., Wickham, R., Harte, N., Schnoor, D., Purl, S., Rehwalt, M., Kopp, P., Manson, S., Coveny, S., McHale, M., & Cahill, M. (1991). Correlates of fatigue in people with breast or lung cancer. *Oncology Nursing Forum, 18,* 81–87.

Bliwise, D. L. (1993). Sleep in normal aging and dementia. *Sleep, 16,* 40–81.

Bloem, B., Lagaany, A., vanBeek, W., Haan, J., Roos, R., & Wintzen, A. (1990). Prevalence of subjective dysphagia in commuunity residents aged over 87. *British Medical Journal, 300,* 721–722.

Blustein, J., & Weiss, L. (1998). The use of mammography by women aged 75 and older: Factors related to health, functioning, and age. *Journal of the American Geriatrics Society, 46,* 941–946.

Boland, C. S. (1998). Parish nursing. Addressing the significance of social support and spirituality for sustained health-promoting behaviors in the elderly. *Journal of Holistic Nursing, 16,* 355–368.

Bonder, B. R. (1993). *Dressing in individuals with Alzheimer's disease. Final report NIA RO1-AG10646-02.*

Bonica, J. J. (1990). *The management of pain* (2nd ed.). Philadelphia: Delea and Febiger.

Bookbinder, M., Coyle, N., & Thaler, H. (in press). Implementing national standards for cancer pain management. *Journal of Pain and Symptom Management.*

Borgquist, L., Ceder, L., & Thorngren, K. (1990). Function and social status 10 years after hip fracture. *Acta Orthopaedica Scandinavica, 61,* 404–410.

Borum, M. L. (1998). Does age influence screening for colorectal cancer? *Age Ageing, 27,* 509–511.

Bossé, R., Aldwin, C., Levenson, M., Spiro, A., & Mroczek, D. (1993). Change in social support after retirement: Longitudinal findings from the normative aging study. *Journal of Gerontology: Psychological Sciences, 48,* P210–217.

Bots, M. L., Hofman, A., de Bruyn, A. M., de Jong, P. T., & Grobbee, D. E. (1993). Isolated systolic hypertension and vessel wall thickness of the carotid artery. The Rotterdam Elderly Study. *Arteriolsclerosis & Thrombosis Journal, 13,* 64–67.

Boult, C., Murphy, J., Sloane, P., & Drone, C. (1991). The relation of dizziness to functional decline. *Journal of the American Geriatrics Society, 39,* 858–861.

Bourgeois, M. S., Burgio, L. D., Schulz, R., Beach, S., & Palmer, B. (1997). Modifying repetitive verbalizations of community dwelling patients with AD. *The Gerontologist, 37*(1), 30–39.

Bowers, B. J. (1989). Continuing care retirement communities' response to residents aging in place: The reluctantly accommodating model. *Journal of Housing for the Elderly, 5,* 65–81.

Boyle, D. M., Engelking, C., Blesch, K. S., Dodge, J., Sarna, L., & Weinrich, S. (1992). Oncology Nursing Society Position Paper on Cancer and Aging: The mandate for Oncology Nursing. *Oncology Nursing Forum, 19,* 913–933.

Brady, P. F. (1987). Labeling confusion in the elderly. *Journal of Gerontological Nursing, 13*(6), 29–32.

Braithwaite, V. (1986). The burden of home care: How is it shared? *Community Health Studies, 10,* S7–11.

Braithwaite, V. (1992). Caregiving burden: Making the concept scientifically useful and policy relevant. *Research on Aging, 14,* 3–27.

Braithwaite, V. (1998). Institutional respite care: Breaking chores of breaking social bonds. *The Gerontologist, 38,* 610–617.

Branch, L. G., Wettle, T. T., Scherr, P. H., Cook, N. R., Evans, D. H., Hebert, L. E., Masland, E. N., Keough, M. E., & Taylor, J. O. (1988). A prospective study of incident comprehensive medical home use among the elderly. *American Journal of Public Health, 78,* 255–259.

Braun, J., Wykle, M., & Cowling, R. (1988). Failure to thrive in older persons: a concept derived. *The Gerontologist, 28,* 809–813.

Braun, K. L., Horwitz, K. J., & Kaku, J. M. (1988, Winter). Successful foster caregivers of geriatric patients. *Health and Social Work, 13,* 25–34.

Braun, K. L., & Rose, C. L. (1986). The Hawaii geriatric foster care experiment: Impact evaluation and cost analysis. *The Gerontologist, 26*(5), 516–524.

Braun, K. L., & Rose, C. L. (1987). Geriatirc patient outcomes and costs in three settings: Nursing home, foster family, and own home. *Journal of American Geriatric Society, 35*, 387–397.

Braun, K. L., Suzuki, K. M., Cusick, K. E., & Howard-Carhart, K. (1997). Developing and testing training materials on elder abuse and neglect for nurse aides. *Journal of Elder Abuse & Neglect, 9*, 1–15.

Brennan, M. R. (1994). *Spirituality in the homebound elderly.* Unpublished doctoral dissertation, The Catholic University of America, Washington, D.C.

Brennan, P. L., Moos, R. H., & Lemke, S. (1988). Preferences of older adults and experts for physical and architectural features of group living facilities. *The Gerontologist, 28*, 84–90.

Brewster, A. C., Karlin, B. G., Hyde, L. A., Jacobs, C. M., Bradbury, R. C., & Chae, Y. A. (1985). MEDISGRPS: A clinically-based approach to classifying hospital patients at admission. *Inquiry, 22*, 377.

Bridges-Parlet, S., Knopman, D., & Thompson, T. (1994). A descriptive study of physically aggressive behavior in dementia by direct observation. *Journal of the American Geriatrics Society, 42*, 192–197.

Brock, A. M. (1984). From wife to widow: A changing lifestyle. *Journal of Gerontological Nursing, 10*, 8–15.

Brod, M., Mendelsohn, G. A., & Roberts, B. (1998). Patients' experience of Parkinson's disease. *Journals of Gerontology Series B-Psychological Sciences & Social Sciences, 53B*, 213–222.

Brod, M., Stewart, A. L., & Sands, L. (1999). Conceptualization of quality of life in dementia. *Journal of Mental Health and Aging, 5*, 7–20.

Brod, M., Stewart, A. L., Sands, L., & Walton, P. (1999). Conceptualization and measurement of quality of life in dementia: The dementia quality of life instrument (DQoL). *The Gerontologist, 39*(1), 25–35.

Brody, E. (1971). Excess disabilities of mentally impaired aged: Impact of individualized treatment. *Gerontologist, 25*, 124–133.

Brody, E. (1981). Women in the middle and family help to old people. *The Gerontologist, 22*, 471–480.

Brookshire, R. H. (1997). *Introduction to Neurogenic Communication Disorders* (5th ed.) (pp. 73–125). St. Louis: Mosby.

Broos, P. L., Stappaerts, K. H., Lviten, M., & Gruwez, S. (1988). Home-going: Prognostic factors concerning the major goal in treatment of elderly hip fracture patients. *International Surgery, 73*(3), 148–150.

Broos, P. L., & Van Haaften, K. I. (1989). Hip fractures in the elderly: Mortality, functional results and social re-adaptation. *International Surgery, 74*(3), 191–194.

Brooten, D., Brown, L., Hazarck-Munro, B., York, R., Cohen, S., Roncoli, U., & Hollingsworth, A. (1988). Early discharge and specialist transitional care. *Image: Journal of Nursing Scholarship, 20*, 64–68.

Brooten, D., Kumar, S., Brown, L., Butts, P., Finkler, S., Bakewell-Sachs, S., & Gibbons, A. (1986). A randomized clinical trial of early hospital discharge and follow-up of very low birthweight infants. *New England Journal of Medicine, 35*, 934–939.

Brooten, D., & Naylor, M. (1994). Nurses' effect on changing patient outcomes. *Image: Journal of Nursing Scholarship, 27,* 95–99.

Brooten, D., & Naylor, M. D. (1995). Nurses' effect on changing patient outcomes. *Image: Journal of Nursing Scholarship, 27,* 95–99.

Brower, H. T. (1981). Social organization and nurses' attitudes toward older persons. *Journal of Gerontological Nursing, 7,* 293–198.

Brower, H. T. (1985). Do nurses stereotype the aged? *Journal of Gerontological Nursing, 11*(1), 17–28.

Brown, D. R., Ahmed, F., Gary, L. E., & Milburn, N. G. (1995). Major depression in a community sample of African American. *American Journal of Psychiatry, 152,* 373–378.

Brown, S. A., & Grimes, D. E. (1995) A meta-analysis of nurse practitioners and nurse midwives in primary care. *Nursing Research, 44,* 331–339.

Brown, S. A., & Hedges, L. V. (1994). Predicting metabolic control in diabetes: A pilot study using meta-analysis to estimate a linear model. *Nursing Research, 43,* 362–368.

Brown, S. C. (1993b). Revitalizing "handicap" for disability research. *Journal of Disability Policy Studies, 4*(2), 57–75.

Browning, M., & Lewis, E. (1973). *Human sexuality: Nursing implications.* New York: American Journal of Nursing.

Brubaker, E., & Brubaker, T. H. (1995). Critical policy issues. In G. C. Smith, S. S. Tobin, E. A. Robertson-Tchabo, & P. W. Power (Eds.), *Strengthening aging families: Diversity in practice and policy* (pp. 235–247). Thousand Oaks, CA: Sage.

Brush, B. L., & McGee, E. M. (1999). The Expanded Care for Healthy Outcomes (ECHO) Project: Addressing the spiritual care needs of homeless men in recovery. *Clinical Excellence for Nurse Practitioners, 3*(2), 1–7.

Buckwalter, K. C. (1989). Caring and Alzheimer's disease: The nursing perspective. In G. Gilmore, P. Whitehouse, & M. Wykle (Eds.), *Memory, aging and dementia.* New York: Springer Publishing.

Buckwalter, K. C., Gerdner, L. A., Hall, G. R., Kelly, A., Kohout, F., Richards, B., & Sime, M. (in press). Effects of family caregiver home training based on the progressively lowered stress threshold model. *Nursing Monograph Series.* Sigma Theta Tau: Nursing Center Press.

Buckwalter, K. C., Gerdner, L. A., Kohout, F., Hall, G. R., Kelly, A., Richards, B., & Sime, M. (1999). A nursing intervention to decrease depression in family caregivers of persons with dementia. *Archives of Psychiatric Nursing, 13,* 80–88.

Buckwalter, K. C., Hartsock, J., & Gaffney, J. (1985). Music therapy. In G. M. Bulecheck & J. C. McCloskey (Eds.), *Nursing interventions: Treatments for nursing diagnoses* (pp. 58–74). Philadelphia: W. B. Saunders.

Buckwalter, K. C., Maas, M., & Reed, D. (1997). Assessing family and staff caregiver outcomes in Alzheimer disease research. *Alzheimer Disease & Associated Disorders, 11*(Suppl. 6), 105–116.

Buettner, L., & Greenstein, D. (1997). *Simple Pleasures: A multilevel sensorimotor intervention for nursing home residents with dementia* (Research Report): New York State Department of Health.

Bull, M. J. (1992). Managing the transition from hospital to home. *Qualitative Health Research, 2*(1), 27–41.

Bullough, V. L. (1994). *Science in the bedroom: A history of sex research.* New York: Basic Books.

Bullough, V. L., & Bullough, B. (1997). Sex education in American nursing: A historical review. *Nursing History Review, 6,* 199–217.

Burdz, M. P., Eaton, W. O., & Bond, J. B., Jr. (1988). Effect of respite care on dementia and nondementia patients and their caregivers. *Psychology & Aging, 3,* 38–42.

Burge, V., Felts, M., Chenier, T., & Parrillo, A. V. (1995). Drug use, sexual activity, and suicidal behavior in U.S. high school students. *Journal of School Health, 65,* 222–227.

Burgener, S., Jirovec, M., Murrell, L., & Barton, D. (1992). Caregiver and environmental variables related to difficult behaviors in institutionalized, demented elderly persons. *Journal of Gerontology: Psychological Sciences, 47*(4), 242–249.

Burgio, L., Jones, L., Butler, F., & Engel, B. (1988). Behavior problems in an urban nursing home. *Journal of Gerontological Nursing, 14,* 31–34.

Burgio, L., Scilley, K., Hardin, J. M., Hsu, C., & Yancey, J. (1996). Environmental "white noise": An intervention for verbally agitated nursing home residents. *Journal of Gerontology: Psychological Sciences, 51B*(6), P364–P373.

Burdman, G. (1986). *Health Aspects of Aging.* Portland State University, Continuing Education Publication. Portland, OR.

Bureau of Labor Statistics. (1999). Employment projections. Civilian labor force by sex, age, race, and Hispanic origin, 1986, 1996, and projected 2006. Available: http://stats.bls.gov/news.release/ecopro.table1.htm [June 23, 1999].

Burgess, A., Learner, D., D'Agostino, R., Vokonas, P., Hartman, C., & Gaccione, P. (1987). A randomized clinical trial of cardiac rehabilitation. *Social Science and Medicine, 24,* 359–370.

Burggraf, V., & Barry, R. (1998). Gerontological nursing in the 21st century. *Journal of Gerontological Nursing, 24*(6), 29–35.

Burke, W., Housten, M., & Boust, S. (1989). Use of the Geriatric Depression Scale in dementia of the Alzheimer type. *Journal of the American Geriatrics Society, 37,* 856.

Burker, E. J., Wong, H., Sloane, P. D., Mattingly, D., Preisser, J., & Mitchel, C. M. (1995). Predictors of fear of falling in dizzy and nondizzy elderly. *Psychology and Aging, 10,* 104–110.

Burkhardt, M. A. (1989). Spirituality: An analysis of the concept. *Holistic Nursing Practice, 3*(3), 69–77.

Burl, J. B., Bonner, A., Rao, M., & Kahn, A. M. (1998). Geriatric nurse practitioner in long-term care: Demonstration of effectiveness in managed care. *Journal of the American Geriatrics Society, 46,* 506–510.

Burns, A., Rossor, M., Hecker, J., Gauthier, S., Petit, H., H., M. l., Rogers, S. L., & Friedhoff, L. T. (1999). The effects of donepezil in Alzheimer's disease—Results from a multinational trial. *Dementia & Geriatric Cognitive Disorders, 10,* 237–244.

Burns, N., & Grove, S. K. (1993). *The practice of nursing research: Conduct, critique, & utilization* (2nd ed.). Philadelphia, PA: W. B. Saunders.

Burns, P. A. (1995). *A study of the Omnibus Budget Reconciliation Act of 1987 and the amendments of 1989 and 1990. Mandatory education for nursing assistants and their effect on job performance in two counties in Florida.* Unpublished Doctoral Dissertation, University of North Texas.

Burnside, I., & Haight, B. K. (1992). Reminiscence and life review: Analyzing each concept. *Journal of Advanced Nursing, 17,* 855–862.

Burnside, I. M. (1988). *Nursing and the aged: A self-care approach.* New York: McGraw-Hill.

Burns-Tisdal, S., & Goff, W. F. (1989). The geriatric nurse practitioner in home care: Challenges, stresses, and rewards. *Nursing Clinics of North America, 24,* 809–817.

Burnside, I. M. (1980). Wandering behavior. In I. M. Burnside (Ed.), *Psychosocial nursing care of the aged* (2nd ed.) (pp. 298–309). New York: McGraw Hill Book Co.

Burt, B. L., Whelton, P. K., Rocella, E. J., Brown, C., Cutler, J. A., Higgins, M., Horan, M., & Labarthe, D. (1995). Prevalence of hypertension in the U.S. adult population: Results from the third national health and nutrition survey, 1988–1991. *Hypertension, 25,* 305–309.

Burt, M. R. (1996). Homelessness: Definitions and counts. In J. Baumohl (Ed.), *Homeless in America* (pp. 15–23). Phoenix, AZ: Oryx Press.

Burton, L. M. (1992). Black grandparents rearing children of drug-addicted parents: Stressors, outcomes and the social service needs. *The Gerontologist, 32,* 744–751.

Butler, R. (1963). The life review: An interpretation of reminiscence in the aged. *Psychiatry, 26,* 65–76.

Butler, R. (1975). *Why survive: Being old in America.* New York: Harper and Row.

Cain, A. O. (1991). Pets and the family. *Holistic Nursing Practice, 5*(2), 58–63.

Campbell, M. E. (1971). Study of attitudes of nursing personnel toward the geriatric patient. *Nursing Research, 20,* 147–151.

Campbell, T. L., & Patterson, J. M. (1995). The effectiveness of family interventions in the treatment of physical illness. *Journal of Marital and Family Therapy, 21,* 545–583.

Camberg, L., Woods, P., Ooi, W. L., Hurley, A., Volicer, L., Ashley, J., Odenheimer, G., & McIntyre, K. (1999). Evaluation of simulated presence: A personalized approach to enhance well-being in persons with Alzheimer's disease. *Journal of American Geriatrics Society, 47*(4), 446–452.

Campbell, M. K., Bush, T. L., & Hale, W. E. (1993). Medical conditions associated with driving cessation in community-dwelling, ambulatory elders. *Journal of Gerontology, Social Sciences, 48,* S230–S234.

Cantor, S., Spann, S., Volk, R., Cardenas, M., & Warren, M. (1995). Prostate cancer screening: A decision analysis. *The Journal of Family Practice, 41,* 33–41.

Capezuti, E., Evans, L., Strumpf, N., & Maislin, G. (1996). Physical restraint use and falls in nursing home residents. *Journal of the American Geriatrics Society, 44,* 627–633.

Capossela, C., & Warnock, S. (1995). *Share the care: How to organize a group to care for someone who is seriously ill.* New York: Fireside.

Caris-Verhallen, W., Kerkstra, A., & Bensing, J. (1997). The role of communication in nursing care for elderly people: A review of literature. *Journal of Advanced Nursing, 25,* 915–933.

Caris-Verhallen, W., Kerkstra, A., & Bensing, J. (1999). Non-verbal behavior in nurse-elderly patient communication. *Journal of Advanced Nursing, 29*, 808–818.

Caris-Verhallen, W., Kerkstra, A., van der Heijden, P., & Bensing, J. (1998). Nurse-elderly patient communication in home care and institutional care: An explorative study. *International Journal of Nursing Studies, 35*, 95–108.

Carmack, B. J., & Fila, D. (1989). Animal-assisted therapy: A nursing intervention. *Nursing Management, 20*(5), 96–101.

Carney, R. M., Freedland, K. E., Rich, M. W., & Jaffe, A. S. (1995). Depression as a risk factor for cardiac events in established coronary heart disease: A review of possible mechanisms. *Annals of Behavioral Medicine, 17*, 142–149.

Carnoni-Huntley, J., Foley, D., White, L., Suzman, R., Berkman, L., Evans, D., & Wallace, R. (1985). Epidemiology of disability in the oldest old: Methodologic issues and preliminary findings. *Milbank Memorial Fund Quarterly, 63*, 350–376.

Carr, D. B., LaBarge, E., Dunnigan, K., & Storandt, M. (1998). Differentiating drivers with dementia of the Alzheimer type from healthy older persons with a Traffic Sign Naming test. *Journals of Gerontology: Series A, Biological Sciences and Medical Sciences, 53*, M135–M139.

Carrier, V. K., Janson-Bjerklie, S., & Jacobs, S. (1984). The sensation of dyspnea: A review. *Heart and Lung, 13*, 436–447.

Cary, A. H. (1998). Scholar-in-residence program initiates research activities. *Credentialing News, 1*(3), 5.

Casby, J. A., & Holm, M. B. (1994). The effect of music on repetitive disruptive vocalizations of persons with dementia. *The American Journal of Occupational Therapy, 48*, 883–889.

Caserta, M. S., Lund, D. A., & Dimond, M. F. (1990). Understanding the context of perceived health ratings: The case of spousal bereavement in later life. *Journal of Aging Studies, 4*, 231–243.

Casey, D. A. (1991). Suicide in the Elderly: A Two-Year Study of Data from Death Certificates. *Southern Medical Journal, 84*, 1184–1186.

Castor, D., Woods, D., Pigott, K., & Hemmes, R. (1991). Effect of sunlight on sleep patterns of the elderly. *Journal of the American Academy of Physician Assistants, 4*, 321–326.

Caudill, M. (1989). Nursing assistant involvement in patient care planning pays off. *Nursing Management, 20*, 112Y–Z, 1122DD, 112FF.

Caygill, C. P., Charlett, A., & Hill, M. J. (1998). Relationship between the intake of high-fibre foods and energy and the risk of cancer of the large bowel and breast. *European Journal of Cancer Prevention, 7*(Suppl. 2), 11–17.

Ceder, L., Ekelund, L., Inerot, S., Lindbert, L., Odberg, E., & Sjolin, C. (1979). Rehabilitation after hip fracture in the elderly. *Acta Orthopaedica Scandinavica, 50*, 681–688.

Ceder, L., Thorngren, K., & Wallden, B. (1980). Prognostic indicators and early home rehabilitation in elderly patients with hip fractures. *Clinical Orthopaedics and Related Research, 152*, 173–184.

Centers for Disease Control. (1996c). *HIV/AIDS surveillance report: U.S. HIV and AIDS cases reported through June 1996.* Atlanta: Centers for Disease Control, Center for Infectious Disease.

Chaisson, C. M. (1980). Life cycle: A social simulation game to improve attitudes and response to the elderly. *Journal of Gerontological Nursing, 6,* 587–592.

Champion, V. (1991). The relationship of selected variables to breast cancer detection behaviors in women 35 and older. *Oncology Nursing Forum, 18,* 733–739.

Champion, V. L. (1995). Results of a nurse-delivered intervention on proficiency and nodule detection with breast self-examination. *Oncology Nursing Forum, 22,* 819–824.

Chandler, J. D., & Chandler, J. E. (1988). The prevalence of neuropsychiatric disorders in a nursing home population. *Journal of Geriatric Psychiatry & Neurology, 1,* 761–76.

Chang, B. L. (1999). Cognitive-behavioral intervention for homebound caregivers of persons with dementia. *Nursing Research, 48,* 173–182.

Chapey, R. (1994). Introduction to language intervention strategies in adult aphasia. In R. Chapey (Ed.), *Language intervention strategies in adult aphasia* (3rd ed.) (pp. 3–4). Baltimore, MD: Williams & Wilkins.

Chapman, S. B., & Ulatowska, H. K. (1991). Aphasia and aging. In D. Ripich (Ed.), *Geriatric communication disorders* (pp. 241–254). Austin, TX: Pro-Ed.

Chassagne, P., Landrin, I., Neveu, C., Czernichow, P., Bouaniche, M., Doucet, J., Denis, P., & Bercoff, E. (1999). Fecal incontinence in the institutional elderly: Incidence, risk factors, and prognosis. *American Journal of Medicine, 106,* 185–190.

Chemerinski, E., Petracca, G., Tesón, A., Sabe, L., Leiguarda, R., & Starkstein, S. (1998). Prevalence and correlates of aggressive behavior in Alzheimer's disease, *Journal of Neuropsychiatry, 10,* 421–425.

Cherkasky, M. (1949). The Montefiore hospital home care program. *American Journal of Public Health and the Nations Health, 39,* 163–166.

Chernoff, R. (1995). Effects of age on nutrient requirements. *Clinical Geriatric Medicine, 11,* 641–651.

Chidester, J. C., & Spangler, A. A. (1997). Fluid intake in the institutionalized elderly. *Journal of American Dietetic Association, 97,* 29–30.

Chlan, L. L. (1998). Music therapy. In M. Snyder & R. Lindquist (Eds.), *Alternative/complementary therapies in nursing.* New York: Springer Publishing.

Choi, E. C. (1986). Unique aspects of Korean-American mothers. *Journal of Obstetric Gynecology Nursing, 15,* 394–400.

Choi, N. G. (1991). Racial differences in the determinants of living arrangements of widowed and divorced elderly women. *The Gerontologist, 31,* 496–504.

Choi, N. G. (1994). Patterns and determinants of social service utilization: Comparison of the childless elderly and elderly parents living with or apart from their children. *The Gerontologist, 34,* 353–362.

Chokroverty, S. (1994). An overview of sleep. In S. Chokroverty (Ed.), *Sleep disorders medicine: Basic science, technical considerations, & clinical aspects* (pp. 7–16). Boston, MA: Butterworth-Heinemann.

Christensen, K., & Dysken, M. (1990). The Geriatric Depression Scale in Alzheimer's disease. *Journal of the American Geriatrics Society, 38,* 724.

Chung, M. K., Bosner, M. S., McKenzie, J. P., Shen, J., & Rich, M. W. (1995). Prognosis of patients > 70 years of age with non-Q-wave acute MI compared with younger patients with similar infarcts and with patients > 70 years of age with Q-wave acute MI. *American Journal of Cardiology, 75,* 18–22.

Chyun, D. (1998). The prognostic importance of diabetes mellitus in elderly patients with myocardial infarction. (Doctoral dissertation, Yale University, 1998). *Dissertation Abstracts International.*

Cimprich, B. (1992). Attentional fatigue following breast cancer surgery. *Research in Nursing and Health, 15,* 199–207.

Clark J. E., Lipe, A. W., & Bilbrey, M. (1998). Use of music to decrease aggressive behaviors in people with dementia. *Journal of Gerontological Nursing, 24*(7), 10–17.

Clark, M. E., Lipe, A. W., & Bilbrey, M. (1998). Use of music to decrease aggressive behaviors in people with dementia. *Journal of Gerontological Nursing, 24*(7), 10–17.

Clark, P. G. (1995). Quality of life, values, and teamwork in geriatric care: Do we communicate what we mean? *The Gerontologist, 35,* 402–411.

Clarke, A. (1994). What is chronic disease? The effects of the re-definition of HIV and AIDS. *Social Science and Medicine, 39,* 591–597.

Claussen, A. H., & Crittenden, P. M. (1991). Physical and psychological maltreatment; Relations among types of maltreatment. *Child Abuse and Neglect: The International Journal, 15,* 5–18.

Clotfelter, C. (1999). The effect of an education intervention on decreasing pain intensity in elderly people with cancer. *Oncology Nursing Forum, 26,* 27–32.

Cobey, J. C., Cobey, J., Conant, L., Weil, U. H., Greenwald, W. F., & Southwick, W. O. (1976). Indicators of recovery from fractures of the hip. *Clinical Orthopaedics and Related Research, 117,* 258–262.

Cohen, C. I. (1999). Aging and homelessness. *The Gerontological Society of America, 39,* 5–14.

Cohen, C. I., & Crane, M. (1996). Old and homeless in London and New York City: A cross-national comparison. In D. Bhugra (Ed.), *Homelessness and mental health* (pp. 150–169). London: Cambridge University Press.

Cohen, C. I., & Sokolovsky, J. (1989). *Old men of the Bowery.* New York: Guilford Press.

Cohen, E., & Cesta, T. (1993). *Nursing Case Management: From Concept to Evaluation.* St. Louis, MO: Mosby Yearbook.

Cohen, S. (1982). Supporting families through respite care. *Rehabilitation Literature, 43,* 1–2, 7.

Cohen, S., & Warren, R. (1985). *Respite Care: Principles, Programs and Policies.* Austin: Pro-Ed.

Cohen-Mansfield, J. (1986). Agitated behaviors in the elderly. *Journal of the American Geriatrics Society, 34,* 722–727.

Cohen-Mansfield, J. (1996). Conceptualization of agitation: Results based on the Cohen-Mansfield Agitation Inventory and the Agitation Behavior Mapping Instrument. *International Psychogeriatrics, 8*(Suppl 3), 309–315.

Cohen-Mansfield, J. (1997). Turnover among nursing home staff: A review. *Nursing Management, 28*(5), 59–64.

Cohen-Mansfield, J. (1999). Measurement of inappropriate behavior associated with dementia. *Journal of Gerontological Nursing, 25*(2), 42–51

Cohen-Mansfield, J., Marx, M. S., & Rosenthal, A. S. (1989). A description of agitation in a nursing home. *Journal of Gerontology, 44*(3), M77–84.

Cohen-Mansfield, J., & Werner, P. (1998a). Predictors of aggressive behavior: A longitudinal study in senior day care centers. *Journal of Gerontology, 53B,* 300–310.

Cohen-Mansfield, J., & Werner, P. (1998b). The effects of an enhanced environment on nursing home residents who pace. *The Gerontologist, 38,* 199–208.

Cohen-Mansfield, J., Werner, P., Culpepper, W. J., Wolfson, M. A., & Bickel, E. (1996). Wandering and aggression. In L. Carstensen, B. Edelstein, & L. Dornbrand (Eds.), *The practical handbook of clinical gerontology* (pp. 374–397). Thousand Oaks, CA: Sage Publications.

Coltharp, W. Jr., Richie, M. F., & Kaas, M. J. (1996). Wandering. *Journal of Gerontological Nursing, 22*(11), 5–10, 49–55.

Cohn, J. (1986). Psychological ramifications of silent myocardial ischemia. *Cardiology Clinics, 4,* 727–734.

Cohn, J. K., & Cohn, P. F. (1983). Patient reactions to the diagnosis of asymptomatic coronary artery disease: Implications for the primary physician and consultant cardiologist. *Journal of the American College of Cardiology, 1,* 95–98.

Cohn, M. D., Horgas, A. L., & Marsiske, M. (1990). Behavior management training for nurse aides: is it effective? *Journal of Gerontological Nursing, 16*(1), 21–25, 39–41.

Collins, C., Liken, M., King, S., & Kokinakis, C. (1993). Loss and grief among family caregivers of relatives with dementia. *Qualitative Nursing Research, 3,* 236–253.

Collins, C., & Ogle, K. (1994). Patterns of predeath service use by dementia patients with a family caregiver. *Journal of the American Geriatrics Society, 42,* 719–722.

Collins, C., Stommel, M., Wang, S., & Given, C. W. (1994). Caregiving transitions: Changes in depression among family caregivers of relatives with dementia. *Nursing Research, 43,* 220–225.

Comana, M. T., Brown, V. M., & Thomas, J. D. (1998). The effect of reminiscence therapy on family coping. *Journal of Family Nursing, 4,* 182–197.

Conn, V. S., Taylor, S. G., & Wiman, P. (1991). Anxiety, depression, quality of life, and self-care among survivors of myocardial infarction. *Issues in Mental Health Nursing, 12*(4), 321–331.

Connelly, C. E. (1987). Self care and the chronically ill patient. *Nursing Clinics of North America, 22,* 621–629.

Connelly, D. M., & Vandervoort, A. A. (1995). Improvement in knee extensor strength of institutionalized elderly women after exercise with ankle weights. *Physiotherapy Canada, 47,* 15–23.

Connelly, D. M., & Vandervoort, A. A. (1996). Improving muscle strength in the frail elderly. *Canadian Nursing Home, 7,* 26–30.

Conrad, N. (1992). Stress and knowledge of suicidal others as factors in suicidal behavior of high school adolescents. *Issues in Mental Health Nursing, 13,* 95–104.

Constantino, R. E. (1981). Bereavement crisis intervention for widows in grief and mourning. *Nursing Research, 30,* 351–353.

Constantino, R. E., & Bricker, P. L. (1996). Nursing post intervention for spousal survivors of suicide. *Issues in Mental Health Nursing, 17,* 151–152.

Cook, J. D. (1981). The therapeutic use of music: A literature review. *Nursing Forum, 20,* 252–266.

Coons, D. H. (1983). The therapeutic milieu. In W. Reichel (Ed.), *Clinical aspects of aging* (pp. 137–159). Baltimore: Williams & Wilkins.

Corbin, J. M., & Strauss, A. (1991). A nursing model for chronic illness management based upon the trajectory framework. *Scholarly Inquiry for Nursing Practice: An International Journal, 5,* 155–174.

Corless, I. B. (1994). Dying well: Symptom control within hospitce care. In J. Fitzpatrick & J. Stevenson (Eds), *Annual Review of Nursing Research* (Vol. 12, pp. 125–146). New York: Springer Publishing.

Coreless, I. B. (1994). Dying well: Symptom control within hospice care. In J. J. Fitzpatrick & J. S. Stevenson (Eds.), *Annual Review of Nursing Research, 12,* 125–146.

Corless, I. B. (1995). A new decade for hospice. In I. B. Corless, B. B. Germino, & M. A. Pittman (Eds.), *A challenge for living: Death, dying, and bereavement* (pp. 77–94). Boston: Jones & Bartlett.

Cornbleth, T. (1977). Effects of a protected hospital ward area on wandering and nonwandering geriatric patients. *Journal of Gerontology, 32,* 573–577.

Costa, P. T. Jr., Williams, T. F., Somerfield, M., et al. (1996). *Early identification of Alzheimer's disease and related dementias: Clinical practice guideline, quick reference guide for clinicians,* No. 19 (AHCPR Publication No. 97-0704). Rockville, MD: U.S. Department of Health and Human Services, Public Health Service, Agency for Health Care Policy and Research.

Cotanch, P., & Strum, S. (1987). Progressive muscle relaxation as antiemetic therapy for cancer patients. *Oncology Nursing Forum, 14*(1), 33–37.

Coupland, N., Coupland, J., Giles, H., & Henwood, K. (1988). Accommodating the elderly: Invoking and extending a theory. *Language in Society, 17,* 1–41.

Cowan, M. J., Kogan, H., Burr, R., Hendershot, S., & Buchanan, L. (1991). Power spectral analysis of heart rate variability after biofeedback training. *Journal of Electrocardiology, 23*(Suppl.), 85–94.

Cowen, M. E., Simpson, S. L., & Vettese, T. E. (1997). Survival estimates for patients with abnormal swallowing studies. *Journal of General Internal Medicine, 12,* 88–94.

Coyne, M. L., & Hoskins, L. (1997). Improving eating behaviors in dementia using behavioral strategies. *Clinical Nursing Research, 6,* 275–290.

Crane, M. (1992). Elderly, homeless, and mentally ill: A study. *Nursing Standard, 7,* 35–38.

Crane, M. (1994). Elderly homeless people: Elusive subjects and slippery concepts. *Aging and Society, 14,* 631–40.

Crane, M. (1998). The association between mental illness and homelessness among older people: An exploratory study. *Aging and Mental Health, 2,* 171–180.

Crane, M. (1999). For safety's sake. *Spectrum: The Journal of State Government, 72,* 5–8.

Criqui, M. H., & Denenberg, J. O. (1998). The generalized nature of atherosclerosis: How peripheral arterial disease may predict adverse event from coronary artery disease. *Vascular Medicine, 3,* 241–5.

Cronin-Stubbs, D. (1996). Delirium intervention research in acute care settings. In J. J. Fitzpatrick & J. Norbeck (Eds.), *Annual review of nursing research* (Vol. 14, pp. 57–73). New York: Springer Publishing.

Crosby, F. E., Ventura, M. R., Frainier, M. A., & Wu, Y. B. (1993). Well being and concerns of patients with peripheral arterial occlusive disease. *Journal of Vascular Nursing, 2*, 5–11.

Crosby, L. J., & Parsons, L. C. (1992). Cerebrovascular response of closed head-injured patients to a standardized endotracheal tube suctioning and manual hyperventilation procedure. *Journal of Neuroscience Nursing, 24*, 40–49.

Crowley, M. (1996). Exercise restores seniors' strength and spirits. *Health Progress, 6*, 42–44.

Crum, R., Anthony, J., Bassett, S., & Folstein, M. (1993). Population-based norms for the Mini-Mental State Examination by age and educational level. *Journal of the American Medical Association, 269*, 2386–2391.

Crutchfield, D. B. (1999). Medication Challenges in the assisted living facility. *Journal of the American Pharmaceutical Association 39*, 222–225.

Cugliari, A. M., Miller, T., & Sobol, J. (1995). Factors promoting completion of advance directives in the hospital. *Archives of Internal Medicine, 155*, 1893–1898.

Cumming, E., & Henry, W. (1961). *Growing old: The process of disengagement.* New York: Basic Books.

Curb, J. D., Masaki, K., Rodriguez, B. L., Abbott, R. D., Burchfiel, C. M., Chen, R., Petrovitch, H., Sharp, D., & Yano, K. (1996). Peripheral artery disease and cardiovascular risk factors in the elderly. The Honolulu Heart Program. *Arteriosclerotic-Thrombotic Vascular Biology, 12*, 1495–1500.

Cutler, W., Friedman, E., & Genovese-Stone, E. (1993). Prevalence of kyphosis in a healthy sample of pre- and postmenopausal women. *American Journal of Physical Medicine and Rehabilitation, 72*, 219–225.

Czeisler, C. A., Dumont, M., Duffy, J. F., Steinberg, J. D., Richardson, G. S., Brown, E. N., Sanches, R., Rios, C. D., & Ronda, J. M. (1992). Association of sleep-wake habits in older people with changes in output of circadian pacemaker. *The Lancet, 340*, 933–936.

Dahl, E. (1980). Mortality and life expectancy after hip fractures. *Acta Orthopaedica Scandinavica, 51*, 163–170.

Daltroy, L. H., & Laing, M. H. (1993). Arthritis education: Opportunities and state of the art. *Health Education Quarterly, 20*, 3–16.

Daly, E., & Futrell, M. (1989). Retirement attitudes and health status. *Journal of Gerontological Nursing, 15*, 29–32.

Damron-Rodriguez, J., Frank, J., Heck, E., Liu, D., Sragow, S., Cruise, P., & Osterweil, D. (1998). Physician knowledge of community-based care: What's the score? *Annals of Long-Term Care, 6*, 112–121.

Damrosch, S., & Strasser, J. A. (1988). The homeless elderly in America. *Journal of Gerontological Nursing, 14*(10), 26–29.

Danford, S. (1982). Therapeutic design for aging. In A. M. Horton (Ed.), *Mental health interventions for aging* (pp. 163–169). South Hadley, MA: J. F. Bergin.

Dannefer, D. (1988). What's in a name: An account of the neglect of variability in the study of aging. In J. E. Birren & V. L. Bengtson (Eds.), *Emergent theories of aging* (pp. 356–384). New York: Springer.

Dart, A., Jerums, G., Nicholson, G., d'Emden, M., Hamilton-Craig, I., Tallis, G., Best, J., West, M., Sullivan, D., Bracs, P., & Black, D. (1997). A multicenter, double-blind, one-year study comparing safety and efficacy of atorvastatin versus simvastatin in patients with hypercholesterolemia. *The American Journal of Cardiology, 80,* 39–44.

D'Avanzo, C. E. (1992). Barriers to health care for Vietnamese refugees. *Journal of Professional Nursing, 8,* 245–253.

Davis, L. L. (1997). Family conflicts around dementia home care. *Family Systems Medicine, 15,* 85–95.

Davis, R. (1982). You *can* go home again. *Geriatric Nursing, 1,* 238–240.

Dawe, D., & Moore-Orr, R. (1995). Low-intensity, range-of-motion exercise: Invaluable nursing care for elderly patients. *Journal of Advanced Nursing, 21,* 675–681.

Decker, S. D., & Young, E. (1991). Self-perceived needs of primary caregivers of home-based hospice clients. *Journal of Community Heath Nursing, 8*(3), 147–154.

De Geest, S., Abraham, I., Moons, P., Dunbar-Jacob, J., & Vanhaecke, J. (1998). Use of structured interviews in assessing compliance. The Fifth International Congress of Behavioral Medicine, 19-22 August 1998; Copenhagen, Denmark. Abstract 60-2.

De Geest, S., Abraham, I., Moons, P., Vandeputte, M., Van Cleemput, J., Evers, G., Daenen, W., & Vanhaecke, J. (1998). Late acute rejections and subclinical noncompliance with cyclosporine-therapy in heart transplant patients. *Journal of Heart and Lung Transplantation, 17,* 854–863.

De Geest, S., Borgermans, L., Gemoets, H., Abraham, I., Vlaminck, H., Evers, G., & Vanrenterghem, Y. (1995). Incidence, determinants, and consequences of subclinical noncompliance with immunosuppressive therapy in renal transplant recipients. *Transplantation, 59,* 340–347.

DeLeon, M. J., Potegal, M., & Gurland, B. (1984). Wandering and parietal signs in senile demential of Alzheimer's type. *Neuropsychobiology, 11,* 155–157.

Delgado, J., & Estrada, L. (1993). Improving data collection strategies. *Public Health Reports, 108,* 540–545.

Delieu, J., & Keady, J. (1997). The biology of dementia due to Parkinson's disease. *British Journal of Nursing, 6,* 806–810.

Dellefield, K. S., & McDougall, G. J. (1996). Increasing metamemory in community elderly. *Nursing Research, 45,* 284–290.

DeLoach, L. J., Higgins, M. S., Caplan, A. B., & Stiff, J. L. (1998). The visual analog scale in the immediate postoperative period: Intrasubject variability and correlation with a numeric scale. *Anesthesia Analg, 86,* 102–106.

DeMallie, D. A., North, C. S., & Smith E. M. (1997). Psychiatric disorders among the homeless: A comparison of older and younger groups. *The Gerontologist, 37,* 61–66.

Dement, W., Richardson, G., Prinz, P., Carskadon, M., Kripke, D., & Czeisler, C. (1985). Changes of sleep and wakefulness with age. In C. E. Finch & E. L. Schneider (Eds.), *Handbook of the biology of aging* (2nd ed.) (pp. 692–720). New York: Van Nostrand Reinhold Company.

Demi, A., Bakeman, R., Sowell, R., Moneyham, L., & Seals, B. (1996, October). Suicidality among HIV-infected women. Paper presented at Ninth Annual Association of Nurses in AIDS Care, Chicago, IL.

Demi, A. S., & Miles, M. S. (1986). Bereavement. In H. H. Werley, J. J. Fitzpatrick, & R. L. Taunton (Eds.), *Annual Review of Nursing Research* (Vol. 4, pp. 105–123). New York: Springer.

Demi, A. S., & Miles, M. S. (1986). Bereavement. *Annual Review of Nursing Research, 4,* 105–123.

Demitrack, M. A., Dale, J. K., Straus, S. E., Laue, L., Listwak, S. J., Kruesi, M. J., Chrousos, G. P., & Gold, P. W. (1991). Evidence for impaired activation of the hypothalamic-pituitary-adrenal axis in patients with chronic fatigue syndrome. *Journal of Clinical Endocrinology and Metabolism, 73,* 1224–1234.

Dempsey, M., & Baago, S. (1998). Latent grief: The unique and hidden grief of carers of loved ones with dementia. *American Journal of Alzheimer's Disease, 13,* 84–91.

Denham, S. A. (1999). Part 2: Family health during and after death of a family member. *Journal of Family Nursing, 5,* 160–183.

Dennis, K. E., & Goldberg, A. P. (1993). Differential effects of body fatness and body fat distribution on risk factors for cardiovascular disease in women: Impact of weight loss. *Arteriosclerosis and Thrombosis, 13,* 1487–1494.

Dennis, K. E., & Goldberg, A. P. (1996). Weight control self- efficacy types and positive transitions affect weight loss in obese women. *Addictive Behaviors, 21,* 103–116.

D'Eramo-Melkus, G., Wylie-Rosett, J., & Hagan, J. (1992). Metabolic impact of education in NIDDM. *Diabetes Care, 15,* 864–869.

Derogatis, L. R. (1983). *SCL-90 administration, scoring, and procedures manual-II.* Towson, MD: Clinical Psychometric Research.

Desgranges, B., Eustache, F., Rioux, P., De La Sayette, V., & Lechevalier, B. (1996). Memory disorders in Alzheimer's disease and the organization of human memory. *Cortex, 32,* 387–412.

deVillers, A. S., Russell, V. A., Carstens, M. E., Aalbers, C., Gagiano, C. A., Chalton, D. O., & Taljaard, J. J. F. (1987). Noradrenergic function and hypothamamic-pituitary-adrenal axis activity in primary unipolar major depressive disorder. *Psychiatry Research, 22,* 127–140.

Diabetes Control and Complications Trial (DCCT) Research Group. (1993). The effect of intensive treatment of diabetes on the development and progression of long-term complications in insulin-dependent diabetes mellitus. *New England Journal of Medicine, 329,* 977–986.

Diamond, M., Caserta, M., & Lund, D. (1994). Understanding depression in older adults. *Clinical Nursing Research, 3,* 253–268.

Dilorio, C. (1990). An analysis of trends in neuroscience nursing research. *Journal of Neuroscience Nursing, 22,* 139–146.

Dimond, M. (1981). Bereavement and the elderly: A critical review with implications for nursing practice and research. *Journal of Advanced Nursing, 6,* 461–470.

Dimond, M., Caserta, M., & Lund, D. (1994). Understanding depression in bereaved older adults. *Clinical Nursing Research, 3,* 253–268.

Dimond, M., Lund, D. A., & Caserta, M. S. (1987). The role of social support in the first two years of bereavement in an elderly sample. *The Gerontologist, 27,* 599–604.

Diokno, A., McCormick, K. A., Colling, J., Fantl, J. A., Loughery, R., Newman, D. K., Ouslander, J., Pearson, B., Raz, S., Resnick, N. M., Rohner, R. J., Schnelle, J., Tries, J., Urich, V., & Vernon, M. (1992). *Urinary incontinence in adults: AHCPR Clinical Practice Guideline* (Publication No. 92-0038). Rockville, MD: U.S. Department of Health and Human Services, Public Health Service, Agency for Health Care Policy and Research.

Dionne-Proulz, J., & Pepin, R. (1993). Stress management in the nursing profession. *Journal of Nursing Management, 1,* 75–81.

Dirks, J. F., Wunder, J., Kinsman, R., McElhinny, J., & Jones, N. F. (1993). A pain rating scale and a pain behavior checklist for clinical use: Development, norms, and the consistency score. *Psychotherapeutics and Psychosomatics, 59,* 41–49.

Dishman, R. K. (1994). Motivating older adults to exercise. *Southern Medical Journal, 87,* S79–S82.

Dobbs, A. R., Heller, R. B., & Schopflocher, D. (1998). A comparative approach to identify unsafe older drivers. *Accident Analysis and Prevention, 30,* 363–370.

Dock, L. (1910). *Hygiene and morality: A manual for nurses and others.* New York: Putnam.

Donahue, D. M. (1999). Career corner. About certification options. *Massachusetts Nurse, 69,* 10.

Donaldson, C., Tarrier, N., & Burns, A. (1998), Determinants of carer stress in Alzheimer's disease. *International Journal of Geriatric Psychiatry, 13,* 248–256.

Donovan, J. M., & Syngal, S. (1998). Colorectal cancer in women: an underappreciated but preventable risk. *Journal of Womens Health, 7,* 45–48.

Dorfman, L. (1989). Retirement preparation and retirement satisfaction in the rural elderly. *The Journal of Applied Gerontology, 8,* 432–450.

Dossey, L. (1997). The healing power of pets. A look at animal-assisted therapy. *Alternative Therapies, 3*(4), 8–16.

Doughty, D. B., & Jackson, D. B. (1993). Constipation teaching guide. *Gastrointestinal Disorders.* St. Louis, MO: Mosby.

Dowdell, E. B. (1995). Caregiver burden: Grandmothers raising their high risk grandchildren. *Journal of Psychosocial Nursing, 33,* 27–30.

Drachman, D. A. (1998). A 69-year-old man with chronic dizziness. *Journal of the American Medical Association, 280,* 2111–2118.

Drachman, D. S., Swearer, J. M., O'Donnell, B. F., Mitchell, A. L., & Maloon, A. (1992) The Caretaker Obstreperous Behavior Rating Assessment (COBRA) scale. *Journal of the American Geriatrics Society, 40,* 463–480.

Dracup, K., & Moser, D. K. (1991). Treatment-seeking behavior among those with signs and symptoms of acute myocardial infarction. *Heart and Lung, 20,* 570–575.

Dressel, P. L., & Barnhill, S. K. (1994). Reframing gerontological thought and practice: The case of grandmothers with daughters in prison. *The Gerontologist, 34,* 685–691.

Drinka, T. (1999, April). Leadership in interdisciplinary health care education and practice: How can we cultivate leaders? Paper presented at the *Interdisciplinary Team Training Institute in Geriatrics and Primary Care,* Newport, RI.

Drossman, D. A., Funch-Jensen, P., Janssens, J., Talley, N. J., Thompson, W. G., & Whitehead, W. E. (1990). Identification of subgroups of functional disorders. *Gastroenterology International, 3,* 159–172.

Drossman, D. A., Li, Z., Andruzzi, E., Temple, R. D., Talley, N. J., Thompson, W. G., Whitehead, W. E., Janssens, J., Funch- Jensen, P., Corazziari, E., Richter, J. E., & Kock, G. G. (1993). U.S. householder survey of functional gastrointestinal disorders: Prevalence, sociodemography, and health impact. *Digestive Diseases and Sciences, 38,* 1569–1580.

Drossman, D. A., & Thompson, W. G. (1992). The irritable bowel syndrome. *Annals of Internal Medicine, 116,* 1009–1016.

Droste, C., & Roskamm, H. (1983). Experimental pain measurement in patients with asymptomatic myocardial ischemia. *Journal of the American College of Cardiology, 1,* 940–945.

Ducanis, A., & Golin, A. (1979). The Interdisciplinary Health Care Team. London: Aspen Systems.

Duchek, J. M., Hunt, L., Ball, K., Buckles, V., & Morris, J. C. (1998). Attention and driving performance in Alzheimer's disease. *Journal of Gerontology: Psychological Sciences, 53B,* P130–P141.

Duff, J., & Sime, E. (1997). Surgical interventions in the treatment of Parkinson's disease (PD) and Essential Tremor (ET): Medial pallidotomy in PD and chronic deep brain stimulation (DBS) in PD and ET. *AXON, 18,* 85–89.

Dungee-Anderson, D., & Beckett, J. O. (1992). Alzheimer's disease in African-American and White families: A clinical analysis. *Smith College Studies in Social Work, 62*(2), 155–168.

Dunn, H. L. (1961). *High level wellness.* Emmaus, PA: Rodale.

Dupree, L. W., & Schonfeld, L. (1998). Cognitive-behavioral and self-management treatment of older problem drinkers. *Journal of Mental Health and Aging, 4,* 215–231.

Dwyer, J. W., & Coward, R. T. (1992). Gender and family care of the elderly: Research gaps and opportunities. In J. W. Dwyer & R. T. Coward (Eds.), *Gender, families, and elder care* (pp. 151–162). Newbury Park, CA: Sage Publications.

Early Alzheimer's Disease Guideline Panel. (1996). *Recognition and initial assessment of Alzheimer's disease and related dementias* (AHCPR Publication No. 97-0702). Washington, DC: U.S. Government Printing Office.

Eastley, R., & Wilcock, G. (1997). Prevalence and correlates of aggressive behaviors occurring in patients with Alzheimer's disease. *International Journal of Geriatric Psychiatry, 12,* 484–487.

Edelman, C., & Mandle C., (1998). *Health Promotion Throughout the Lifespan.* C. V. Mosby, St. Louis, MO.

Ekman, P., & Friesen, W. V. (1978). *Manual of the Facial Action Coding System.* Palo Alto, CA: Consulting Psychologists Press.

Eisenberg, D. M., Kessler, R. C., Foster, C., Norlock, F. E., Calkins, D. R., & Delbanco, T. L. (1993). Unconventional medicine in the United States: Prevalence, costs, and patterns of use. *New England Journal of Medicine, 32,* 246–252.

Ellershaw, J. E., Sutcliffe, J. M., & Saunders, C. M. (1995). Dehydration and the dying patient. *Journal of Pain Symptom Management, 10,* 192–197.

Ellis, M. R., Vinson, D. C., & Ewigman, B. (1999). Addressing spiritual concerns of patients: Family physicians' attitudes and practices. *Journal of Family Practice, 48,* 105–109.

Eng, C., Pedulla, J., Eleazer, G. P., McCann, R., & Fox, N. (1997). Progam of all-inclusive care for the elderly (PACE): an innovative model of integrated geriatric care and financing. *Journal of the American Geriatrics Society, 45,* 223–32.

Eng, M. A. (1993). The hospice interdisciplinary team: A synergistic approach to the care of dying patients and their families. *Holistic Nurse Practitioner, 7,* 49–56.

Erickson, E. H. (1982). *The life cycle review.* New York: WW Norton & Co.

Erkert, J. D. (1988). Dehydration in the elderly. *Journal of the American Academy of Physician Assistants, 1*(4), 261–269.

Ersek, M., Ferrell, B. R., Hassey Dow, K., & Melancon, C. H. (1997). Quality of life in women with ovarian cancer. *Western Journal of Nursing Research, 19,* 334–350.

Ersek, M., Kraybill, B. M., & Hansberry, J. (1999). Investigating the educational needs of licensed nursing staff and certified nursing assistants in nursing homes regarding end-of-life care. *American Journal of Hospice and Palliative Care, 16,* 573–582.

Estes, C. L. (1979). *The aging enterprise.* San Francisco, CA: Josey Bass.

Estes, C. L., Binney, E. A., & Culbertson, R. A. (1992). The gerontological imagination: Social influences on the development of gerontology, 1945–present. *International Journal of Aging and Human Development, 35,* 49–65.

Estes, C., Linkins, K., & Binney, E. (1996). The political economy of aging. In R. H. Binstock & L. K. George (Eds.), *Handbook of aging and the social sciences.* San Diego: Academic Press.

Estes, M. (1998). *Health assessment and physical examination.* New York: Delmar Publishers.

Evans, B. D., & Rogers, A. E. (1994). 24-hour sleep/wake patterns in healthy elderly persons. *Applied Nursing Research, 7,* 75–83.

Evans, D. A., Scherr, P. A., Cook, N. R., Albert, M. S., Funkenstein, H H., Smith, L. A., Hebert, L. E., Wetle, T. T., Branch, L. G., Chown, M., Hennekens, C. H., & Taylor, J. O. (1990). Estimated prevalence of Alzheimer's disease in the United States. *The Milbank Quarterly, 68,* 267–289.

Evans, L. K. (1987). Sundown syndrome in institutionalized elderly. *Journal of the American Geriatrics Society, 35,* 101–108.

Evans, L. K. (1994). Overcoming institutional challenges to collaborative practice. In E. L. Sieglar & F. W. Whitney (Eds.), *Nurse-Physician Collaboration: Care of adults and the Elderly* (pp. 33–42). New York: Springer Publishing Co.

Evans, L. K. (1996). Knowing the patient: The route to individualized care. *Journal of Gerontological Nursing, 22*(3), 15–19.

Evans, L., & Strumpf, N. (1989). Tying down the elderly: A review of the literature on physical restraint. *Journal of the American Geriatrics Society, 37,* 65–74.

Evans, L., & Strumpf, N. (1990). Myths about elder restraint. *Image: Journal of Nursing Scholarship, 22,* 124–128.

Evans, L., Strumpf, N., Allen-Taylor, S., Capezuti, E., Maislin, G., & Jacobson, B. (1997). A clinical trial to reduce restraints in nursing homes. *Journal of the American Geriatrics Society, 45,* 675–681.

Evans, L., Strumpf, N., Williams, C., Williams, T., Middleton, W., Jacobsen, B., Allen-Taylor, S., & Capezuti, E. (1993). A comparison of physical restraints in American and European nursing homes. *Gerontologist, 34*(Special issue 1), 271.

Evans, W. B., White, G. L., Wood, S. D., Hood, S. B., & Bailey M. B. (1998). Managing dysphagia: Fundamental of primary care. *Clinician Reviews, 8*(8), 47–54, 57–59, 63–64, 69–71.

Fahey, V. A. (1999). *Vascular nursing* (3rd ed.). Philadelphia: W. B. Saunders Company.

Falck, K., Grohn, P., Sorsa, M., Vanio, H., Heinonen, E., & Holsti, L. R. (1979). Mutagenicity in urine of nurses handling cytostatic drugs. *Lancet, 1,* 1250–1251.

Famularo, R., Kinscherff, R., Bunshaft, D., Spivak, G., & Fenton, T. (1989). Parental compliance to court ordered treatment interventions in cases of child maltreatment. *Child Abuse and Neglect, 13,* 507–514.

Fantl, J. A., Newman, D. K., Colling, J., DeLancey, J. O. L., Keeys, C., Loughery, R., McDowell, B. J., Norton, P., Ouslander, J., Schnelle, J., Staskin, D., Tries, J., Urich, V., Vitousek, S. H., Weiss, B. D., & Whitmore, K. (1996). *Urinary incontinence in adults: Acute and chronic management: AHCPR Clinical Practice Guideline* (Publication No. 96-0682). Rockville, MD: U.S. Department of Health and Human Services, Public Health Service, Agency for Health Care Policy and Research.

Farmer, M., White, L. R., Brody, J., & Bailey, K. R. (1984). Race and sex differences in hip fracture incidence. *American Journal of Public Health, 74,* 1374–1380.

Farran, C. J., Keane-Hagerty, E., Salloway, S., Kupferer, S., & Wilken, C. S. (1991). Finding meaning: An alternate paradigm for Alzheimer's disease caregivers. *The Gerontologist, 31,* 483–489.

Federman, D. G., Trent, J. T., Froelich, C. W., Demirovic, J., & Kirsner R. S. (1998). Epidemiology of peripheral vascular disease: a predictor of systemic vascular disease. *Ostomy Management, (5),* 58–60.

Feetham, S. (1993). Family outcomes: Conceptual and methodological issues. In P. Moritz (Ed.), *Patient outcomes research: Examining the effectiveness of nursing practice.* Bethesda, MD: National Center for Nursing Research.

Fehring, R. J., Miller, J. F., & Shaw, C. (1997). Spiritual well-being, religiosity, hope, depression, and other mood states in elderly people coping with cancer. *Oncology Nursing Forum, 24*(4), 63–71.

Feig, L. (June, 1997). Informal and formal kinship care: Findings from national and state data. U. S. Department of Health and Human Services, Office of the Assistant Secretary for Planning and Evaluation.

Feinberg, L. F., & Kelly, K. A. (1995). A well-deserved break: Respite programs offered by California's Statewide System of Caregiver Resource Centers. *The Gerontologist, 35,* 701–705.

Feldman, M. J., Ventura, M. R., & Crosby, F. (1987). Studies of nurse practitioner effectiveness. *Nursing Research, 36,* 303–306.

Feldstein, M. A., & Gemma, P. B. (1995). Oncology nurses and chronic compounded grief. *Cancer Nursing, 18,* 228–236.

Feldstein, P. J. (1994). *Health policy and issues: An economic perspective on health reform.* Ann Arbor, MI: AUPHA Press/Health Administration Press.

Feldt, K. S. (1996). Treatment of pain in cognitively impaired versus cognitively intact post hip fractured elders (Doctoral dissertation, University of Minnesota, 1996). *Dissertation Abstracts International, 57-09B,* 5574.

Feldt, K. S., Ryden, M. B., & Miles, S. (1998). Treatment of pain in cognitively impaired compared with cognitively intact older patients with hip fracture. *Journal of the American Geriatrics Society, 46,* 1079–1085.

Feldt, K., Warne, M., & Ryden, M. (1998). Examining pain in aggressive cognitively impaired older adults. *Journal of Gerontological Nursing, 24*(11), 14–22.

Felson, D. T., Kiel, D. P., Anderson, J. J., & Kamel, W. B. (1988). Alcohol consumption and hip fractures: The Framingham study. *American Journal of Epidemiology, 128,* 1102–1110.

Fengler, A., & Goodrich, N. (1979). Wives of elderly disabled men: the hidden patients. *The Gerontologist, 19,* 175–183.

Fenton, M. V., & Brykczynski, K. A. (1993). Qualitative distinctions and similarities in the practice of clinical nurse specialists and nurse practitioners. *Journal of Professional Nursing, 9,* 313–26.

Ferrans, C. E., & Powers, M. J. (1992). Psychometric assessment of the quality of life index. *Research in Nursing and Health, 15,* 29–38.

Ferrell, B. A. (1993). The assessment and control of pain in the nursing home. In L. Z. Rubenstein & D. Weilan (Eds.), *Improving care in the nursing home* (pp. 241–250). London: Sage Publications.

Ferrell, B. A., Ferrell, B. R., & Osterweil, D. (1990). Pain in the nursing home. *Journal of the American Geriatrics Society, 38,* 409–414.

Ferrell, B. A., Ferrell, B. R., & Rivera, L. (1995). Pain in cognitively impaired nursing home patients. *Journal of Pain and Symptom Management, 10,* 591–598.

Ferrell, B. R., & Hassey Dow, K. (1997). Quality of life in long-term cancer survivors. *Oncology, 11,* 565–571.

Ferrell, B. R., Hassey Dow, K., Leigh, S., Ly, J., & Gulasekaram, P. (1995). Quality of life among long-term cancer survivors. *Oncology Nursing Forum, 22,* 915–922.

Ferrell, B. R., Wisdom, C., & Wenzel, C. (1989). Quality of life as an outcome variable in management of cancer pain. *Cancer, 63,* 2321–2327.

Fiatarone, M. A., O'Neill, E. F., Ryan, N. D., Clements, K. M., Solares, G. R., Nelson, M. E., Roberts, S. B., Kehayias, J. J., Lipsitz, L. A., & Evans, W. J. (1994). Exercise training and nutritional supplementation for physical frailty in very elderly people. *The New England Journal of Medicine, 330,* 1769–1775.

Fick, D. (1997). Recognition and management of delirium superimposed on dementia in hospitalized elders [Special Issue 1]. *The Gerontologist, 37,* 79.

Fick, D., & Foreman, M. D. (in press). The consequences of not recognizing delirium superimposed on dementia in hospitalized elders. *Journal of Gerontological Nursing.*

Finlayson, R. E. (1998). Prescription drug dependence in the elderly: The clinical pathway to recovery. *Journal of Mental Health and Aging, 4*(2), 233–249.

Finnick, M., Reis, J., & Drobits, K. (1990). How nurse aides perceive quality of care. *Nursing Homes, 39*(3/4), 12–16.

Fishbein, M., & Ajzen, I. (1975). *Belief, attitude, intention, and behavior: An introduction to theory and research.* Reading, MA: Addison-Wesley.

Fitzgerald, J. F., Moore, P. S., & Dittus, R. S. (1988). The care of elderly patient with hip fracture: Changes since implementation of the prospective payment system. *New England Journal of Medicine, 319,* 1392–1397.

Fitzgerald, J. F., & Dittus, R. S. (1990). Institutionalized patients with hip fractures: Characteristics associated with returning to community dwelling. *Journal of General Internal Medicine, 5,* 298–303.

Fitzpatrick, J. J., & Whall, A. L. (1996). *Conceptual models of nursing: Analysis and application* (3rd ed.). Stamford, CT: Appleton & Lange.

Fleming, C. M., & Scanlon, C. (1994). The role of the nurse in the Patient Self Determination Act. *Journal of the New York State Nurses Association, 25,* 19–23.

Fleming, M. F., & Barry, J. L.. (1992). *Addictive disorders.* St. Louis: Mosby.

Flint, A. (1995). Effects of respite care on patients with dementia and their caregivers. *International Psychogeriatrics, 7,* 505–517.

Floyd, F., Haynes, S., Doll, E., Winemiller, D., Lemsky, C., Burgy, T., Werle, M., & Heilman, N. (1992). Assessing retirement satisfaction and perceptions of retirement experiences. *Psychology and Aging, 7,* 609–621.

Folstein, M. (1998). Mini-mental and son. *International Journal of Geriatric Psychiatry, 13,* 290–294.

Folstein, M., Folstein, S., & McHugh, P. (1975). Mini-mental state: A practical method for grading the cognitive state of patients for the clinician. *Journal of Psychiatric Research, 12,* 189–198.

Folta, J. R. (1965). The perception of death. *Nursing Research, 14,* 232–235.

Forbes, C. S. (1997). The concepts and benefits of dementia specific programming within an assisted living setting. *American Journal of Alzheimer's Disease, January/February,* 16–22.

Forbes, D. A. (1998). Strategies for managing behavioral symptoms associated with dementia of the Alzheimer's type: A systematic overview. *Canadian Journal of Nursing, 30,* 67–86.

Forbes, E. J. (1994). Spirituality, aging, and the community-dwelling caregiver and care recipient. *Geriatric Nursing, 15,* 297–302.

Ford, M., Fox, J., Fitch, S., & Donovan, A. (1987). Psychiatric skills: Light in the darkness. The environment of patients with Alzheimer's disease. *Nursing Times, 83,* 26–29.

Foreman, M. D. (1993). Acute confusion in the elderly. In J. J. Fitzpatrick & J. S. Stevenson (Eds.), *Annual review of nursing research* (Vol. 11, pp. 3–30). New York: Springer Publishing.

Fortinsky, R., & Hathaway, T. (1990). Information and service needs among active and former family caregivers of person with Alzheimer's disease. *The Gerontologist, 30,* 604–609.

Fowler, S. B. (1997). Hope and a health-promoting lifestyle in persons with Parkinson's disease. *Journal of Neuroscience Nursing, 29,* 111–116.

Fox, S. D., & Wold, J. E. (1996). Baccalaureate gerontological nursing experiences: Raising consciousness levels and affecting attitudes. *Journal of Nursing Education, 35,* 348–355.

Francis, G. M. (1991). "Here comes the puppies": The power of the human-animal bond. *Holistic Nursing Practice, 5*(2), 38–41.

Franklin, S. S., Sutton-Tyrell, K., Belle, S. H., Weber, M. A., & Kuller, L. H. (1997). The importance of pulsatile components of hypertension in predicting carotid stenosis in older adults. *Journal of Hypertension, 15,* 1143–50.

Frasure-Smith, N., Lesperance, F., & Talajic, M. (1993). Depression following myocardial infarction: Impact on 6-month survival. *Journal of the American Medical Association, 270,* 1819–1825.

Frazier-Smith, N., Lesperance, F., & Talajic, M. (1993). Depression following myocardial infarction: Impact on 6 month survival. *Journal of the American Medical Association, 270*(15), 1819–1825.

Freedland, K. E., Carney, R. M. Lustman, P. J., Rich, M. W., & Jaffe, A. S. (1992). Major depression in coronary artery disease patients with or without a prior history of depression. *Psychosomatic Medicine, 54,* 416–421.

Freeman, L. (1995). Home-sweet-home health care. *Monthly Labor Review, 118*(3), 3–11.

Frengley, J. D., & Mion, L. C. (1998). Physical restraints in the acute care setting: Issues and future direction. *Clinics in Geriatric Medicine, 14,* 727–743.

Freud, S. (1957). *Mourning and melancholia: Standard edition of the complete psychological works of Sigmund Freud* (Vol. 14). London: Hogarth Press.

Fried, L. P., Kronmal, R. A., Newman, A. B., Bild, D. E., Mittelmark, M. B., Polak, J. F., Robbins, J. A., & Gardin, J. M., Cardiovascular Health Study Collaborative Research Group. (1998). Risk factors for 5-year mortality in older adults. *Journal of the American Medicine Association, 279,* 585–592.

Friedland, R. P., Koss, E., Kumar, A., Gaine, S., Metzler, D., Haxby, J. V., & Moore, A. (1988). Motor vehicle crashes in dementia of the Alzheimer type. *Annals of Neurology, 24,* 782–786.

Friedman, E., & Havighurst, R. (Eds.) (1954). *The meaning of work and retirement.* Chicago: University of Chicago Press.

Friedmann, E., Katcher, A. H., Lynch, J. J., & Thomas, S. A. (1980). Animal companions and one-year survival of patients after discharge from a coronary care unit. *Public Health Reports, 95,* 307–312.

Friedman, M. M. (1993). Social support sources and psychological well-being in older women with heart disease. *Research in Nursing and Health, 16,* 405–413.

Frumkin, N. L., Palumbo, C. L., & Naeser, M. A. (1994). Brain imaging and its applications to aphasia rehabilitation: CT and MRI. In R. Chapey (Ed.), *Language Intervention Strategies in Adult Aphasia* (3rd ed.) (pp. 47–49, 76). Baltimore, MD: Williams & Wilkins.

Fucile, S., Wright, P. M., Chan, I., Yee, S., Langlais, M., & Gisel, E. G. (1998). Functional oral-motor skills: Do they change with age? *Dysphagia, 13,* 195–201.

Fukuda, K., Straus, S. E., Hickie, I., Sharpe, M. C., Dobbins, J. G., Komaroff, A., & the International Chronic Fatigue Syndrome Study Group. (1994). The chronic fatigue syndrome: A comprehensive approach to its definition and study. *Annals of Internal Medicine, 121,* 953–959.

Fulmer, T. (1991). The geriatric nurse specialist role: a new model. *Nursing Management, 22,* 91–93.

Fulmer, T., & Abraham, I. L. (1998). Rethinking geriatric nursing. *Nursing Clinics of North America, 33,* 387–394.

Fulmer, T., & Edelman, C. L. (1991). *Adult Day Care,* Management and Care of the Elderly, Psychosocial Perspectives, Harper, Mary S. (ed), Sage Publications, 269–289.

Fulmer, T., & Gurland, B. J. (1996). Restriction as elder mistreatment: Differences between caregiver and elder perceptions. *Journal of Mental Health and Aging, 2,* 89–100.

Fulmer, T., Mion, L. C., & Bottrell, M. M. (1996). Pain management protocol. *Geriatric Nursing, 17,* 222–226.

Fulmer, T., Hollander, Feldman, P., Kim, T. S., Carty, B., Beers, M., Molina, M., & Putnam, M. (1999). An intervention study to enhance medication compliance in community-dwelling elderly individuals. *Journal of Gerontological Nursing, 25*(8), 6–14.

Funk, S., Tornquist, E., Champagne, M., & Wiese, R. (Eds.). (1993). *Key aspects of caring for the chronically ill.* New York: Springer Publishing.

Futrell, M., & Jones, W. (1977). Attitudes of physicians, nurses, and social workers toward the elderly and health maintenance service for the aged implications for health manpower policy. *Journal of Gerontological Nursing, 3,* 42–46.

Galindo-Ciocon, D. J., Ciocon, J. B., & Galindo, D. J. (1995). Gait training and falls in the elderly. *Journal of Gerontological Nursing, 21*(6), 11–17.

Gallagher, D., Lovett, S., & Zeiss, A. (1989). Interventions with caregivers of frail elders: Current research status and future research directions. In M. Ory & K. Bond (Eds.), *Aging and health care: Social science and policy perspectives* (pp. 167–190). New York: Routledge.

Gallagher-Thompson, D., & Powers, D. V. (1997). Primary stressors and depressive symptoms in caregivers of dementia patients. *Aging & Mental Health, 1,* 248–255.

Gallo, A. M., Breitmayer, B. J., & Knafl, K. A. (1992). Well siblings of children with chronic illnesses: Parents' reports of their psychological adjustment. *Pediatric Nursing, 18,* 23–27.

Garnick, M., & Fair, W. (1998). Combating prostate cancer. *Scientific American, 279*(6), 75–83.

Garstecki, D., & Erler, S. (1998). Hearing loss, control, and demographic factors influencing hearing aid use among older adults. *Journal of Speech, Language, and Hearing Research, 41,* 527–537.

Gaspar, P. M. (1988). What determines how much patients drink? *Geriatric Nursing, 9,* 221–224.

Gass, K. A. (1987a). Coping strategies of widows. *Journal of Gerontological Nursing, 13*(8), 29–33.

Gass, K. A. (1987b). The health of conjugally bereaved older widows: The role of appraisal, coping and resources. *Research in Nursing & Health, 10,* 39–47.

Gass, K. A. (1988). Aged widows and widowers: Similarities and differences in appraisal, coping, resources, type of death, and health dysfunction. *Archives of Psychiatric Nursing, 2,* 200–210.

Gass, K. A., & Chang, A. S. (1989). Appraisals of bereavement, coping, resources, and psychosocial health dysfunction in widows and widowers. *Nursing Research, 38,* 31–36.

Gaston, E. T. (1951). Dynamic music factors in mood change. *Music Educators Journal, 3,* 42–44.

Gastrin, G., Miller, A. B., To, T., Aronson, K. J., Wall, C., Hakama, M., Louhivuori, K., & Pukkala, E. (1994). Incidence and mortality from breast cancer in the Mama program for breast screening in Finland, 1973–1986. *Cancer, 73,* 2168–2174.

Gates, D. M., Fitzwater, E., & Meyer, U. (1999). Violence against caregivers in nursing homes: expected, tolerated and accepted. *Journal of Gerontological Nursing 25*(4), 12–22.

Gelberg, L., Linn, L. S., & Mayer-Oakes, S. A. (1990). Differences in health status between older and younger homeless adults. *Journal of the American Geriatrics Society, 38,* 1220–1229.

George, L. K., & Gwyther, L. P. (1986). Caregiver well-being: A multidimensional examination of family caregivers of demented adults. *Gerontologist, 26,* 253–259.

Gerdner, L. A. (in press). Effects of individualized vs. Classical "relaxation" music on the frequency of agitation in elderly persons with Alzheimer's disease and related disorders. *International Psychogeriatrics.*

Gerdner, L. A., & Swanson, L. (1993). Effects of individualized music on elderly patients who are confused and agitated. *Archives of Psychiatric Nursing, 7,* 282–291.

Giasson, M., & Bouchard, L. (1998). Effect of therapeutic touch on the well-being of persons with terminal cancer. *Journal of Holistic Nursing, 16,* 383–398.

Gibbons, P., Gannon, M., & Wrigley, M. (1997). A study of aggression among referrals to a community-based psychiatry of old age service. *International Journal of Geriatric Psychiatry, 12,* 384–388.

Giebel, G. D., Lefering, R., Triold, H., & Blochl, H. (1998). Prevalence of fecal incontinence: What can be expected? *International Journal of Colorectal Disease, 13,* 73–77.

Gift, A. (1989). Validation of a vertical visual analogue scale as a measure of clinical dyspnea. *Rehabilitation Nursing, 14,* 323–325.

Gift, A., Moore, T., & Soeken, K. (1992). Relaxation to reduce dyspnea and anxiety in COPD patients. *Nursing Research, 41,* 242–246.

Gilbert, M., Counsell, C. M., & Snively, C. (1996). Pallidotomy: A surgical intervention for control of Parkinson's disease. *Journal of Neuroscience Nursing. 28,* 215–216, 221.

Gilford, D. M. (Ed.). (1998). The aging population in the twenty-first century. *Statistics for Health Policy.* Washington, DC: National Academy Press.

Gill, T. M., Williams, C. S., Mendes de Leon, C. F., & Tinetti, M. E. (1997). The role of change in physical performance in determining risk of dependence in ADLs among nondisabled community-living elderly persons. *Journal of Clinical Epidemiology, 60,* 765–772.

Gilliss, C., & Knafl, K. (1997). Nursing care of families in non-normative transitions: The state of science and practice. In A. S. Hinshaw, S. L. Feetham, & J. Shaver (Eds.), *Handbook of clinical nursing research.* Thousand Oaks, CA: Sage.

Gilmour, J., & Penny, S. (1991). Hydration & Ageing. *New Zealand Journal of Nursing, November,* 15–17.

Givens, B. A., & Givens, C. W. (1991). Family caregiving for the elderly. In J. J. Fitzpatrick & J. S. Stevenson (Eds.), *Annual review of nursing research* (Vol. 9, pp. 77–92). New York: Springer Publishing.

Glaser, B. G., & Strauss, A. L. (1965). *Awareness of dying.* Chicago: Aldine.

Glaser, B. G., & Strauss, A. L. (1968). *Time for dying.* Chicago: Aldine.

Glazier, J. J., Chierchia, S., Brown, M. J., & Maseri, A. (1986). Importance of generalized defective perception of painful stimulus as a cause of silent myocardial ischemia in chronic stable angina pectoris. *The American Journal of Cardiology, 58,* 667–672.

Glick, O. J., & Tripp-Reimer, T. (1996). The Iowa conceptual model of gerontological nursing. In E. A. Swanson & T. Tripp-Reimer (Eds.), *Advances in gerontological nursing* (Vol. 1, pp. 11–55). New York: Springer Publishing.

Goddaer, J., & Abraham, I. L. (1994). Effects of relaxing music on agitation during meals among nursing home residents with severe cognitive impairment. *Archives of Psychiatric Nursing, 8,* 150–158.

Goldberg, R. J., Gore, J. M., Gurwitz, J. H., Alpert, J. S., Brady, P., Strohsnitter, W., Chen, Z., & Dalen, J. E. (1989). The impact of age on the incidence and prognosis of initial acute MI: The Worcester Heart Attack Study. *American Heart Journal, 117,* 543–549.

Goldsmith, S. M., Hoeffer, B., & Rader, J. (1995). Problematic wandering behavior in the cognitively impaired elderly. *Journal of Psychosocial Nursing, 33*(2), 6–12.

Goodman, C. C., Pynoos, J., & Stevenson, L. M. (1988). Board and care castaways: Older adults outside the long term care continuum. *Social Work in Health Care, 13*(4), 65–79.

Goodridge, D. M., Johnston, P., & Thomson, M. (1996). Conflict and aggression as stressors in the work environment of nursing assistants: Implications for institutional elder abuse. *Journal of Elder Abuse & Neglect, 8,* 49–67.

Gordon, M. (1994). *Nursing diagnosis: Process and application* (3rd ed.). St. Louis: Mosby.

Gosnell, D. (1973). An assessment tool to identify pressure sores. *Nursing Research, 22,* 5–59.

Gottlieb, S. S., McCarter, R. J., & Vogel, R. A. (1998). Effect of beta-blockade on mortality among high-risk and low-risk patients after myocardial infarction. *New England Journal of Medicine, 339,* 489–497.

Grabbe, L., Demi, A., Camann, M., & Potter, L. (1997). The health status of elderly persons in the last year of life: A comparison of deaths by suicide, injury, and natural causes. *American Journal of Public Health, 87,* 434–437.

Grafman, J., Weingartner, H., Newhouse, P. A., Thompson, K., Lalonde, F., Litvan, I., Molchan, S., & Sunderland, T. (1990). Implicit learning in patients with Alzheimer's disease. *Pharmacopsychiatry, 32,* 94–101.

Graham, J. D. (1995). Licensing standards for elderly drivers. *Consumers' Research Magazine, 78*(12), 18–22.

Grammas, P., Moore, P., & Weigel, P. H. (1999). Microvessels from Alzheimer's disease brains kill neurons in vitro. *American Journal of Pathology, 154,* 337–342.

Grant, L. A., & Sommers, A. R. (1998). Adapting living environments for persons with Alzheimer's disease. *Geriatrics, 53*(Supp. 1), S61–S65.

Grant, M., & Nolan, G. (1994). Informal carers: Sources and concomitants of satisfaction. *Health and Social Care, 1,* 147–159.

Greene, M., Adelman, R., Friedmann, E., & Charon, R. (1994). Older patient satisfaction with communication during an initial medical encounter. *Social Science Medicine, 38,* 1279–1288.

Greipp, M. E. (1992). Undermedication for pain: An ethical model. *Advances in Nursing Science, 15,* 44–53.

Grey, M., Cameron, M. E., Lipman, T. H., & Thurber, F. W. (1995). Psychosocial status of children with diabetes over the first two years. *Diabetes Care, 18,* 1330–1336.

Grimby, A., & Rosenhall, U. (1995). Health-related quality of life and dizziness in old age. *Gerontology, 41,* 286–298.

Grimm, R. J. (1996). Dizziness. *Nurse Practitioner Forum, 7,* 160–166.

Groher, M. (1997). Nature of the problem. In M. Groher (Ed.), *Dysphagia: Diagnosis and management* (3rd ed.) (pp. 1–6). Boston: Butterworth-Heinemann.

Groher, M., & McKaig, T. N. (1995). Dysphagia and dietary levels in skilled nursing facilities. *Journal of the American Geriatrics Society, 43,* 528–532.

Groom, D. (1993). Elder care. A diagnostic model for failure to thrive. *Journal of Gerontological Nursing, 19,*(6), 12–16.

Grzeczkowski & Knapp (1988). The gerontological nurse practitoners as director of nursing n the long-term facility. *Nursing Management, 19,* 64B-D, 64F.

Gu, X., & Belgrade, M. J. (1993). Pain in hospitalized patients with medical illnesses. *Journal of Pain & Symptom Management, 8,* 17–21.

Gudwin, A. L., & Padussis, C. J. (1994). Smoking, age, and sex in carotid artery artheroscleerosis: a review of 3,865 carotid duplex scans. *Maryland Medicine, 43,* 265–268.

Gunter, L., & Estes, C. (1979). *Education for gerontic nursing.* New York: Springer Publishing.

Gurnack, A. M. (1996). *Older adults' misuse of medicines, alcohol, and other drugs.* New York: Springer Publishing Company.

Gurnack, A. M., & Schonfeld, L. (1998). Substance misuse among older adults. *Journal of Mental Health and Aging, 4,* 195–196.

Guzzetta, C. E. (1988). Music therapy: Hearing the melody of the soul. In B. M. Dossey, L. Keegan, C. E. Guzzetta, & L. G. Kolkmeier (Eds.), *Holistic nursing: A handbook for practice* (pp. 263–288). Rockville, MD: Aspen.

Gwyther, L., Ballard, E., & Hinman-Smith, E. (1990). *Overcoming Barriers for Appropriate Service Use: Effective Individualized Strategies for Alzheimer's Care.* Durham, NC: Duke University, Center for Study of Aging and Human Development.

Haapanen-Neimi, N., Vuori, I., & Pasanen, M. (1999). Public health burden of coronary heart disease risk factors among middle-aged and elderly men. *Preventive Medicine, 28,* 343–348.

Haas, G., & Sakr, W. (1997). Epidemiology of prostate cancer. *CA: A Cancer Journal for Clinicians, 47,* 273–287.

Haber, L. C., Fagan-Pryor, E. C., & Allen, M. (1997). Comparison of registered nurses' and nursing assistants' choices of interventions for aggressive behaviors. *Issues in Mental Health Nursing, 18,* 113–124.

Hackett, T. P. (1985). Depression following myocardial infarction. *Psychosomatics, 26,* 23–28.

Hagen, B. F., & Sayers, D. (1995). When caring leaves bruises: The effects of staff education on resident aggression. *Journal of Gerontological Nursing, 21*(11), 7–16.

Haight, B., Christ, M. A., & Dias, J. (1994). Does nursing education promote ageism? *Journal of Advanced Nursing, 20,* 382–390.

Hak, E, van Essen, G. A., Stalman, W. A., & de Melker, R. A. (1998). Improving influenza vaccination coverage among high-risk patients: A role for computer-supported prevention strategy? *Family Practice, 15*(2), 138–143.

Hales, D. (1981). *The complete book of sleep.* Reading, MA: Addison Wesley Publishing Company.

Hall, G. R., & Buckwalter, K. C. (1987). Progressively lowered stress threshold: A conceptual model for care of adults with Alzheimer's disease. *Archives of Psychiatric Nursing, 1,* 399–406.

Hall, G. R., Gerdner, L., Zwycart-Stauffacher, M., & Buckwalter, K. C. (1995). Principles of nonpharmacological management: Caring for people with Alzheimer's disease using a conceptual model. *Psychiatric Annals, 25,* 432–440.

Hall, G., Kirschling, M. V., & Todd, S. (1986). Sheltered freedom: An Alzheimer's unit in an ICF. *Geriatric Nursing, 7,* 132–137.

Hall, N. (1997). Health maintenance & promotion. In R. Ham & P. Sloane (Eds.), *Primary Care Geriatrics.* New York: C. V. Mosby Co.

Hampton, F. R. (1992). The encyclopedia of aging and the elderly.

Hamric, A. B., Spross, J. A., & Hanson, C. M. (1996). *Advanced practice nursing: An integrated approach.* Philadelphia: W. B. Saunders.

Handley, M., & Stuart, M. (1994). The use of prostate specific antigen for prostate cancer screening: A managed care perspective. *The Journal of Urology, 152,* 1689–1692.

Hanly, P. J., & Zuberi-Khokhar, N. (1996). Periodic limb movements during sleep in patients with congestive heart failure. *Chest: the Cardiopulmonary Journal, 109,* 1497–1502.

Happ, M. B., Williams, C. C., Strumpf, N. E., & Burger, S. G. (1996). Individualized care for frail elders: Theory and practice. *Journal of Gerontological Nursing, 22*(3), 7–14.

Harper, M. S., & Lacey, B. M. (1993). Mental health/mental illness of the elderly who are homeless. *ABNF Journal, 4*(2), 45–9.

Harrington, C., Carillo, H., Thollaug, S. C., & Summers, P. R. (1996). Nursing facilities, staffing, residents, and facility deficiencies, 1991-95. San Francisco: Department of Social and Behavioral Sciences, School of Nursing, University of California.

Harris, J. L., & Williams, L. K. (1991). Universal self-care requisites as identified by homeless elderly men. *Journal of Gerontological Nursing, 17*(6), 39–43.

Harris, K. A., Ameli, F. M., Lally, M., Provan, J. W., Goldberg, M. R., Johnston, & Walker, P. M. (1986). Abdominal aortic aneurysm resection in patients more than 80 years old. *Surgical Gynecology, 162,* 5368.

Harris, M. D., Rinehart, J. M., & Gerstman, J. (1993). Animal-assisted therapy for the homebound elderly. *Holistic Nurse Practice, 8,* 27–37.

Hart, B. D., & Wells, D. L. (1997). The effects of language used by caregivers on agitation in residents with dementia. *Clinical Nurse Specialist, 11,* 20–23.

Hassey, D., Ferrell, B. R., Leigh, S., & Melancon, C. (in press). The cancer survivor as co-investigator: The benefits of collaborative research with advocacy groups. *Cancer Practice.*

Hathaway, D., Abell, T., Cardoso, S., Hartwig, M., Elmer, D., Horton, J., Lawrence, D., Gaber, L., & Gaber, A. O. (1993). Improvement in autonomic function following pancreas-kidney versus kidney-alone transplantation. *Transplantation Proceedings, 25*(1 Pt. 2), 1306–1308.

Hawley, D. J. (1995). Psycho-educational interventions in the treatment of arthritis. *Bailliere's Clinical Rheumatology, 9,* 803–823.

Hazlett, R. L., Tusa, R. J., & Waranch, H. R. (1995). Development of an inventory for dizziness and related factors. *Journal of Behavioral Medicine, 19,* 75–85.

Hegge, M. (1991). A qualitative retrospective study of coping strategies of newly widowed elderly: Effects of anticipatory grieving on the caregiver. *American Journal of Hospice & Palliative Care, 8*(4), 28–34.

Heidrich, S. M. (1998). Health promotion in old age. *Annual Review of Nursing Research, 16,* 173–195.

Heinemann, G. D., Schmitt, M. H., Farrell, M. P., & Brallier, S. A. (1999). Development of an attitudes toward health care teams scale. *Evaluating Health Professionals, 22*(1), 123–142.

Heitkemper, M. M., Jarrett, M., Cain, K., Shaver, J. F., Bond, E. F., Woods, N. F., & Walker, E. (1996). Increased urine catecholamines and cortisol in women with irritable bowel syndrome. *American Journal of Gastroenterology, 91,* 906–913.

Heitkemper, M. M., Levy, R., Jarrett, M., & Bond, E. F. (1995). Interventions for irritable bowel syndrome: A nursing model. *Gastroenterology Nursing, 18,* 224–230.

Held-Warmkessel, J. (1998). Colon cancer: Prevention and detection strategies. *Advance Nurse Practice, 6*(7), 42–45.

Henderson, V. (1961) *Basic Principles of Nursing Care.* London: International Council of Nurses.

Henderson, V., & Nite, G. (1978). *Principles and practice of nursing* (6th ed.). New York: National League of Nursing.

Henretta, J., O'Rand, A., & Chan, C. (1993). Gender differences in employment after spouse's retirement. *Research on Aging, 15,* 148–169.

Herr, K. A., & Mobily, P. R. (1991). Complexities of pain assessment in the elderly. *Journal of Gerontological Nursing, 17,* 12–18.

Herr, K. A., & Mobily, P. R. (1993). Comparison of selected pain assessment tools for use with the elderly. *Applied Nursing Research, 6,* 39–46.

Herth, K. (1990). Relationship of hope, coping styles, concurrent losses, and setting to grief resolution in the elderly widow(er). *Research in Nursing and Health, 13,* 109–117.

Herth, K. (1990a). Relationship of hope, coping styles, concurrent losses, and setting to grief resolution in the elderly widow(er). *Research in Nursing & Health, 13,* 109–117.

Herth, K. (1990b). Fostering hope in terminally-ill people. *Journal of Advanced Nursing, 15,* 1250–1259.

Heumann, L. F. (1991). A cost comparison of congregate housing and long term care facilities for elderly residents with comparable support needs in 1985 and 1990. *Journal of Housing for the Elderly, 7,* 75–97.

Hewawasam, L. (1996). The use of two-dimensional grid patterns to limit hazardous ambulation in elderly patients with Alzhiemer's disease. *Nt Research, 1,* 217–228.

Hibbard, J. (1995). Women's employment history and their post-retirement health and resources. *Journal of Women & Aging, 7*(3), 43–54.

Higgins, M., Enright, P., Kronmal, R., Schenker, M., Anton-Culver, H., & Lyles, M. (1993). Smoking and lung function in elderly men and women: The cardiovascular health study. *Journal of the American Medical Association, 269,* 2741–2748.

Highfield, M. F., & Cason, C. (1983). Spiritual needs of patients: Are they recognized? *Cancer Nursing, 6,* 187–192.

Hildebrand, J., Joos, S., & Lee, M. (1997). Use of the diagnosis "failure to thrive" in older veterans. *Journal of the American Geriatrics Society, 45,* 1113–1117.

Hill, M. N., & Becker, D. M. (1995). Role of nurses and health care workers in cardiovascular health promotion. *American Journal of the Medical Sciences, 310,* S123–S126.

Hirst, S. T., & Metcalf, B. J. (1989). Whys and whats of wandering. *Geriatric Nursing, 10,* 237–238.

Hoch, C. C., Buysse, D. J., Monk, T. H., & Reynolds, C. F. (1992). Sleep disorders and aging. In J. E. Birren, R. B. Sloane, & G. D. Cohen (Eds.). *Handbook of Mental Health and Aging* (2nd ed.) (pp. 557–581). New York: Academic Press Inc.

Hoeffer, B. (1987a). A casual model of loneliness among older single women. *Archives of Psychiatric Nursing, 1,* 366–373.

Hoeffer, B. (1987b). Predictors of life outlook of older single women. *Research in Nursing & Health, 10,* 111–117.

Hoeffer, B., Rader, J., McKenzie, D., Lavelle, M., & Stewart, B. (1997). Reducing aggressive behavior during bathing cognitively impaired nursing home residents. *Journal of Gerontological Nursing, 23,* 16–23.

Hoenig, H., Sloane, R., & Kahn, K. (1998). Hip fracture rehabilitation. *Archives of Internal Medicine, 158,* 100.

Hogstel, M. O., & Nelson, N. (1992). Anticipation and early detection can reduce bowel elimination complications. *Geriatric Nursing, 13*(1), 28–33.

Hogue, C. C. (1984). Falls and mobility in late life: An ecological model. *Journal of the American Geriatrics Society, 32,* 858–861.

Hogue, C. C., Studenski, S., & Duncan, P. (1990). Assessing mobility: the first step in preventing falls. In S. G. Funk, E. M. Tornquist, M. T. Champagne, L. A. Copp, & R. A. Wiese (Eds.), *Key aspects of recovery: Improving nutrition, rest, and mobility* (pp. 275–280). New York: Springer Publishing Company.

Holmberg, S. K. (1997). Evaluation of a clinical intervention for wanderers on a geriatric nursing unit. *Archives of Psychiatric Nursing, 11,* 21–28.

Holohan-Bell, J., & Brummel-Smith, K. (1999). Impaired mobility and deconditioning. In J. Stone, J. Wyman, & S. Salisbury (Eds.), *Clinical gerontological nursing: A guide to advanced practice* (pp. 267–287). Philadelphia, PA: W. B. Saunders.

Holstein, J., Chatellier, G., Piette, F., & Moulias, R. (1994). Prevalence of associated diseases in different types of dementia among elderly institutionalized patients: Analysis of 3447 records. *Journal of the American Geriatric Society, 42*(9), 972–977.

Hopman-Rock, M., deBock, G. H., Bijlsma, J. W., Springer, M. P., Hofman, A., & Kraaimaat, F. W. (1997). The pattern of health care utilization of elderly people with arthritic pain in the hip or knee. *International Journal of Quality Health Care, 9,* 129–137.

Hopp, F. P. (1999). Patterns and predictors of formal and informal care. *Gerontologist,* *39*(2), 167–176.

Horn, S., Ashton, C., & Tracy, D. (1994). Prevention and treatment of pressure ulcers by protocol. In S. Horn & D. Hopkins (Eds.), *Clinical practice improvement: A new technology for developing cost-effective quality health care.* New York: Faulkner & Gray.

Hopper, K., & Milburn, N. G. (1996). Homelessness among African Americans: A historical contemporary perspective. In J. Baumohl (Ed.), *Homelessness in America* (pp. 123–131). Phoenix, AZ: Oryx Press.

Horowitz, A. (1985). Family caregiving to the frail elderly. In C. Eisdorfer (Ed.), *Annual review of gerontology* (Vol. 5, pp. 194–246). New York: Springer Publishing.

Horowitz, A. (1992). Methodological issues in the study of gender within family caregiving relationships. In J. W. Dwyer & R. T. Coward (Eds.), *Gender, families, and elder care* (pp. 132–150). Newbury Park, CA: Sage.

Hubbard, P., Muhlenkamp, A. F., & Brown, N. (1984). The relationship between social support and self-care practices. *Nursing Research, 33,* 266–270.

Hudson, M. F. (1989). Analysis of the concepts of elder mistreatment: Abuse and neglect. *Journal of Elder Abuse and Neglect, 1*(1), 5–25.

Hudson, M. F. (1991). Elder mistreatment: A taxonomy with definitions by Delphi. *Journal of Elder Abuse and Neglect, 3*(2), 1–20.

Hudson, M. F. (1994). Elder abuse: Its meaning to middle-aged and older adults: Part 2. Pilot results. *Journal of Elder Abuse and Neglect, 6*(1), 55–83.

Hudson, M. F., & Carlson, J. (1994). Elder abuse: Its meaning to middle-aged and older adults: Part 1. Instrument development. *Journal of Elder Abuse and Neglect, 6*(1), 29–55.

Hugo, M. (1992). Left or right, up or down: A case for positioning of unconscious head-injured patients. *Curationis: South African Journal of Nursing, 15*(1), 1–7.

Hull, M. M. (1992). Coping strategies of family caregivers in hospice home care. *Oncology Nursing Forum, 19,* 1179–1187.

Hungelmann, J., Kenkel-Rossi, E., Klassen, L., & Stollenwerk, R. (1996). Focus on spiritual well-being: Harmonious interconnectedness of mind-body-spirit-use of the JAREL spiritual well-being scale. *Geriatric Nursing, 17,* 262–266.

Hunt, L., Carr, D., Duchek, J. M., Grant, E., Buckles, V., & Morris, J. C. (1997). Reliability and validity of the Washington University Road Test: A performance-based assessment for drivers with dementia of the Alzheimer type. *Archives of Neurology, 54,* 707–712.

Hunt, L., Morris, J. C., Edwards, D., & Wilson, B. S. (1993). Driving performance in persons with mild senile dementia of the Alzheimer type. *Journal of the American Geriatric Society, 41,* 747–753.

Hunter, S. (1992). Adult Day Care: Promoting Quality of Life for the Elderly. *Journal of Gerontological Nursing, 18,* 17–20.

Hurley, A., Volicer, B., Hanrahan, P., Houde, S., & Volicer, L. (1992). Assessment of discomfort in advanced Alzheimer patients. *Research in Nursing and Health, 15,* 367–377.

Hurley, A. C., Volicer, L., Camberg, L., Ashley, J., Woods, P., Odenheimer, G., Ooi, W. L., McIntyre, K., & Mahoney, E. K. (1999). Measurement of observed agitation in patients with Alzheimer's disease. *Journal of Mental Health and Aging, 5,* 117–133.

Hurley, A. C., Volicer, B. J., Mahoney, M. A., & Volicer, L. (1993). Palliative fever management in Alzheimer patients: Quality plus fiscal responsibility. *Advances in Nursing Science, 16*(1), 21–32.

Hurley, A. C., Volicer, B., & Volicer, L. (1996). Effect of fever management strategy on the progression of dementia of the Alzheimer type. *Alzheimer Disease and Associated Disorders, 10*(1), 5–10.

Hurley, R. (1991). The continuing care retirement community executive: A manager for all seasons. *Hospital and Health Services Administration, 36,* 365–381.

Hussain, N. A., & Warshaw, G. (1996). Utility of clysis for hydration in nursing home residents. *Journal of the American Geriatric Society, 44,* 969–973.

Hustins, K. (1993). Gender differences and bereavement. *Canadian Nurse, 89*(3), 48.

Hutchinson, S. A., & Wilson, H. S. (1998). The Theory of Unpleasant Symptoms and Alzheimer's disease. *Scholarly Inquiry for Nursing Practice: An International Journal, 12,* 143–157.

Hwang, S. W., Orav, J., O'Connell, J. J., Lebow, J. M., & Brennan, T. A. (1997). Causes of death in homeless adults in Boston. *Annals of Internal Medicine, 126,* 625–628.

Hyer, K. (1998). The John A. Hartford Foundation Geriatric Interdisciplinary Team Training Program. In Siegler, E. L., Hyer, K., Fulmer, T., & Mezey, M. (Eds.), *Geriatric interdisciplinary team training* (pp. 3–12). New York: Springer Publishing.

Ide, B. A., Tobias, C., Kay, M., Monk, J., & de Zapien, J. G. (1990). A comparison of coping strategies used effectively by older Anglo and Mexican-American widows: A longitudinal study. *Health Care for Women International, 11,* 237–249.

Inouye, S., Acampora, D., Miller, R., Fulmer, T., Hurst, L., & Cooney, L. (1993). The Yale Geriatric Care Program: A model of care to prevent functional decline in hospitalized elderly patients. *Journal of the American Geriatric Society, 41,* 1342–1352.

Inouye, S. K., Wagner, D. R., Acampora, D., Horwitz, R. I., Cooney, L. M. Jr, & Tinetii, M. E. (1993). A controlled trial of a nursing-centered intervention in hospitalized elderly medical patients: The Yale Geriatric Care Program. *Journal of the American Geriatric Society, 41,* 1353–1360.

Institute of Medicine (1991). *Enhancing Lives, Extending Lives: Report of the Committee for a National Research Agenda on Aging.* Washington, DC, National Academy Press.

Institute of Medicine. (1997). *Approaching Death: Improving Care at the End of Life.* Washington: National Academy Press.

International Association for the Study of Pain. (1986). Pain terms: The current list with definitions and notes on usage. *Pain, 3,* S216–S221.

International Continence Society Committee for the Standardisation of Terminology of the Lower Urinary Tract Function. (1990). *British Journal of Obstetrics and Gynaecology,* (Suppl. 6), 1–16.

International Council of Nurses. (1999). *International Classification for Nursing Practice Beta–1.* Geneva: Author

Irvine, D. M., Vincent, L., Bubela, N., Thompson, L., & Graydon, J. (1991). A critical appraisal of the research literature investigating fatigue in the individual with cancer. *Cancer Nursing, 14,* 188–199.

Isaacson, J. E., & Rubin, A. M. (1999). Otolaryngologic management of dizziness in the older patient. *Clinics in Geriatric Medicine, 15,* 179–192.

Isaia, D., Parker, V., & Murrow, E. (1999). Spiritual well-being among older adults. *Journal of Gerontological Nursing, 25*(8), 15–21.

Jacob, L. (1994). *Adult Aphasia: Understanding the Disability* (3rd ed.). Cambridge, MA: Youville Hospital and Rehabilitation Center.

Jacob, S. R. (1996). The grief experience of older women whose husbands had hospice care. *Journal of Advanced Nursing, 24,* 280–286.

Jacobs, J. (1995, Fall). Statement of purpose for the Alternative and Complementary Health Section of the American Public Health Association. *SPIG Newsletter, APHA,* pp. 2–3.

Jacobs, S. R. (1996). The grief experience of older women whose husbands had hospice care. *Journal of Advanced Nursing, 24,* 280–286.

Jacobson, A. F. (1998). Assessing dizziness in the elderly. *American Journal of Nursing, 98,* 22.

Jacobson, G. P., & Newman, C. W. (1990). The development of the Dizziness Handicap Inventory. *Archives of Otolaryngology and Head and Neck Surgery, 116,* 424–427.

Jacox, A. K., Carr, D. B, Payne, R., Berde, C. B., Brietbart, W., Cain, J. M., Chapman, C. R., Cleeland, C. L., McGavery, C. L., Miaskowski, C. A., Mulder, D. S., Paice, J. A., Shapiro, B. S., Silberstein, E. B., Smith, R. S., Stover, J., Tsou, C. V., Vecchiarelli, L., & Weissman, D. E. (1994). *Management of cancer pain* (Clinical Practice Guideline No. 9). Rockville, MD: Agency for Health Care Policy and Research.

Jalowiec, A. (1993). Coping with illness: Synthesis and critique of the nursing literature from 1980–1990. In J. Barnfather & B. Lyon (Eds.), *Stress and coping: State of the science and implications for nursing theory, research and practice.* Indianapolis: Center Nursing Press of Sigma Theta Tau International.

Jambunathan, J., & Stewart, S. (1995). Hmong women in Wisconsin: What are their concerns in pregnancy and childbirth? *Birth, 22,* 204–210.

Janko, K. A., & Shannon, K. M. (1996). Parkinsonism and Parkinson's disease. *Nurse Practitioner Forum, 7,* 174–178.

Jansson, W., Almberg, B., Grafstrom, M., & Winblad, B. (1998). The circle model-support for relatives of people with dementia. *International Journal of Geriatric Psychiatry, 13,* 674–681.

Jarrett, M., Heitkemper, M. M., Cain, K., Tuftin, M., Walker, E., Bond, E., & Levy, R. (in press). The relationship between psychological distress and gastrointestinal symptoms in women.

Jarvis, C. (1996). *Physical Examination and Health Assessment* (2nd ed.). Philadelphia: W. B. Saunders.

Jenkins, J. (1996). Oncology nursing practice. In M. B. Burke, G. Wilkes, & K. Ingwersen (Eds.), *Cancer chemotherapy: A nursing process approach* (2nd ed., pp. 3–19). Boston: Jones and Bartlett.

Jette, A. M., Harris, B. A., Cleary, P. D., & Campion, E. W. (1987). Functional recovery after hip fracture. *Archives of Physical Medicine & Rehabilitation, 68,* 735–740.

Jirovec, M. M. (1991). The impact of daily exercise on the mobility, balance and urine control of cognitively impaired nursing home residents. *International Journal of Nursing Studies, 28,* 145–151.

Johnson, B., & Gross, J. (1982). Handling methotrexate—a safety problem? *American Journal of Nursing, 82,* 1531.

Johnson, J. A., & King, K. B. (1995). Influence of expectations about symptoms on delay in seeking treatment during a myocardial infarction. *American Journal of Critical Care, 4,* 29–35.

Johnson, J. E. (1991). Progressive relaxation and the sleep of older noninstitutionalized women. *Applied Nursing Research, 4,* 165–70.

Johnson, J. E. (1995). Rural elders and the decision to stop driving. *Journal of Community Health Nursing, 12,* 131–138.

Johnson, J. E. (1998a). Nursing assessment of older rural drivers. *Journal of Community Health Nursing, 15,* 217–224.

Johnson, J. E. (1998b). Older rural adults and the decision to stop driving: The influence of family and friends. *Journal of Community Health Nursing, 15,* 205–216.

Johnson, J. E. (1999). *Assessment of older urban drivers by nurse practitioners.* Manuscript submitted for publication.

Johnson, J. E. (in press). Urban elders and the forfeiture of a driver's license. *Journal of Gerontological Nursing.*

Johnson, J. E., Rice, V. H., & Endress, M. P. (1978). Sensory information, instruction in a coping strategy, and recovery from surgery. *Research in Nursing and Health, 1,* 4–17.

Johnson, M. A., & Connelly, J. R. (1990). *Nursing and gerontology: Status report.* Washington, D.C.: Association for Gerontology in Higher Education.

Johnson, M., & Maas, M. (Eds.). (1997). *Nursing outcomes classification (NOC).* St. Louis: Mosby.

Johnson, R. J., Lund, D. A., & Dimond, M. F. (1986). Stress, self-esteem and coping during bereavement among the elderly. *Social Psychology Quarterly, 49,* 273–279.

Johnson, R. J., & Wolinsky, F. D. (1993). The structure of health status among older adults: Disease, disability, functional limitation and perceived health. *Journal of Health and Social Behavior, 34,* 105–121.

Johnston, T. (1990). Retirement: What happens to the marriage. *Issues in Mental Health Nursing, 11,* 347–359.

Joint National Committee. (1993). The fifth report of the Joint National Committee on the Detection, Evaluation and Treatment of High Blood Pressure (JNC V). *Archives of Internal Medicine, 153,* 154–183.

Jones, D., & van Amelsvoort Jones, G. (1986). Communication patterns between nursing staff and the ethnic elderly in a long-term care facility. *Journal of Advanced Nursing, 11,* 265–272.

Jones, D. A., & Peter, T. M. (1992). Caring for elderly dependents: Effects on the carers' quality of life. *Age and Ageing, 21,* 421–428.

Jordan, S., Hardy, B., & Coleman, M. (1999). Medication management: An exploratory study into the role of community mental health nurses. *Journal of Advanced Nursing, 29,* 1068–1081.

Joseph, J. A., Shukitt-Hale, B., Denisova, N. A., Prior, R. L., Cao, G., Martin, A., Taglialatela, G., & Bickford, P. C. (1998). Long-term dietary strawberry, spinach, or vitamin E supplementation retards the onset of age-related neuronal signal-transduction and cognitive behavioral deficits. *Journal of Neuroscience, 18,* 8047–8055.

Journal of Gerontological Nursing (1998). In your practice, what experiences of patients and family members could be classified as a good death" or a positive process of dying? *Journal of Gerontological Nursing, 24*(7), 47–52.

Kahn, D., & Steeves, R. (1993). Spiritual well-being: A review of the research literature. In M. Whedon (Ed.), *Quality of life: A nursing challenge* (pp. 60–64). Philadelphia: Meniscus Ltd.

Kalymun, M. (1990). Toward a definition of assisted-living. *Journal of Housing for the Elderly, 6,* 97–131.

Kanacki, L. S., Jones, P. S., & Galbraith, M. E. (1996). Social support and depression in widows and widowers. *Journal of Gerontological Nursing, 22*(2), 39–45.

Kane, R. A., Caplan, A. L., Urv-Wong, E. K., Freeman, I. C., Aroskar, M. A., & Finch, M. (1997). Everyday matters in the lives of nursing home residents: Wish for and perception of choice and control. *Journal of the American Geriatrics Society, 45,* 1086–1093.

Kane, R. A., Kane, R. L., Arnold, S., Garrard, J., McDermott, S., & Kepferle, L. (1988). Geriatric nurse practitioners as nursing home employees: Implementing the role. *The Gerontologist, 28,* 469–477.

Kane, R. A., Kane, R. L., Illston, L. H., Nyman, J. A., & Finch, M. D. (1991). Adult foster care for the elderly in Oregon. *American Journal of Public Health, 81,* 1113–1120.

Kane, R. A., Kane, R. L., & Ladd, R. C. (1998). Conclusions: The heart of the matter. The heart of long-term care (pp. 285–305). New York: Oxford University Press.

Kane, R. A., & Wilson, K. B. (1993). *Assisted living in the United States: A new paradigm for residential care for frail older persons?* American Association of Retired Persons. Washington, DC.

Kane, R. L., Chen, Q., Finch, M., Blewett, L., Burns, R., & Moskowitz, M. (1998). Functional outcomes of posthospital care for stroke and hip fracture patients under Medicare. *Journal of the American Geriatrics Society, 46,* 1525–1533.

Kane, R., Garrard, J., Buchanan, J., Rosenfeld, A., Skay, C., & McDermott, S. (1991). Improving care in nursing homes. *Journal of American Geriatrics Society, 39,* 359–367.

Kane, R. L., Garrard, J., Skay, C. L., Radosevich, D. M., Buchanan, J. L., McDermott, S. M., & Arnold, S. B. (1989). Effects of a geriatric nurse practitioner on the process and outcomes of nursing home care. *American Journal of Public Health, 79,* 1271–1277.

Kannel, W. B., & Abbott, R. D. (1984). Incidence and prognosis of unrecognized myocardial infarction. *The New England Journal of Medicine, 311,* 1144–1147.

Kannel, W. B., & Wilson, P. W. F. (1995). An update on coronary risk factors. *Medical Clinics of North America, 79,* 951–971.

Kaplan, G. A., & Comacho, T. (1983). Perceived health and mortality: A nine year follow-up of the Human Population Laboratory cohort. *American Journal of Epidemiology, 117,* 292–304.

Kaplan, N. M. (1994). *Clinical hypertension.* Baltimore: Williams and Wilkins.

Karper, W., & Boschen, M. (1993). Effects of exercise on acute respiratory tract infections and related symptoms. *Geriatric Nursing, 14,* 15–18.

Kato, J., Hickson, L., & Worrall, L. (1996). Communication difficulties of nursing home residents: How can staff help? *Journal of Gerontological Nursing, 22*(5), 26–31.

Katz, I., Lesher, E., Kleban, M., Jethanandani, V., & Parmelee, P. (1989). Clinical features of depression in the nursing home. *International Psychogeriatrics, 1,* 5–15.

Katz, P. O. (1998). Gastroesophageal reflux disease. *Journal of the American Geriatric Society, 46,* 1558–1565.

Katz, S. (1983). Assessing self maintenance: Activities of daily living, mobility, and instrumental activities of daily living. *Journal of American Geriatrics Society, 31,* 721–727.

Katz, S., Ford, A. B., Heiple, K. G., & Newill, V. A. (1964). Recovery after fracture of this hip. *Journal of Gerontology, 19,* 285–293.

Katz, S., Ford, A., Moskowitz, R., Jackson, A., & Jaffee, M. (1963). Studies of illness in the aged: The index of ADL: A standardized measure of biological and psychosocial function. *JAMA, 185,* 94–101.

Katz, W. A., & Sherman, C. (1998). Exercise is medicine. Osteoporosis: The role of exercise in optimal management. *Physician & Sportsmedicine, 26,* 39–42.

Kauffman, T., Albright, L., & Wagner, C. (1987). Rehabilitation outcomes after hip fracture in persons 90 years old and older. *Archives of Physical Medicine and Rehabilitation, 68,* 369–371.

Kayser-Jones, J. S. (1981a). Gerontological nursing research review. *Journal of Gerontological Nursing, 7*(4), 217–223.

Kayser-Jones, J. S. (1981b). *Old, alone, and neglected.* Los Angeles, CA: University of California Press.

Kayser-Jones, J. (1996). Mealtime in nursing homes: The importance of individualized care. *Journal of Gerontological Nursing, 22*(3), 26–31.

Kayser-Jones, J. (1997). Inadequate staffing at mealtime: Implication for nursing and health policy. *Journal of Gerontological Nursing, 23*(8), 14–21.

Kayser, J. S., & Minnegerode, F. A. (1975). Increasing nursing students interest in working with aged patients. *Nursing Research, 24,* 23–26.

Kayser-Jones, J., & Pengilly, K. (1999). Dysphagia among nursing home residents. *Geriatric Nursing, 20,* 77–82.

Keating, S. B. (1995). Health promotion and disease prevention in home care. *Geriatric Nursing, 16,* 184–186.

Keddy, B., & Singleton, J. (1991). Women's perceptions of life after retirement. *Activities, Adaptation & Aging, 16,* 57–65.

Keith, P. M. (1986). The social context and resources of the unmarried in old age. *International Journal of Aging and Human Development, 21,* 81–86.

Keith, P. M. (1989). *The unmarried in later life.* New York: Praeger.

Kelley, S. J. (1992). Child maltreatment, stressful life events, and behavior problems in school aged children in residential treatment. *Journal of Child and Adolescent Psychiatric and Mental Health Nursing, 5,* 5–13.

Kelley, S. J. (1993). Caregiver stress in grandparents raising grandchildren. *Image: Journal of Nursing Scholarship, 25*(4), 331–337.

Kelley, S. J., & Damato, E. G. (1995). Grandparents as primary caregivers. *Maternal Child Nursing, 20,* 326–332.

Kelley, S. J., Whitley, D. M., Sipe, T. A., & Yorker, B. C. (in press). Psychological distress in grandmother kinship care providers: The role of resources, social support, and physical health. *Child Abuse and Neglect: The International Journal.*

Kelley, S. J., Yorker, B. C., Whitley, D. M., & Sipe, T. A. (in press). A multi-modal intervention for grandparents raising grandchildren: Results of a pilot study. *Child Welfare.*

Kelley, W. N. (1997). Diseases of the gastrointestinal tract. In W. N. Kelley (Ed.), *Textbook of Internal Medicine* (3rd ed.). Philadelphia: Lippincott-Raven.

Kelsey, J. I., & Hoffman, S. (1987). Risk factors for hip fracture. *The New England Journal of Medicine, 316,* 404–406.

Kenzora, J. E., McCarthy, R. E., Lowell, J. D., & Sledge, C. B. (1984). Hip fracture mortality. *Clinical Orthopaedics and Related Research, 186,* 45–56.

Kerber, K., Enrietto, J. A., Jacobson, K. M., & Baloh, R. W. (1998). *Neurology, 51,* 574–580.

Kerner, D. N., Patterson, T. L., Grant, I., & Kaplan, R. M. (1998). Validity of the quality of well-being scale for patients with Alzheimer's disease. *Journal of Aging & Health, 19,* 44–61.

Kerr, M. E., Rudy, E. B., Brucia, J., & Stone, K. S. (1993). Head-injured adults: Recommendations for endotracheal suctioning. *Journal of Neuroscience Nursing, 25,* 86–91.

Kerr, R. B. (1994). Meanings adult daughters attach to a parent's death. *Western Journal of Nursing Research, 16,* 347–365.

Kiecolt-Glaser, J. (1987). Chronic stress and immunity in family caregivers of Alzheimer's disease victims. *Psychosomatic Medicine, 49,* 523–535.

Kiecolt-Glaser, J. K., Dyer, C. S., & Shuttleworth, E. C. (1988). Upsetting interactions and distress among Alzheimer's disease family caregivers: A replication and extension. *American Journal of Community Psychology, 16,* 825–837.

Kimble, C. S., & Longe, M. D. (1989). Health promotion programs for older adults: *A Planning and Management Guide.* Chicago, IL: AHA/American Hospital Publishing.

Kinzel, T. (1991). Managing lung disease in later life: A new approach. *Geriatrics, 46,* 54–59.

Kirschling, J. M., & Austin, J. K. (1988). Assessing support: The recently widowed. *Archives of Psychiatric Nursing, 2,* 81–86.

Kirschling, J. M., & McBride, A. B. (1989). Effects of age and sex on the experience of widowhood. *Western Journal of Nursing Research, 11,* 207–218.

Kitchen, J., & Rouche, J. (1990). Life-care resident preferences: A survey of the decision-making process to enter a CCRC. In R. D. Chellis & P. J. Grayson (Eds.), *Life Care: A Long Term Solution* (pp. 49–60). Lexington, MA: Lexington.

Kleiger, R. E., Miller, J. P., Bigger, I. T. Jr., Moss, A. L. J., & the Multicenter Postinfarction Research Group. (1987). Decreased heart rate variability and its association with increased mortality after acute myocardial infarction. *American Journal of Cardiology, 59,* 256–262.

Kleiner, S. M. (1999). Water: An essential but overlooked nutrient. *Journal of the American Dietetic Association, 99*, 200–206.

Knebel, A. R., Janson-Bjerklie, S. L., Malley, J. D., Wilson, A. G., & Marini, J. J. (1994). Comparison of breathing comfort during weaning with two ventilatory modes. *American Journal of Respiratory and Critical Care Medicine, 149*, 14–18.

Knight, B. G., Lutzky, S. M., & Macofsky-Urban, F. (1993). A meta-analytic review of interventions for caregiver distress: Recommendations for future research. *Gerontologist, 33*, 240–248.

Knobf, T., & Durivage, H. (1993). Chemotherapy: Principles of therapy. In S. Groenwald, M. Frogge, M. Goodman, & C. Yarbro (Eds.), *Cancer nursing: Principles and practice* (3rd ed., pp. 270–292). Boston: Jones and Bartlett.

Knopman, D. (1991). Long-term retention of implicitly acquired learning in patients with Alzheimer's disease. *Journal of Clinical and Experimental Neuropsychology, 13*, 880–894.

Kocken, P. L., & Voorham, A. J. (1998). Effects of a peer-led senior health education program. *Patient Education & Counseling, 34*, 15–23.

Koenig, H. G., George, L. K., Blazer, D., Pritchett, J. T., & Meador, K. G. (1993). The relationship between religion and anxiety in a sample of community-dwelling older adults. *Journal of Geriatric Psychiatry, 26*, 65–93.

Koenig, H. G., George, L. K., Cohen, H. J., Hays, J. C., Larson, D. B., & Blazer, D. G. (1998). The relationship between religious activities and blood pressure in older adults. *The International Journal of Psychiatry in Medicine, 28*, 180–194.

Koenig, H. G., George, L. K., & Peterson, B. L. (1998). Religiosity and remission of depression in medically ill older patients. *American Journal of Psychiatry, 155*, 536–542.

Koerselman, J., Pursnani, K. G., Peghini, P., Mohiuddin, M. A., Katzka, D., Akkermans, L. M., & Castell, D. O. (1999). Different effects of an oral anticholinergic drug on gastroesophageal reflux in upright and supine position in normal, ambulant subjects: A pilot study. *American Journal of Gastroenterology, 94*, 925–930.

Kolanowski, A., Hurwitz, S., Taylor, L., Evans, L., & Strumpf, N. (1994). Contextual factors associated with disturbing behaviors in institutionalized elders. *Nursing Research, 43*, 73–79.

Kolanowski, A. M. (1995). Disturbing behaviors in demented elders: A concept synthesis. *Archives of Psychiatric Nursing, 9*, 188–194.

Kolanowski, A. M., Strand, G., & Whall, A. (1997). A pilot study of the relation of premorbid characteristics to behavior in dementia. *Journal of Gerontological Nursing, 23*(2), 21–30.

Konu, V. (1977). Myocardial infarction in the elderly: A clinical and epidemiologic study with 1 year follow-up. *Acta Medica Scandinavia, 604*(Suppl. #), 53–68.

Kosloski, K., & Montgomery, R. (1995). The effects of respite on caregivers of Alzheimer's patients: One-year evaluation of the Michigan model respite program. *Journal of Applied Gerontology, 12*, 4–17.

Kositzke, J. A. (1990). A question of balance: Dehydration in the elderly. *Journal of Gerontological Nursing, 16*(5), 4–11.

Kosta, J. C., & Mitchell, C. A. (1998). Current procedures for diagnosing dysphagia in elderly clients. *Geriatric Nursing, 19*, 195–199.

Koss, E., & Gilmore, G. C. (1998). Environmental interventions and functional ability of AD patients. In B. Vellas, J. Fitten, & G. Frisoni (Eds.), *Research and Practice in Alzheimer's Disease* (pp. 186–192). New York: Springer Publishing Co.

Kottke, T. E., Battista, R. N., DeFriese, G. H., & Brekke, M. L. (1988). Attributes of successful smoking cessation interventions in medical practice. A meta-analysis of 39 controlled trials. *Journal of the American Medical Association, 259,* 2883–2889.

Kovach, C. R. (1993). Understanding autobiographical memories: A study of the reminiscences of elderly men. *Journal of Holistic Nursing, 11,* 149–163.

Kovach, C. R., & Weissman, D. (1998). Assessment of discomfort for dementia (ADD) protocol [Special Issue I]. *The Gerontologist, 38,* 126.

Kovach, C. R., Wilson, S. A., & Noonan, P. E. (1996). The effects of hospice interventions on behaviors, discomfort, and physical complications of end-stage dementia nursing home residents. *American Journal of Alzheimer Disease, 11*(4), 7–15.

Kovar, M. G., Fitti, J. E., & Chyba, M. M. (1992). *The Longitudinal Study of Aging; 1984-90.* Hyattsville, MD: National Center for Health Statistics.

Kovarsky, R. S. (1989). Loneliness and disturbed grief: A comparison of parents who lost a child to suicide or accidental death. *Archives of Psychiatric Nursing, 3,* 86–96.

Kovner, C., & Gergen, P. J. (1998). Nurse staffing levels and adverse events following surgery in U. S. hospitals. *Image: Journal of Nursing Scholarship, 30,* 315–321.

Krall, E. A., & Dawson-Huges, B. (1994). Walking is related to bone density and rates of bone loss. *The American Journal of Medicine, 96,* 20–26.

Kramer, A. M., Schlenker, R., Tropea, D., Hrincevich, C., Ahmad, L., & Shaughnessy, P. (1997). Outcomes and costs after hip fracture and stroke. *Journal of the American Medical Association, 277,* 396–404.

Kramer, B. J. (1997). Gain in the caregiving experience: Where are we? What next? *The Gerontologist, 37,* 218–232.

Kramer, J., Yellin, E., & Epstein, W. (1983). Social and economic impacts of four musculoskeletal conditions: A study using national community based data. *Journal of Rheumatology, 26,* 901–907.

Krauskopf, J., Brown, R., Tokarz, K., & Bogutz, A. (1993). *Elderlaw: Advocacy for the Aging.* St. Paul: West Publishing Co.

Krichbaum, K. (1999). APN Care Managers + Care Pathways: The formula for better health outcomes. In M. Snyder & M. Mirr (Eds.), *Advanced Practice Nursing: A Guide to Professional Development* (2nd Edition). New York: Springer Publishing Co.

Kriegsman, D. W., Penninx, B. W. J. H., & van Eijk, J. Th. M. (1995). A criterion-based literature survey of the relationship between family support and incidence and course of chronic disease in the elderly. *Family Systems Medicine, 13,* 39–68.

Krikorian, R. K., Kramer, P. H., & Vacek, J. L (1996). Peripheral angioplasty in the elderly: Safe and beneficial. *Cardiology in the Elderly, 14*(5/6), 207–211.

Kristjanson, L. J., & Ashcroft, T. (1994). The family's cancer journey: A literature review. *Cancer Nursing, 17,* 1–17.

Krumholz, H. M., Radford, M. J., Ellerbeck, E. F., Hennen, J., Meehan, T. P., Petrillo, M., Wang, Y., & Jencks, S. F. (1996). Aspirin for secondary prevention after acute myocardial infarction in the elderly: Prescribed use and outcomes. *Annals of Internal Medicine, 124,* 292–298.

Krumholz, H. M., Seeman, T. E., Merrill, S. S., Mendes de Leon, C., Vaccarino, V., Silverman, D. I., Tsukahara, R., Ostfeld, A. M., & Berkman, L. F. (1994). Lack of association between cholesterol and coronary heart disease mortality and morbidity and all-cause mortality in persons older than 70 years. *Journal of the American Medical Association, 272,* 1335–1340.

Kunik, M., Graham, D. P., Snow-Turek, A. L., Molinari, V., Orengo, C. A., & Workman, R. H. (1998). Contribution of cognitive impairment, depression, and psychosis to the outcome of agitated geropsychiatric inpatients with dementia. *Journal of Nervous and Mental Disease, 186,* 299–303.

Kutza, E. A., & Keigher, S. M. (1991). The elderly "new homeless": An emerging population at risk. *Social Work, 36,* 288–293.

Kynette, D., & Kemper, S. (1986). Aging and the loss of grammatical forms: A cross sectional study of language performance. *Language and Communication, 6,* 43–49.

Lacroix, A. Z., Leveille, S. G., Hecht, J. A., Grothaus, L. C., & Wagner, E. H. (1996). Does walking decrease the risk of cardiovascular disease hospitilizations and death in older adults? *Journal of the American Geriatrics Society, 44,* 113–120.

Laffrey, S. C. (1986). Development of a health conception scale. *Research in Nursing and Health, 9,* 107–113.

Lafluente, C. R., & Lane, P. L. (1995). The lived experience of homeless men. *Journal of Community Health Nursing, 12,* 211–219.

Lalonde, M. (1974). *A new perspective on the Health of Canadians.* Ottawa, Government of Canada, 1974.

Lambert, H. C., & Gisel, E. G. (1996). The assessment of oral, pharyngeal and esophageal dysphagia in elderly persons. *Physical and Occupational Therapy in Geriatrics, 14*(4), 1–25.

Landefeld, C., Palmer, R., Kresevic, D., Fortinsky, R., & Kowal, J. (1995). A randomized trial of care in a hospital medical unit especially designed to improve the functional outcomes of acutely ill older patients. *New England Journal of Medicine, 332,* 1338–44.

Landis, S., Murray, T., Bolden, S., & Wingo, P. (1999). *Cancer statistics, 1999. CA: A Cancer Journal for Clinicians, 49,* 8–31.

Lange, P. (1994). Future studies in localized prostate cancer. What should we think? What can we do? *Journal of Urology, 152,* 1932–1938.

Langmore, S. E., & Miller, R. M. (1994). Behavioral treatment for adults with oropharyngeal dysphagia. *Archives of Physical Medicine and Rehabilitation, 75,* 1154–1160.

Langmore, S. E., Terpenning, M. S., & Schork, A. (1998). Predictors of aspiration pneumonia: how important is dysphagia? *Dysphagia, 13,* 69–81.

Lantz, M. S., Buchalter, E. N., & McBee, L. (1997). The wellness group: A novel intervention for coping with disruptive behavior in elderly nursing home residents. *The Gerontologist, 37,* 551–556.

Lanza, M. (1983). Origins of aggression. *Journal of Psychosocial Nursing Mental Health Services, 12,* 11–16.

Lareau, S., Carrieri-Kohlman, V., Janson-Bjerklie, S., & Roos, P. (1994). Development and testing of the pulmonary functional status and dyspnea questionnaire (PFSDQ). *Heart & Lung: Journal of Acute & Critical Care, 23*, 242–250.

Lareau, S., Meek, P., Press, D., Anholm, J., & Roos, P. (1999). Dyspnea in patients with chronic obstructive pulmonary disease: Does dyspnea worsen longitudinally in the presence of declining lung function? *Heart & Lung: Journal of Acute & Critical Care, 28*, 65–73.

Larkin, J. P., & Hopcroft, B. M. (1993). In-hospital respite as a moderator of caregiver stress. *Health and Social Work, 18*, 132–138.

Larson, E., & Ropka, M. (1991). An update on nursing research and HIV infection. *Image: Journal of Nursing Scholarship, 23*, 4–12.

Larson, O. J., & Ferketich, S. L. (1993). Patient satisfaction with nurses' caring during hospitalization. *Western Journal of Nursing Research, 15*, 690–707.

Larsson, B., Svardsudd, K., Welin, L., Wilhelmsen, L., Bjorntorp, P., & Tibblin, G. (1984). Abdominal adipose tissue distribution, obesity and risk of cardiovascular disease and death: 13 year follow-up of participants in the study of men born in 1913. *British Medical Journal, 288*, 1401–1404.

Lauver, D. (1992). Psychosocial variables, race, and intentions to seek care for breast cancer symptoms. *Nursing Research, 41*, 236–241.

Lavie, C., & Milani, R. V. (1995). Effects of cardiac rehabilitation programs on exercise capacity, coronary risk factors, behavioral characteristics, and quality of life in a large elderly cohort. *American Journal of Cardiology, 76*, 177–179.

Lavie, C. J., Milani, R. V., & Littman, A. B. (1993). Benefits of cardiac rehabilitation and exercise training in secondary coronary prevention in the elderly. *Journal of the American College of Cardiology, 22*, 678–683.

Lawrence, R. H., & Jette, A. M. (1996). Disentangling the disablement process. *Journals of Gerontology: Social Sciences, 51*, S173–S182.

Lawson, J., Fitzgerald, J., Birchall, J., Aldren, C. P., & Kenny, R. A. (1999). Diagnosis of geriatric patients with severe dizziness. *Journal of the American Geriatrics Society, 47*, 12–17.

Lawton, M. (1975). Competence, environmental press and the adaptation of older people. In P. Windley, T. Byerts, & F. Ernst (Eds.), *Theory development in environments and aging* (pp. 13–83). Washington, DC: Gerontological Society.

Lawton, M. P. (1991). A multidimensional view of quality of life in frail elders. In J. E. Birren, J. C. Rowe, & D. E. Deutchman (Eds.), *The concept and measurement of quality of life in the frail and elderly* (pp. 4–27). San Diego, CA: Academic Press.

Lawton, M. P. (1994). Quality of life in Alzheimer's disease. *Alzheimer Disease Association and Disorders, 8*, 138–150.

Lawton, M. P., Haitsma, K. V., & Klapper, J. (1996). Observed affect in nursing home residents with Alzheimer's disease. *Journals of Gerontology Series B-Psychological Sciences & Social Sciences, 51B*(1), P3–14.

Lawton, M. P., Moss, M., & Grimes, M. (1985). The changing service needs of older tenants in planned housing. *The Gerontologist, 25*, 258–264.

Lawton, M. P., Van Haitsman, K. V., & Klapper, J. (1996). Observe affect in nursing home residents with Alzheimer's disease. *Journal of Gerontology, 51B*, 3–14.

Lebowitz, B. (1978). Old age and family functioning. *Journal of Gerontological Social Work, 1,* 111–118.

Lee, G., & Shehan, C. (1989). Retirement and marital satisfaction. *Journal of Gerontology: Social Sciences, 44,* S226–S230.

Lee, G. R., Willetts, M. C., & Seccombe, K. (1998). Widowhood and depression: Gender differences. *Research on Aging, 20,* 611–630.

Leetun, M. C. (1996). Wellness spirituality in the older adult. *Nurse Practitioner, 21*(8), 60–70.

Leidy, N. (1994). Functional status and the forward progress of merry-go-rounds: Toward a coherent analytical framework. *Nursing Research, 43,* 196–202.

Lempert, T., Wolsey, C., Davies, R., Gresty, M., & Bronstein, A. (1997). Three hundred sixty-degree rotation of the posterior semicircular canal for treatment of benign positional vertigo: A placebo-controlled trial. *Neurology, 49,* 729–733.

Lenz, E. R., Pugh, L. C., Milligan, R. A., Gift, A., & Suppe, F. (1997). The middle-range theory of unpleasant symptoms: An update. *Advances in Nursing Science, 19*(3), 14–27.

Leon, J., Cheng, C-K., & Neumann, P. J. (1998). Alzheimer's Disease Care: Costs and Potential Saving. *Health Affairs, 17,* 206–216.

Lernfelt, B., Wikstrand, J., & Svanborg, A. (1991). Aging and left ventricular function in elderly healthy people. *American Journal of Cardiology, 68,* 547–549.

Lesher, E., & Berryhill, J. (1994). Validation of the Geriatric Depression Scale-Short Form among inpatients. *Journal of Clinical Psychology, 50,* 256–260.

Letvak, S. (1997). Relational experiences of elderly women living alone in rural communities: A phenomenologic inquiry. *Journal of the New York State Nurses Association, 28*(2), 20–25.

Levi, S. (1997). Posthospital setting, resource utilization, and self-care outcome in older women with hip fracture. *Archives of Physical Medicine and Rehabilitation, 78,* 973–979.

Levkoff, S. E., Besdine, R. W., & Wetle, T. (1986). Acute confusional states (delirium) in the hospitalized elderly. In C. Eisdorfer (Ed.), *Annual review of geriatrics and gerontology* (pp. 1–26). New York: Springer Publishing.

Levy, R., Jarrett, M. J., Cain, K., & Heitkemper, M. M. (1997). The relationship between daily life stress and gastrointestinal symptoms in women. *Journal of Behavioral Medicine, 20,* 177–193.

Lewis, D. J., & Robinson, J. A. (1986). Assessment of coping strategies of ICU nurses in response to stress. *Critical Care Nurse, 6*(6), 38–43.

Lewis, R. R., Padayachee, T. S., Ariyanayagam, R. P., & Gosling, R. G. (1988). Prevalence of severe intenal carotid artery disease in hypertensive elderly pateints. *Journal of Hypertension, 6,* S33–S36.

Li, G. (1995). The interaction effect of bereavement and sex on the risk of suicide in the elderly: An historical cohort study. *Social Science & Medicine, 40,* 825–828.

Libman, E., Fichten, C. S., Weinstein, N., Tagalakis, V., Amsel, R., Brender, W., & Creti, L. (1998). Improvement and deterioration in sleep status of "younger" and "older" seniors: A longitudinal study. *Journal of Mental Health & Aging, 4,* 183–192.

Liehr, P., & Smith, M. J. (1999). Middle range theory: Spinning research and practice to create knowledge for the new millennium. *Advances in Nursing Science, 21*(4), 81–91.

Lierman, L., Kaspryzk, D., & Benoliel, J. (1991). Understanding adherence to breast self-examination in older women. *Western Journal of Nursing Research, 13,* 46–61.

Light, E., Niederehe, G., & Lebowitz, B. D. (Eds.). (1994). *Stress effects on family caregivers of Alzheimer's patients: Research and interventions.* New York: Springer Publishing.

Lindgren, C. L. (1996). Chronic sorrow in persons with Parkinson's and their spouses. *Scholarly Inquiry for Nursing Practice, 10,* 351–370.

Linn, M. W., Klett, C. J., & Caffey, E. M. (1980). Foster home characteristics and psychiatric patient outcome. *Archives of General Psychiatry, 37,* 129–132.

Linton, A. D., Matteson, M. A., & Byers, V. (1997). The relationship between premorbid life-style and wandering behaviors in institutionalized people with dementia. *Aging: Clinical and Experimental Research, 9,* 415–418.

Litwin, M., & deKernion, J. (1994). Editorial: Perspectives on the problem of prostate cancer. *Journal of Urology, 152,* 1680–1681.

Liukkonen, A. (1995). Life in a nursing home for frail elderly. *Clinical Nursing Research, 4,* 358–372.

Logemann, J. A. (1995). Dysphagia. In G. Maddox (Ed.). *Encyclopedia of aging* (2nd ed.) (pp. 297–298). New York: Springer.

Lonergan, E. (Ed.). (1996). *Geriatrics.* Stamford: Appleton & Lange.

Long, A., & Reid, W. (1996). An exploration of nurses attitudes to the nursing care of the suicidal patient in an acute psychiatric ward. *Journal of Psychiatric and Mental Health Nursing, 3,* 29–37.

Longman, A. J., Saint-Germain, M. A., & Modiano, M. (1992). Use of breast cancer screening by older Hispanic women. *Public Health Nursing, 9,* 118–124.

Longstreth, G. F., & Wolde-Tsadik, G. (1993). Irritable bowel–type symptoms in HMO examinees: Prevalence, demographics, and clinical correlates. *Digestive Diseases and Sciences, 38,* 1581–1589.

Lorig, K. (1996). *Patient education: A practical approach.* Thousand Oaks, CA: Sage.

Lorig, K., Stewart, A., Ritter, P., Gonzalez, V., Laurent, D., & Lynch, J. (1996). *Outcome measures for health education and other health care interventions.* Thousand Oaks, CA: Sage.

Lovell, B. B., Ancoli-Israel, S., & Gevirtz, R. (1995). Effect of bright light treatment on agitated behavior in institutionalized elderly subjects. *Psychiatry Research, 57,* 7–12.

Lubkin, I. M. (1995). *Chronic illness impact and interventions.* Boston: Jones and Bartlett.

Lucas-Blaustein, M. J., Filipp, L., Dungan, C., & Tune, L. (1988). Driving in patients with dementia. *Journal of the American Geriatric Society, 36,* 1087–1091.

Lueckenotte, A. (1996). *Gerontologic nursing.* St. Louis: Mosby.

Lueckenotte, A. G. (1996). *Gerontologic nursing.* St. Louis: C. V. Mosby.

Lugger, K. E. (1994). Dysphagia in the elderly stroke patient. *Journal of Neuroscience Nursing, 26,* 78–84.

Lund, D. A., Caserta, M. S., & Dimond, M. F. (1986). Gender differences through two years of bereavement among the elderly. *Gerontologist, 26,* 314–320.

Lund, D. A., Caserta, M. S., Van Pelt, J., & Gass, K. A. (1990). Stability of social support networks after later-life spousal bereavement. *Death Studies, 14,* 53–73.

Lund, D. A., Hill, R. D., Caserta, M. S., & Wright, S. D. (1995). Video respite™: An innovative resource for family, professional caregivers, and persons with dementia. *The Gerontologist, 35,* 683–687.

Lund, D. A., Johnson, R., Baraki, H. N., & Dimond, M. F. (1984). Can pets help the bereaved? *Journal of Gerontological Nursing, 10,* 8–12.

Lusiani, L., Perrone, A., Pesevanto, R., & Conte, G. (1994). Prevalence, clinical features, and acute course of atypical myocardial infarction. *Angiology, 41,* 49–55.

Lyketsos, C. G., Steele, C., Galik, E., Rosenblatt, A., Steinberg, M., Warren, A., & Sheppard, J. M. (1999). Physical aggression in dementia patients and its relationship to depression. *American Journal of Psychiatry, 156,* 66–71.

Lyness, J., Noel, T., Cox, C., King, D., Conwell, Y., & Caine, E. (1997). Screening for depression in elderly primary care patients. A comparison of the Center for Epidemiologic Studies-Depression Scale and the Geriatric Depression Scale. *Archives of Internal Medicine, 157,* 449–54.

Lyon, B. (1993). Summary and preliminary synthesis. In J. S. Barnfather & B. L. Lyon (Eds.), *Stress and coping: State of the science and implications for nursing theory, research and practice.* Indianapolis: Sigma Theta Tau.

Lyon, B. L. (1996). *Conquering stress in changing times.* Research Triangle Park, NC: Glaxo Wellcome Inc.

Lyon, B. L., & Werner, J. S. (1987). Stress. In J. J. Fitzpatrick & R. L. Taunton (Eds.), *Annual Review of Nursing Research* (Vol. 5, pp. 3–22). New York: Springer Publishing.

Maas, M., & Buckwalter, K. (1990). *Nursing evaluation research: Alzheimer's care unit. Final report.* Rockville, MD: National Institutes of Health, National Center for Nursing Research.

Maas, M. L., & Buckwalter, K. C. (1991). Alzheimer's disease. In J. J. Fitzpatrick & J. S. Stevenson (Eds.), *Annual review of nursing research* (Vol. 9, pp. 19–55). New York: Springer Publishing.

Maas, M., Buckwalter, K. C., Swanson, E., Specht, J., Tripp-Reimer, T., & Hardy, M. (1994). The caring partnership: Staff and families of persons institutionalized with Alzheimer's disease. *American Journal of Alzheimer's Care and Related Disorders and Research, 9*(6), 21–30.

Maas, M., & Swanson, E. (1991). Family Involvement in Care. Grant funded in part by the National Center for Nursing Research.

Maas, M., Swanson, E., Reed, D., & Specht, J. (1996, November). *Nursing staff perceptions of family involvement in care in SCUs.* Paper presented at the 49th Annual Meeting of the Gerontological Society of America, Washington, DC.

MacDonald, J. B. (1984). Presentation of acute myocardial infarction in the elderly. *Age and Ageing, 13,* 196–200.

MacDonald, M., Remus, G., & Laing, G. (1994). The link between housing and health in the elderly. *Journal of Gerontological Nursing, 20*(7), 5–10.

MacKenzie, T. D., Bartecchi, C. E., & Schrier, R. W. (1994). The human costs of tobacco use. *New England Journal of Medicine, 330,* 975–980.

Maddox, M. A. (1992). The Role of the Nurse Practitioner in Adult Day Care. *Journal of American Academy of Nurse Practitioners, 4*(3), 107–110.

Magaziner, J., Simonsick, E., Kashner, T. M., Hebel, J. R., & Kenzora, J. E. (1989). Survival experience of aged hip fracture patients. *American Journal of Public Health, 79*(3), 274–278.

Mahon, S. (1991). Managing the psychosocial consequences of cancer recurrence: Implications for nurses. *Oncology Nursing Forum, 18,* 577–583.

Mahoney, D. F. (1994). Appropriateness of geriatric prescribing decisions made by nurse practitioners and physicians. *Image: Journal of Nursing Scholarship, 26,* 41–46.

Mahoney, E. K., Hurley, A. C., Volicer, L., Bell, M., Gianotis, P., Harsdhorn, M., Lane, P., Lesperance, R., MacDonald, S., Novakoff, L., Rheaume, Y., Timms, R., & Warden, V. (1999). Development and testing of the resistiveness to care scale. *Research in Nursing and Health, 22,* 27–38.

Manson, J. E., Colditz, G. A., Stampfer, M. J., Willett, W. C., Rosner, B., Monson, R. R., Speizer, F. E., & Hennekens, C. H. (1990). A prospective study of obesity and risk of coronary heart disease in women. *New England Journal of Medicine, 322,* 882–889.

Marcus, F. I., Friday, K., McCans, J., Moon, T., Hahn, E., Cobb, L., Edwards, J., & Kuller, L. (1990). Age related prognosis after acute myocardial infarction. The Multicenter Diltiazem Postinfarction Trial. *American Journal of Cardiology, 65,* 559–566.

Mark, B. A., Salyer, J., Geddes, N., & Smith, C. (1998). The Outcomes Research in Nursing Administration Project: Methodological issues in implementation. *Outcomes Management Nursing Practice, 2*(3), 111–116.

Marks, R. M., & Sachar, E. G. (1973). Undertreatment of medical in patients with narcotic analgesics. *Annals of Internal Medicine, 78,* 173–181.

Markson, L. J., Kern, D. C., Annas, G. J., & Glantz, L. H. (1994). Physician assessment of patient competence. *Journal of the American Geriatrics Society, 42,* 1074–1080.

Marottoli, R. A., Ostfeld, A. M., Merrill, S. S., Perlman, G. D., Foley, D. J., & Cooney, L. M. (1993). Driving cessation and changes in mileage driven among elderly individuals. *Journal of Gerontology: Social Sciences, 48,* S255–S260.

Marshall, F. (1994). Editorial: Risk factors for urinary incontinence after radical prostatectomy. *Journal of Urology, 156,* 1724.

Martinson, I. M. (1995). Pediatric hospice nursing. In J. Fitzpatrick & J. Stevenson (Eds.), *Annual review of nursing research* (Vol. 13, pp. 195–214). New York: Springer Publishing.

Martinson, I. M., Armstrong, G. D., Geis, D. P., Anglim, M. A., Gronseth, E. C., MacInnis, H., Kersey, J. H., & Nesbitt, M. E. (1978). Home care for children dying of cancer. *Pediatrics, 62,* 106–113.

Martocchio, B. C. (1980). *Living while dying.* Bowie, MD: Robert J. Brady.

Marzinski, L. R. (1991). The tragedy of dementia: Clinically assessing pain in the confused nonverbal elderly. *Journal of Gerontological Nursing, 17,* 25–28.

Master, R. J., Feltin, M., Joainchill, J., Mark, R., Kavesh, W. N., Rabkin, M. T., Turner, B., Bachrach, S., & Lennox, S. (1980). A continuum of care for the inner city—assessement of its benefits for Boston's elderly and high-risk populations. *The New England Journal of Medicine, 302*(26), 1434–1440.

Masterman, D. L., & Cummings, J. L. (1998). Parkinson's disease update. Part I: clinical features, neuropathology, and treatment. Neuropsychiatric aspects. *Clinical Geriatrics, 6*(2), 61–71.

Masters, M., & Shontz, F. C. (1989). Identification of problems and strengths of the hospice client by clients, caregivers, and nurses: Implication for nursing. *Cancer Nursing, 12*(4), 226–235.

Matteson, M., McConnell, E. S., & Linton, A. D. (1997a). Nursing diagnosis related to physiological alterations. In A. C. Gaw (Ed.), *Gerontological nursing* (2nd ed.) (pp. 423–435). Philadelphia: W. B. Saunders Company.

Matteson, M., McConnell, E. S., & Linton, A. D. (1997b). *Gerontological nursing: Concepts and practice.* Philadelphia: W. B. Saunders Company.

Matteson, M. A., & Linton, A. D. (1996). Wandering behaviors in institutionalized persons with dementia. *Journal of Gerontological Nursing, 22*(9), 39–46.

Matteson, M. A., Linton, A. D., Cleary, B. L., Barnes, S. J., & Lichtenstein, M. J. (1997). Management of problematic behavioral symptoms associated with dementia: A cognitive developmental approach. *Aging: Clinical and Experimental Research, 9,* 342–355.

Matthews, E. A., Farrell, G. A., & Blackmore, A. M. (1996). Effects of an environmental manipulation on agitation and sleep in dementia sufferers in a nursing home. *Journal of Advanced Nursing, 24,* 439–447.

Maurer, J. D., Rosenberg, H. M., & Keemer, J. B. (1990). Deaths of Hispanic origin: 15 reporting states, 1979–1981. *Vital Health Statistics, 20*(18) (DHHS Publication No. 91-1855). Washington, DC: U.S. Government Printing Office.

Mayer-Oakes, S. A., Oye, R. K., & Leake, B. (1991). Predictors of mortality in older patients with acute pulmonary edema and normal ejection fraction after acute myocardial infarction. *Journal of the American Geriatric Society, 39,* 862–868.

Maxfield, M. C., Lewis, R. E., & Cannon, S. (1996). Training staff to prevent aggressive behavior of cognitively impaired elderly patients during bathing and grooming. *Journal of Gerontological Nursing, 22*(1), 37–43.

McAiney, C. A. (1998). The development of the empowered aide model: an intervention for long-term care staff who care for Alzheimer's residents. *Journal of Gerontological Nursing, 24*(1), 17–22, 58–64.

McCance, K., & Huether, S. (1990). *Pathophysiology: The biologic basis for disease in adults and children.* St. Louis, MO: C. V. Mosby.

McCance, K. L., & Huether, S. E. (1998). Structure and function of the digestive system. In A. C. Gaw (Ed.), *Pathophysiology: The biologic basis for disease in adults and children* (3rd ed.) (pp. 1314–1320). St. Louis, MO: Mosby.

McCloskey, J. C., & Bulechek, G. M. (Eds.). (1996). *Nursing Interventions Classification (NIC)* (2nd ed.). St. Louis, MO: Mosby.

McConnell, E. A. (1998). Managing patient falls and wandering. *Nursing Management, 29,* 75–77.

McCorkle, M. D. (1934). *A curriculum study in social hygiene for nurses.* New York: American Social Hygiene Association and NLNE.

McCormick, W., Inui, T., & Roter, D. (1996). Interventions in physician-elderly patient interactions. *Research On Aging, 18,* 103–136.

McCowan, D. E., & Davies, B. (1995). Patterns of grief in young children following the death of a sibling. *Death Studies, 19,* 41–53.

McCracken, A. L. (1994). Women, aging, and nursing[editorial]. *Journal of Gerontological Nursing, 20*(7), 3–4.

McCracken, A. L., & Torgersen, D. (1994). The role of the nursing home in nursing research of the elderly. *Director, 2,* 68–70.

McDonald, D., Freeland, M., Thomas, G., & Moore, J. (1999). *The effect of an intervention teaching preoperative older adults pain management knowledge and pain communication skills.* Manuscript submitted for publication.

McDonald, D., & Sterling, R. (1998). Acute pain reduction strategies used by well older adults. *International Journal of Nursing Studies, 35,* 265–270.

McDougall, G. J. (1990). A review of screening instruments for assessing cognition and mental status in older adults. *Nurse Practitioner, 15,* 18–28.

McDougall, G. (1995). A critical review of research on cognitive function/impairment in older adults. *Archives of Psychiatric Nursing, 9,* 22–33.

McDowell, B. J., Martin, D. C., Snustad, D. G., & Flynn, W. (1986). Comparison of the clinical practice of a geriatric nurse practitioner and two internist at a geriatric ambulatory care center. *Public Health Nursing 3,* 140–146.

McEvoy, C. L., & Patterson, R. L. (1986). Behavioral treatment of deficit skills in dementia patients. *The Gerontologist, 26,* 475–478.

McGee, H. M., O'Boyle, C. A., Hickey, A., O'Malley, K., & Joyce, C. R. B. (1991). Individual quality of life in patients undergoing hip replacement. *Lancet, 339,* 1088–1091.

McGinty, D., Littner, M., & Stern, N. (1987). Sleep-Related breathing disorders in aging. In W. Emser, D. Kurz, & W. B. Webb (Eds.), *Interdisciplinary topics in gerontology: Sleep, aging and related disorders* (pp. 13–36). New York: Karger.

McHugh, M., West, P., Assatly, C., Duprat, L., Howard, L., Niloff, J., Waldo, K., Wandel, J., & Clifford, J. (1996). Establishing an interdisciplinary patient care team. *Journal of Nursing Administration, 26,* 21–27.

McKhann, G., Drachman, D., Folstein, M., Katzman, R., Price, D., & Stadian, E. (1984). Clinical diagnosis of Alzheimer's disease: Report of the NINCDS-ADRDA work group. *Neurology, 34,* 939–944.

McLaughlin, C. (1994). Casualty nurses' attitudes toward attempted suicide. *Journal of Advanced Nursing, 20,* 1111–1118.

McLendon, B. M., & Doraiswamy, P. M. (1999). Defining meaningful change in Alzheimer's disease trials: The donepezil experience. *Journal of Geriatric Psychiatry & Neurology, 12,* 39–48.

McMahon, M., & Rhudick, P. (1961). Reminiscence. *Archives of General Psychiatry, 10,* 292–298.

McMillan, S. C. (1996). Pain and pain relief experienced by hospice patients with cancer. *Cancer Nursing, 19,* 298–307.

McMillan, S. C., & Mahon, M. (1994). The impact of hospice services on the quality of life of primary caregivers. *Oncology Nursing Forum, 21,* 1189–1195.

Meara, J., Mitchelmore, E., & Hobson, P. (1999). Use of the GDS–15 geriatric depression scale as a screening instrument for depressive symptomatology in patients with Parkinson's disease and their carers in the community. *Age & Ageing, 28,* 35–38.

Meehan, M. (1994). National pressure ulcer prevalence survey. *Advanced Wound Care, 7*(3), 27–30, 34, 36–38.

Mcck, P. A., & Lareau, S. C. (1997). Comparison of actual and recalled rating of dyspnea and fatigue. *American Journal of Respiratory and Critical Care Medicine, 155,* A200.

Meek, S. S. (1993). Effects on slow stroke back massage on relaxation in hospice clients. *Image: Journal of Nursing Scholarship, 25,* 17–21.

Meijer, W. T., Hoes, A. W., Rutgers, D., Bots, M. L., Hofman, A. & Grobbee, D. E. (1998). Peripheral arterial disease in the elderly: The Rotterdam Study. *Arterioscrosis, Thrombosis & Vascular Biology, 18,* 185–192.

Meiner, S. E. (1997). Polypharmacy in the elderly: Early intervention can prevent complications. *ADVANCE for Nurse Practitioners, 5*(7), 28–34.

Meischke, H., Eisenberg, M. S., & Larsens, M. P. (1993). Prehospital delay interval for patients who use emergency medical services: The effect of heart-related medical conditions and demographic variables. *Annals of Emergency Medicine, 22,* 1597–1601.

Meleis, A. I. (1997). *Theoretical nursing: Development and progress* (3rd ed.). Philadelphia: Lippincott.

Melillo, K. D., & Futrell, M. (1998). Wandering and technology devices. *Journal of Gerontological Nursing, 29*(8), 32–38.

Meltzer, H. Y. (1990). The role of serotonin in depression. In P. M. Whitaker-Asmitia & S. J. Peroutka (Eds.), The nueorpharmacology of serotonin. *Annals of New York Academy of Science, 600,* 486–500.

Melzack, R. (1975). The McGill pain questionnaire: Major properties and scoring methods. *Pain, 1,* 277–299.

Melzack, R., Abbott, F. V., Zackon, W., Mulder, D. S., & Davis, M. W. (1987). Pain on a surgical ward: A survey of the duration and intensity of pain and the effectiveness of medication. *Pain, 29*(1), 67–72.

Melzack, R., Ofiesh, J. G., & Mount, B. M. (1976). The Brompton mixture: Effects on pain in cancer patients. *Canadian Medical Association Journal, 115,* 125–128.

Melzack, R., & Wahl, P. D. (1965). Pain mechanisms: A new theory. *Science, 150,* 971–979.

Mendel, B., Lutzen, K., Bergenius, J., & Bjorvell, H. (1997). Living with dizziness: An exploratory study. *Journal of Advanced Nursing, 26,* 1134–1141.

Mendoza, F. S., Ventura, S. J., Valdez, R. B., Castillo, R. O., Salvidar, L. E., Baisden, K., & Martorell, R. (1991). Selected measures of health status for Mexican-American, mainland Puerto Rican, and Cuban-American children. *Journal of the American Medical Association, 265,* 227–232.

Meraviglia, M. (1999). Critical analysis of spirituality: Its empirical indicators. *Journal of Holistic Nursing, 17,* 18–33.

Messenger, T., & Roberts, K. T. (1994). The terminally ill: Serenity nursing interventions for hospice clients. *Journal of Gerontological Nursing, 20*(11), 17–22.

Mettlin, C., Murphy, G., Lee, F., Litrup, P., Chesley, A., Babaian, R., Badalament, R., Kane, R., Mostofi, F., & Investigators of the American Cancer Society-National

Prostate Cancer Detection Project. (1994). Characteristics of prostate cancer detected in the American Cancer Society-National Prostate Cancer Detection Project. *Journal of Urology, 152,* 1737–1740.

Meyer, H. (1990). The bottom line on assisted living. *Hospitals & Health Networks,* July 20,1998, 22–26.

Meyer, H. (1998). The bottom line on assisted living. [Journal Article. *Hospitals & Health Networks, 72*(14), 22–26.

Meyer, L. (1956). *Emotion and meaning in music.* Chicago: University of Chicago Press.

Meyers, B. S., & Bruce, M. L. (1998). The depression-dementia conundrum: Integrating clinical and epidemiological perspectives. *Archives of General Psychiatry, 55,* 1082–1083.

Mezey, M. D. (1988). Strategies for attracting staff and faculty in long-term care. *NLN Publications, 20-2231,* 85–97.

Mezey, M., & Fulmer, T. (1998). Quality care for the frail elderly. *Nursing Outlook, 46,* 291–292.

Mezey, M. D., Lynaugh, J. E., & Cartier, M. M. (1988). The teaching nursing home program, 1982-87: A report card. *Nursing Outlook, 36,* 285–288.

Mezey, M., Mitty, E., Rappaport, M., & Ramsey, G. (1997). Implementation of the Patient Self Determination Act in nursing homes in New York City. *Journal of the American Geriatric Society, 45,* 43–49.

Mezey, M., Ramsey, G., Mitty, E., & Leitman, R. (1995, October–November). *The Patient Self Determination Act: Cultural and socio-economic differences among recently discharged hospital patients.* Paper presented at the American Public Health Association, 123rd annual meeting, San Diego, CA.

Mezey, M. D., Stokes, S., & Rauckhurst, L. (1995). *Health assessment in the older adult.* New York: Springer Publishing.

Mezey, M. D., Teresi, J., Mitty, E., Ramsey, G., & Goldstein, T. (1997). *Determination of decision-making capacity sufficient to execute a health care proxy.* Manuscript submitted for publication.

Miceli, B. V. (1999). Nursing unit meal management maintenance program. *Journal of Gerontological Nursing, 25*(8), 22–36.

Midanik, L., Soghikian, K., Ransom, L., & Tekawa, S. (1995). The effect of retirement on mental health and health behaviors: The Kaiser Permanente Retirement Study. *Journal of Gerontology: Social Sciences, 50B,* S59–61.

Michaelsson, E., Norberg, A., & Samuelsson, S. M. (1987). Assessment of thirst among severely demented patients in the terminal phase of life. Exploratory interviews with ward sisters and enrolled nurses. *International Journal of Nursing Studies, 24,* 87–93.

Middleton, J. I., Richardson, J. S., Berman, E. (1997). An assessment and intervention study of aggressive behavior in cognitively impaired institutionalized elderly. *American Journal of Alzheimer's Disease, 12,* 24–29.

Middleton, J. I., Stewart, N. J., & Richardson, J. S. (1999). Caregiver distress related to disruptive behaviors on special care units versus tradtional long-term care units. *Journal of Gerontological Nursing, 25*(3), 11–19.

Milisen, K., Foreman, M. D., Godderis, J., Abraham, I. L., & Broos, P. L. O. (1998). Delirium in the hospitalized elderly: Nursing assessment and management. *Nursing Clinics of North America, 33,* 417–433.

Miller, C. W. (1978). Survival and ambulation following hip fracture. *Journal of Bone and Joint Surgery [AM], 60,* 930–934.

Miller, J., Neelon, V., Dalton, J., Ng'andu, N., Bailey, D. Jr., Layman, E., & Hosfeld, A. (1996). The assessment of discomfort in elderly confused patients: A preliminary study. *Journal of Neuroscience Nursing, 28,* 175–182.

Miller, N. H., Smith, P. M., DeBusk, R. F., Sobel, D. S., & Taylor, C. B. (1997). Smoking cessation and hospitalized patients: Results of a randomized trial. *Archives of Internal Medicine.*

Miller, S. K. (1997). Impact of a gerontological nurse practitioner on the nursing home elderly in the acute care setting. *AACN Clinical Issues: Advanced Practice in Acute & Critical Care, 8,* 609–615.

Millison, M. B. (1988). Spirituality and the caregiver. Developing an underutilized facet of care. *American Journal of Hospice Care, 5*(2), 37–44.

Millison, M. (1995). A review of research on spiritual care and hospice. *The Hospice Journal, 10,* 3–18.

Minkler, M., & Roe, K. M. (1993). *Grandmothers as caregivers: Raising children of the crack cocaine epidemic.* Newbury Park, CA: Sage.

Minkler, M., Roe, K. M., & Robertson-Beckley. (1994). Raising grandchildren from crack-cocaine households: Effects on family and friendship ties of African-American women. *American Journal of Orthopsychiatry 64,* 20–29.

Minnick, A. F., Mion, L. C., Leipzig, R., Lamb, K., & Palmer, R. M. (1998). Prevalence and patterns of physical restraint use in the acute care setting. *Journal of Nursing Administration, 28*(11), 19–24.

Minors, D., Atkinson, G., Bent, N., Rabbitt, P., & Waterhouse, J. (1998). The effects of age upon some aspects of lifestyle and implications for studies on circadian rhythmicity. *Age & Ageing, 27,* 67–72.

Mishima, K., Okawa, M., Hishikawa, Y., Hozumi, S., Hori, H., & Takahashi, K. (1994). Morning bright light therapy for sleep and behavior disorders in elderly patients with dementia. *Acta Psychiatrica Scandinavica, 89,* 1–7.

Miskella, C., & Avis, M. (1998). Care of the dying person in the nursing home: Exploring the care assistants' contribution. *European Journal of Oncology Nursing 2,* 80–88.

Mitchell, P. H., Kirkness, C., Burr, R., March, K., & Newell, D. W. (in press). Waveform predictors of adverse responses to nursing care. *Acta Neurochirurgica.*

Mittleman, M. S., Ferris, S. H., Shulman, E., Steinberg, G., & Levin, B. (1996). A family intervention to delay nursing home placement of patients with Alzheimer's disease: A randomized controlled trial. *The Journal of the American Medical Association, 276,* 1725–1731.

Mittleman, M., Ferris, S., Steinberg, G., Schulman, E., Mackell, J., Ambinder, A., & Cohen, J. (1995). A comprehensive support program: Effect on depression in spouse-caregivers of AD patients. *The Gerontologist, 35,* 792–802.

Mitchell, R. B., Gingrich, D., & Jones, R. L. (1994). The Biology of aging. *Journal of the American Academy of Physician Assistants, 7,* 210–215.

Mobily, K., Lemke, J., & Gisin, G. (1991). The idea of leisure repertoire. *The Journal of Applied Gerontology, 10,* 208–223.

Mock, V., Hassey Dow, K., Meares, C., Grimm, P., Dieneman, J., Haisfield-Wolfe, M., Quitasol, W., Mitchell, S., Chakravarthy, A., & Gage, I. (1997). Effects of exercise on fatigue, physical functioning, and emotional distress during radiation therapy for breast cancer. *Oncology Nursing Forum, 24.*

Monahan, R. S., & McCarthy, S. (1992). Nursing home employment: The nurse aide's perspective. *Journal of Gerontological Nursing, 18*(2), 13–16.

Monsour, N., & Robb, S. S. (1982). Wandering behavior in old age: A psychosocial study. *Social Work, 27,* 411–416.

Montgomery, C. (1994). Swimming upstream: The strengths of women who survive homelessness. *Advanced Nursing Science, 16*(3), 34–45.

Montgomery, R. (1986). Researching respite: Beliefs, facts, and questions. In R. Montgomery & J. Prothero (Eds.), *Developing respite services for the elderly* (pp. 18–32). USA: University of Washington Press.

Montgomery, R. (1988). Respite care: Lessons from a controlled design study. *Health Care Financing Review, 9,* S133–S138.

Montgomery, R. J. V. (1996). Next steps for social and behavioral research related to Alzheimer's disease. *International Psychogeriatrics, 8,* 103–107.

Montgomery, R., & Borgatta, E. (1989). The effects of alternative support strategies on family caregiving. *The Gerontologist, 29,* 457–464.

Moody, L. E. (1999). Living longer, dying longer: Nursing's opportunity to make a difference. *Nursing Outlook, 47,* 41–42.

Moore, J. (1998). CCRCs shine in the shadows. *Contemporary Long Term Care, 21,* 39–40.

Moore, K. (1999). A review of the anatomy of the male continence mechanism and the cause of urinary incontinence after prostatectomy. *Journal of Wound, Ostomy and Continence Nursing, 26,* 86–93.

Moos, R., & Billings, A. (1986). Conceptualizing and measuring coping resources and processes. In L. Goldberger & S. Breynitz (Eds.), *Handbook of stress; theoretical and clinical perspectives.* New York: Free Press.

Mor, V., Sherwood, S., & Gutkin, C. (1986). A national study of residential care for the aged. *The Gerontologist, 26,* 405–417.

Morey, M. C., Crowley, G. M., Robbins, M. S., Cowper, P. A., & Sullivan, J. R. (1994). The gerofit program: A VA innovation. *Southern Medical Journal, 87,* S83–S87.

Morley, J. E., & Silver A. J. (1995). Nutritional issues in nursing home care. *Annals of Internal Medicine, 123,* 850–859.

Morris, L. E. H. (1996). A spiritual well-being model: Use with older women who experience depression. *Issues in Mental Health Nursing, 17,* 439–455.

Morrison, R. S., Ahronheim, J. C., Morrison, G. R., Darling, E., Baskin, S. A., Morris, J., Choi, C., & Meier, D. (1998). Pain and discomfort associated with common hospital procedures and experiences. *Journal of Pain and Symptom Management, 15,* 91–101.

Mosier, R., Nusser-Gurlach, B., Manz, B., & Bergstrom, N. (1998). Pain assessment in cognitively impaired and non-impaired elderly. Presented at 22nd Annual Midwest Nursing Research Society, Columbus, OH.

Mossey, J. M., Knott, K., & Craik, R. L. (1990). The effects of persistent depressive symptoms on hip fracture recovery. *Journal of Gerontology, 45,* M163–M168.

Mossey, J., Mutran, E., Knott, K., & Craik, R. (1989). Determinants of recovery 12 months after hip fracture: The importance of psychosocial factors. *American Journal of Public Health, 72*, 279–286.

Mossey, J. M., & Shapiro, E. (1982). Self-rated health: A predictor of mortality among the elderly. *American Journal of Public Health, 72*, 800–808.

Mudd, S. A., Boyd, C. J., Brower, K. J., Young, J. P., & Blow, F. C. (1994). Alcohol withdrawal and related nursing care in older adults. *Journal of Gerontological Nursing, 20*(10), 17–26.

Mujic, V. R, & Rao, S. S. (1999). Recognizing atypical manifestations of GERD. Asthma, chest pain, and otolaryngologic disorders may be due to reflux. *Postgraduate Medicine, 105*, 53.

Muller, R. T., Gould, L. A., Betzu, R., Vacek, T., & Pradeep, V. (1990). Painless myocardial infarction in the elderly. *American Heart Journal, 199*, 202–203.

Murphy, E., & Fenton, M. S. (1991). An analysis of theory-research linkages in published gerontologic nursing studies, 1983–1989. *Advances in Nursing Science, 13*(4), 1–13.

Murray, R., & Zentner, J. (1997). *Health assessment promotion strategies throughout the life span* (6th ed.). Stamford, CT: Appleton & Lange.

Musick, M. A., Koenig, H. G., Hays, J. C., & Cohen, H. J. (1998). Religious activity and depression among community-dwelling elderly persons with cancer: The moderating effect of race. *Journal of Gerontology, 53B*, 218–227.

Myers, A., Robinson, E., van Natta, M., Michaelson, J., Collins, K., & Parker, S. (1991). Hip fractures among the elderly: Factors associated with in-hospital mortality. *American Journal of Epidemiology, 134*, 1128–1137.

Myers, D. (1991). Work after cessation of career job. *Journal of Gerontology: Social Sciences, 46*, S93–102.

Nadelman, J., Frishman, W. H., Ooi, W. L., Tepper, D., Greenberg, S., Guzik, H., Lazar, E. J., Heiman, M., & Aronson, M. (1990). Prevalence, incidence, and prognosis of recognized and unrecognized myocardial infarction in persons aged 75 years and older: The Bronx Aging Study. *The American Journal of Cardiology, 66*, 533–537.

Naegle, M. A. (1995). Education, research, and theory development. In E. J. Sullivan (Ed.), *Nursing care of clients with substance abuse*. St. Louis: Mosby.

Nagi, S. Z. (1991). Disability concepts revisited. In A. M. Pope & A. R. Tarlov (Eds.), *Disability in America: Toward a national agenda for prevention* (pp. 309–327). Washington, DC: National Academy Press.

Nagley, S. (1984). *Prevention of confusion in hospitalized elderly persons.* Unpublished doctoral dissertation, Case Western Reserve University, Cleveland OH.

Nam, R., Fleshner, N., Rakovitch, E., Klotz, L., Trachtenberg, J., Choo, R., Morton, G., & Danjoux, C. (1999). Prevalence and patterns of the use of complementary therapies among prostate cancer patients: An epidemiologic analysis. *The Journal of Urology, 161*, 1521–1524.

Namazi, K. H., Gwinnup, P. B., & Zadorozny, C. A. (1994). A low intensity exercise/movement program for patients with Alzheimer's disease: The TEMP-AD Protocol. *Journal of Aging and Physical Activity, 2*, 80–92.

Namazi, K. H., Rosner, T. T., & Calkins, M. P. (1989). Visual barriers to prevent ambulatory Alzheimer's patients from exiting through an emergency door. *The Gerontologist, 29,* 699–702.

Narain, P., Rubenstein, L. Z., Wieland, A. D., Rushbrook, R., Strome, L. S., Pietrusaka, F., & Mosley, J. E. (1988). Predictors of immediate and 6 month outcomes in hospitalized elderly patients. The importance of functional status. *Journal of the American Geriatric Society, 36,* 775–873.

Narayanasamy, A. (1993). Nurses' awareness and educational preparation in meeting their patients' spiritual needs. *Nurse Education Today, 13,* 196–201.

National Center for Health Statistics (1998). Advanced Report & Mortality.

National Chronic Care Consortium, Chronic care networks for Alzheimer's Disease, April 13, 1999, http://www.ncccresourcecenter.org/about/an/Alzheimers.html.

National Institute on Aging (1999). Alzheimer's disease: Unraveling the mystery. [Announcement posted on the World Wide Web]. Washington, DC: Author. Retrieved May 6, 1999 from the World Wide Web: http://test.jbs1.com/adear/unravel.html

National Institute on Alcohol Abuse and Alcoholism (NIAAA). (1993). *Eighth special report to US Congress: Alcohol and health* (DHHS Publication No. ADM 281-88-003). Alexandria, VA: Editorial Experts.

National Institute of Health. (1995). *Progress Report of Alzheimer's Disease 1994.* Bethesda: Author.

National Institute Health Consensus Development Panel. (1992). Diagnosis and treatment of depression in late life. *Journal of the American Medical Association, 268,* 1018–1024.

National Institute of Nursing Research. Opening Statement. http://www.nih.gov/ninr/openingstatement99.htm

National Kidney and Urologic Diseases Advisory Board. (1994). *Barriers to rehabilitation of persons with end-stage renal disease or chronic urinary incontinence* (Workshop summary report). Bethesda, MD: Author.

National sample survey of registered nurses. (1997). Washington, DC: Division of Nursing, Bureau of Health Professions, Health Resources and Services Administration.

Naylor, M. (1990). Comprehensive discharge planning for hospitalized elderly: A pilot study. *Nursing Research, 39*(3), 156–161.

Naylor, M., Brooten, D., Campbell, R., Jacobsen, B., Mezey, M., Pauly, M., & Schwartz, J. S. (1999). Comprehensive discharge planning and home follow-up of hospitalized elders. *Journal of the American Medical Association, 281*(7), 613–620.

Naylor, M., Brooten, D., Jones, R., Lavizzo, O., Mourey, R., Mezey, M., & Pauly, M. (1994). Comprehensive discharge planning for hospitalized elderly. *Annals of Internal Medicine, 120,* 999–1006.

Naylor, M. D., Munro, B. H., & Brooten D. A. (1991). Measuring the effectiveness of nursing practice. *Clinical Nurse Specialist, 5,* 210–215.

Neale, A. V., Tilley, B. C., & Vernon, S. W. (1986). Marital status, delay in seeking treatment and survival from breast cancer. *Social Science and Medicine, 23,* 305–312.

Neelon, V. J., & Champagne, M. T. (1992). Managing cognitive impairment: The current bases for practice. In S. G. Funk, E. M. Tornquist, M. T. Champagne, & R. A. Wiese (Eds.), *Key aspects of elder care: Managing falls, incontinence, and cognitive impairment* (pp. 239–250). New York: Springer Publishing.

Negri, E., Franceschi, S., Parpinel, M., & LaVecchia, C. (1998). Fiber intake and risk of colorectal cancer. *Cancer Epidemiol Biomarkers Prevention, 7*, 667–771.

Neidlinger, S., Scroggins, K., & Kennedy, L. (1987). Cost evaluation of discharge planning for hospitalized elderly. *Nursing Economics, 5*, 225–230.

Nelson, R., Furner, S., & Jesudason, V. (1998). Fecal incontinence in Wisconsin nursing homes: Prevalence and association. *Disease of the Colon Rectum, 41*, 1226–1229.

Nemcek, M. (1989). Factors influencing Black women's breast self-examination practice. *Cancer Nursing, 12*, 339–343.

Newbern, V., & Krowchuk, H. (1994). Failure to thrive in elderly people: A conceptual analysis. *Journal of Advanced Nursing, 19*, 840–849.

Newman, M. A. (1994). *Health as expanding consciousness* (2nd ed.). New York: National League for Nursing.

The Niche Project Faculty. (1994). Geriatric models of care: Which one's right for your institution? *American Journal of Nursing, 94*, 21–23.

Nicholas, M., Connor, L. T., Obler, L. K., & Albert, M. L. (1998). Aging, language, and language disorders. In M. T. Sarno (Ed.), *Acquired aphasia* (3rd ed.) (pp. 413–439). San Diego, CA: Academic Press.

Nicholson, S. (1997). Certification groups pass NCSBN audit. *Clinician News, 1*(2), 10–11.

Nicolosi, L., Harryman, E., & Kresheck, J. (1989). *Terminology of communication disorders: Speech, language and hearing* (3rd ed.) (p. 9). Baltimore, MD: Williams & Wilkins.

Nightingale, F. (1860). *Notes on nursing: What it is and what it is not.* London: Harrison and Sons.

Nightingale, F. (1969). *Notes on nursing* (p. 103). New York: Dover Publications. (Original work published 1860).

Noble-Adams, R. (1995). Dehydration: Subcutaneous fluid administration. *British Journal of Nursing, 4*, 492–494.

Nolen, N. R., & Garrard, J. (1988). Predicting dependent feeding behaviors in the institutionalized elderly. *Journal of Nutrition for the Elderly, 7*(3), 17–25.

Normand, S. T., Glickman, M. E., Sharma, R. G. V. R. K., & McNeil, B. J. (1996). Using admission characteristics to predict short-term mortality from myocardial infarction in elderly patients. *Journal of the American Medical Association, 275*, 1322–1328.

North American Nursing Diagnosis Association. (1994). *Taxonomy I revised—1990, with official nursing diagnoses.* St. Louis, MO: Author.

Northouse, L. (1981). Mastectomy patients and the fear of cancer recurrence. *Cancer Nursing, 4*, 213–220.

Northouse, L. (1995). The impact of cancer in women on the family. *Cancer Practice, 3*, 134–142.

Northridge, M. E., Nevitt, M. C., Kelsey, J. L., & Link, B. (1995). Home hazards and falls in the elderly: The role of health and functional status. *American Journal of Public Health, 85,* 509–515.

Norton, D., McLaren, R., & Exton-Smith, A. N. (1975). *An investigation of geriatric nursing problems in hospital.* London: Churchill Livingstone. (Original work published in 1962)

Nugent, E. (1995). Reminiscence as a nursing intervention. *Journal of Psychosocial Nursing, 33*(11), 7–11.

Nursing Home Reform Law. Omnibus Budget Reconciliation Act of 1987. (PL–100–203).

Nyman, J. A., Finch, M., Kane, R. A., Kane, R. L., Illston, L. H. (1997). The substitutability of adult foster care for nursing home care in Oregon. *Medical Care, 35,* 801–813.

Nystrom, A. E. M. (1995). The concept of cogiation. *Journal of Advanced Nursing, 21,* 364–370.

Office of Alternative Medicine. (1992). *Alternative medicine: Expanding medical horizons. A report to the National Institutes of Health on alternative medical systems and practices in the United States* (NIH Publication No.94-066). Washington, DC: U.S. Government Printing Office.

Office of Disease Prevention & Health Promotion (1987). *Publications List U.S. Government Printing Office;* Washington, DC.

Office of Technology Assessment. (1987). *Losing a million minds: Confronting the tragedy of Alzheimer's disease and other dementias.* Washington, DC: U.S. Government Printing Office.

Office of Technology Assessment, U.S. Congress, HCS 37, (1986). *Nursing Practitioners, Physician Assistants, and Certified Nurse-Midwives: A Policy Analysis.* [hereinafter OTA Study] citing definitions adopted by the American College of Nurse-Midwives.

Ogilvie-Harris, D. J., Botsford, D., & Worden Hawker, R. (1993). Elderly patients with hip fracture: Improved outcome with the use of care maps with high quality medical and nursing protocols. *Journal of Orthopedic Trauma,*(7), 428–437.

Ohori, M., Wheeler, T., Dunn, J., Stamey, T., & Scardino, P. (1994). The pathological features and prognosis of prostate cancer detectable with current diagnostic tests. *Journal of Urology, 152,* 1714–1720.

Oktay, J. S., & Volland, P. J. (1987). Foster home care for the frail elderly as an alternative to nursing home care: An experimental evaluation. *American Journal of Public Health, 77,* 1505–1510.

Oktay, J., & Volland, P. (1990). Post-hospital support program for the frail elderly and their caregivers: A quasi-experimental evaluation. *American Journal of Public Health, 80,* 39–45.

Oliver, S., & Redfern, S. (1991). Interpersonal communication between nurses and elderly patients: Refinement of an observation schedule. *Journal of Advanced Nursing, 16,* 30–38.

O'Loughlin, G., & Shanley, C. (1998). Swallowing problems in the nursing home: A novel training approach. *Dysphagia, 13,* 172–183.

Olsson, C., & Goluboff, E. (1994). Detection and treatment of prostate cancer: Perspective of the urologist. *Journal of Urology, 152,* 1695–1699.

O'Mahoney, D., & Foote, C. (1998). Prospective evaluation of unexplained syncope, dizziness, and falls among community-dwelling elderly adults. *Journal of Gerontology, 53A,* M435–440.

Omnibus Budget Reconciliation Act of 1987 (public law 100–203). §100

Omnibus Budget Reconciliation Act of 1990. (1991). *Patient Self Determination Act* (Pub.L. No. 101-508 [4206, 4751, codified in scattered sections of 42 U.S.C., esp. 1395cc, 1396a], West Supp.).

O'Neill, D. P., & Kenny, E. K. (1998). Spirituality and chronic illness. *Image: Journal of Nursing Scholarship, 30,* 275–280.

Opie, N. (1992). Childhood and adolescent bereavement. In J. Fitzpatrick & J. Stevenson (Eds.), *Annual review of nursing research* (Vol. 10, pp. 127–141). New York: Springer Publishing.

Osato, E., Takano, S., Phillips, L., & Winne, D. (1993). Clinical manifestations. Failure to thrive in the elderly. *Journal of Gerontological Nursing, 19*(8), 28–34.

Osborn, C. L., & Marshall, M. J. (1993). Self-feeding performance in nursing home residents. *Journal of Gerontological Nursing, 19*(3), 7–14.

Osterweil, D., Martin, M., & Syndulko, K. (1995). Predictors of skilled nursing placement in a multilevel long-term-care facility. *Journal of the American Geriatric Society, 43,* 108–12.

Ouslander, J. G., & Schnelle, J. F. (1993). Assessment, treatment and management of urinary incontinence in the nursing home. In L. Rubenstein & D. Wieland (Eds.), *Improving care in the nursing homes. Comprehensive review of clinical research.* Newbury Park, CA: Sage Publications Inc.

Ouellet, L. L., & Rush, K. L. (1996). A study of nurses' perceptions of client mobility. *Western Journal of Nursing Research, 18,* 565–579.

Ouellet, L. L., & Rush, K. L. (1998). Conceptual model of client mobility. *Journal of Orthopaedic Nursing, 2*(3), 132–135.

Owsley, C., Ball, K., McGwin, G., Sloane, M. E., Roenker, D. L, White, M. F., & Overly, E. T. (1998). Visual processing impairment and risk of motor vehicle crash among older adults. *The Journal of the American Medical Association, 279,* 1083–1088.

Padilla, G. V., Presant, C., Grant, M. M., Metter, G., Lipsett, J., & Heide, F. (1983). Quality of life index for patients with cancer. *Research in Nursing and Health, 6,* 117–126.

Paier, G., & Strumpf, N. E. (1999). Meeting the health care needs of older adults. In M. Mezey & D. O. McGivern (Eds.), *Nurses, nurse practitioners: Evolution to advanced practice.* New York: Springer Publishing Co.

Palmateer, L. M., & McCartney, J. R. (1985). Do nurses know when patients have cognitive deficits? *Journal of Gerontological Nursing, 11*(2), 6–16.

Palmer, A. C., & Withee, B. M. (1996). Dementia care: Effects of behavioral intervention training on staff perceptions of their work in veterans' nursing home. *Geriatric Nursing, 17,* 137–140.

Palmer, M. H. (1996). *Urinary continence: Assessment and promotion.* Gaithersburg, MD: Aspen Publications.

Palmer, R. M., Landefeld, C. S., Kresevic, D., & Kowal, J. (1994). A medical unit for the acute care of the elderly. *Journal of the American Geriatrics Society, 45,* 545–552.

Paloutzian, R. F., & Ellison, C. W. (1982). Loneliness, spiritual well-being and the quality of life. In L. A. Peplau & D. Pearlman (Eds.), *Loneliness: A sourcebook of current theory, research and therapy* (pp. 224–37). New York: Wiley and Sons.

Pals, J. K., Weinberg, A. D., Beal, L. F., Levesque, P. G., Cunningham, T. J., & Minaker, K. L. (1995). Clinical triggers for detection of fever and dehydration: Implications for long-term care nursing. *Journal of Gerontological Nursing, 21*(4), 13–19.

Panel for the Prediction and Prevention of Pressure Ulcers in Adults. (1992). *Pressure ulcers in adults: Prediction and prevention.* Clinical practice guideline No. 3 (AHCPR Publication No. 92-0047). Rockville, MD: U.S. Department of Health and Human Services, Agency for Health Care Policy and Research.

Parke, B. (1992). Pain in the cognitively impaired elderly. *Canadian Nurse, 88,* 17–20.

Parker, L. D., Cantrell, C., & Demi, A. S. (1997). Older adults' attitudes toward suicide: Are there race and gender differences? *Death Studies, 21,* 289–298.

Parker, S., Tong, T., Bolden S., & Wingo, S. (1997). Cancer statistics 1996. *CA: A Cancer Journal for Clinicians, 47*(1), 5–27.

Parkin, D., Pisani, P., & Ferlay, J. (1999). Global cancer statistics. *CA: A Cancer Journal for Clinicians, 49,* 33–64.

Parmelee, P., Katz, I., & Lawton, M. (1989). Depression among institutionalized aged: Assessment and prevalence estimation. *Journal of the American Geriatric Society, 44,* M22–29.

Parmelee, P., & Katz, I. (1990). Geriatric Depression Scale. *Journal of the American Geriatrics Society, 38,* 1379–1380.

Parmelee, P., Katz, I., & Lawton, M. (1991). Incidence of depression in long-term care settings. *Journal of Gerontology, 47,* M189–M196.

Parmelee, P., Kleban, M., Lawton, M., & Katz, I. (1991). Depression and cognitive change among institutionalized aged. *Psychology of Aging, 6,* 504–11.

Parmelee, P. A., Smith, B., & Katz, I. R. (1993). Pain complaints and cognitive status among elderly institution residents. *Journal of the American Geriatrics Society, 41,* 517–522.

Parr, J., Green, S., & Behncke, C. (1989). What people want, why they move, and what happens after they move: A summary of research in retirement housing. *Journal of Housing for the Elderly, 5,* 7–33.

Parshall, M. (1999). Adult emergency visits for chronic cardiorespiratory disease: Does dyspnea matter? *Nursing Research, 48*(2), 62–70.

Parsons, L. C., & Wilson, M. M. (1984). Cerebrovascular status of severe closed head injured patients following passive position changes. *Nursing Research, 33,* 68–75.

Pathy, M. S. (1967). Clinical presentation of myocardial infarction in the elderly. *British Heart Journal, 29,* 190–199.

Peacock, E., & Talley, W. (1985). Developing leisure competence: A goal for late adulthood. *Educational Gerontology, 11,* 261–276.

Pearson, J., Teri, L., Wagner, A., Truax, P., & Logsdon, R. (1993). The relationship of problem behavior in dementia patients to the depression and burden of caregiving spouses. *The American Journal of Alzheimer's Disease and Related Disorders & Research, 8,* 15–22.

Pehl, C., Waizenhoefer, C. D., Wendl, B., Schmidt, T., Schepp, W., & Pfeiffer, A. (1999). Effect of low and high fat meals on lower esophageal sphincter motility and gastroesophageal reflux in healthy subjects. *American Journal of Gastroenterology, 94,* 1192–1196.

Pender, N. (1985). Effects of progressive muscle relaxation training on anxiety and health locus of control among hypertensive adults. *Research in Nursing and Health, 8,* 67–72.

Pendergast, J. (1998). Government affairs. Michigan board of nursing approves new nursing rules. *Michigan Nurse, 71*(9), 7.

Penner, L. A., Ludenia, K., & Mead, G. (1984). Staff attitudes: Image or reality. *Journal of Gerontological Nursing, 10,* 110–117.

Pepine, C. J. (1986). Silent myocardial ischemia: Definition, magnitude and scope of the problem. *Cardiology Clinics, 4,* 577–581.

Perkins, K. (1992). Psychosocial implications of women and retirement. *Social Work, 37,* 526–532.

Pernenkil, R., Vinson, J. M., Shah, A. S., Beckham, V., Wittenberg, C., & Rich, M. W. (1997). Course and prognosis in patients > 70 years of age with congestive heart failure and normal versus abnormal left ventricular ejection fraction. *American Journal of Cardiology, 79,* 216–219.

Persson, D. (1993). The elderly driver: Deciding when to stop. *The Gerontologist, 33,* 88–91.

Peterman, B. A., Springer, P., & Farnsworth, J. (1995). Analyzing job demands and coping techniques. *Nursing Management, 26*(2), 51–53.

Petit, J. (1994). Continuing care retirement communities and the role of the wellness nurse. *Geriatric Nursing, 15,* 28–31.

Pfeffer, R., Afifi, A., & Chance, J. (1987). Prevalence of Alzheimer's disease in a retirement community. *American Journal of Epidemiology, 125,* 420–436.

Phillips, C. D., Sloane, P. D., Hawes, C., Koch, G., Han, J., Spry, K., Dunteman, G., & Williams, R. L. (1997). Effects of residence in Alzheimer disease special care units on functional outcomes. *JAMA, 278,* 1340–1344.

Phillips, D. M., Kruse, J. E., Wesley, R. M., & Gail, D. (1999). Comparison of OBRA surveys of long-term care facilities in two states. *Annals of Long Term Care, 7*(7), 258–262.

Phillips, R. M., & Baldwin, B. A. (1997). Teaching psychosocial care to long-term care nursing assistants. *Journal of Continuing Education in Nursing, 28,* 130–134.

Picot, S. J. (1995). Rewards, costs, and coping of African American caregivers. *Nursing Research, 44*(3), 147–152.

Pienta, K., & Esper, P. (1993). Risk factors for prostate cancer. *Annals of Internal Medicine, 118,* 793–803.

Pienta, K., Goodson, J., & Esper, P. (1996). Epidemiology of prostate cancer: Molecular and environmental clues. *Urology, 48,* 676–683.

Pierson, D., & Kacmarek, R. (Eds.). (1992). *Foundations of Respiratory Care.* New York: Churchill Livingstone.

Pilch, J. J. (1988). Wellness: Wellness spirituality. *Health Values, 12*(3), 28–31.

Pillemer, K. A., & Finkelhor, D. A. (1988). The prevalence of elder abuse: A random sample survey. *Gerontologist, 28,* 51–57.

Piotrowski, M. M. (1978). Aphasia: Providing better nursing care. *Nursing Clinics of North America, 13,* 543–553.

Piper, B. F. (1989). Fatigue: Current bases for practice. In S. G. Funk, E. M. Tornquist, M. T. Champagne, L. A. Copp, & R. Wiese (Eds.), *Key aspects of comfort* (pp. 187–240). New York: Springer Publishing.

Platakis, J. (1987). Promoting Health and Wellness in the Elderly. *Nursing Administration Quarterly, 11,* 42–43.

Platt, W., Bell, B., & Kozak, J. (1998). Physiotherapy Functional Mobility Profile: A tool for measuring functional outcome in chronic care clients. *Canadian Journal of Physiotherapy, 50,* 47–52.

Pollack, S. E. (1993). Adaptation to chronic illness: A program of research for testing nursing theory. *Nursing Science Quarterly, 6,* 86–92.

Pollak, C. P., & Stokes, P. E. (1997). Circadian rest-activity rhythms in demented and nondemented older community residents and their caregivers. *Journal of the American Geriatrics Society, 45,* 446–452.

Porter, A., Zimmerman, J., Ruffin, M., Chernew, M., Callaghan, C., Davis, R., Lee, F., Montie, J., Swanson, G., & Oesterling, J. (1996). Recommendations of the first Michigan conference on prostate cancer. *Urology, 48,* 519–533.

Porter, E. J. (1994a). Older widows' experience of living alone at home. *Image: Journal of Nursing Scholarship, 26,* 19–24.

Porter, E. J. (1994b). "Reducing my risks": A phenomenon of older widows' lived experience. *Advances in Nursing Science, 17,* 54–65.

Porter, E. J. (1995a). The life-world of older widows: The context of lived experience. *The Journal of Women & Aging, 7*(4), 31–46.

Porter, E. J. (1995b). Non-equilibrium systems theory: Some applications for gerontological nursing practice. *Journal of Gerontological Nursing, 21*(6), 24–31.

Porter, E. J. (1998a). Older widows' intention to keep the generations separate. *Health Care of Women International, 19,* 395–410.

Porter, E. J. (1998b). "Staying close to shore": A context for older rural widows' use of health care. *Journal of Women & Aging, 10*(4), 25–39.

Post, S. G., & Whitehouse, P. J. (1995). Fairhill guidelines on ethics of the care of people with Alzheimer's disease: A clinical summary. *Journal American Geriatrics Society, 43,* 1423–1429.

Potempa, K. M. (1993). Chronic fatigue. In J. J. Fitzpatrick & J. S. Stevenson (Eds.), *Annual review of nursing research* (Vol. 11, pp. 57–76). New York: Springer Publishing.

Prevost, S., Wilson, E., & Gerber, D. (1991). Acute care nurses' knowledge and attitudes related to aging. *Heart and Lung—Journal of Critical Care, 20,* 359–363.

Price, J. F., Mowbray, P. I., Lee, A. J., Rumley, A., Lowe, G. D., & Fowkes, F. G. (1999). Relationship between smoking and cardiovascular risk factors in the development of peripheral arterial disease and coronary artery disease: Edinburgh Artery Study. *European Heart Journal, 20,* 344–353.

Price, J. L., Stevens, H. O., & LaBarre, M. C. (1995). Spiritual caregiving in nursing practice. *Journal of Psychosocial Nursing, 33*(12), 5–9.

Prochaska, J. O., Velicer, W. F., Rossi, J. S., Goldstein, M. G., Marcus, B. H., Rakowski, W., Fiore, C., Harlow, L. L., Redding, C. A., Rosenblook, D., & Rossi, S. R. (1994). Stages of change and decisional balance for 12 problem behaviors. *Health Psychology, 13,* 39–46.

Province, M. A., Hadley, E. C., Hornbrook, M. C., Lipsitz, L. A., Miller, J. P., Mulrow, C. D., Ory, M. G., Sattin, R. W., Tinetti, M. E., & Wolf, S. L. (1995). The effects of exercise on falls in elderly patients. A preplanned meta-analysis of the FICSIT trials. *Journal of the American Medical Association, 273,* 1381–1383.

Puentes, W. J. (1999). Effect of reminiscence learning on nurses' attitudes and empathy with other adults. *Image: Journal of Nursing Scholarship, 31,* 94.

Quayhagen, M. P., & Quayhagen, M. (1996). Discovering life quality in coping with dementia. *Western Journal of Nursing Research, 18,* 120–135.

Quint, J. (1967). *The Nurse and the Dying Patient.* New York: McMillan.

Rader, J., Doan, J., & Schwab, M. (1985). How to decrease wandering, a form of agenda behavior. *Geriatric Nursing, 6,* 196–199.

Radloff, L. (1977). The CES-D Scale: A self-report depression scale for research in the general population. *Applied Psychological Measurement, 1,* 385–401.

Ragneskog, H., Kihlgren, M., Karlsson, I., & Norberg, A. (1996). Dinner music for demented patients. *Clinical Nursing Research, 5,* 262–282.

Raina, P., Waltner-Toews, D., Bonnett, B., Woodward, C., & Abernathy, T. (1999). Influence of companion animals on the physical and psychological health of older people: An analysis of a one-year longitudinal study. *Journal of American Geriatrics Society, 47,* 323–329.

Rains, J. W., & Ray, D. W. (1995). Participatory action research for community health promotion. *Public Health Nursing, 12,* 256–261.

Rakowski, W., Dube, C., Marcus, B. H., Prochaska, J. O., Velicer, W., & Abrams, D. (1992). Assessing elements of women's decisions about mammography. *Health Psychology, 11,* 111–118.

Ramirez, M., Teresi, J. A., Holmes, D., & Fairchild, S. (1998). Ethnic and racial conflict in relation to staff burnout, demoralization, and job dissatisfaction in SCUs and non-SCUs. *Journal of Mental Health & Aging, 4,* 459–479.

Ramsay, J. A., McKenzie, J. K., Fish, D. G. (1982). Physicians and nurse practitioners: Do they provide equivalent care? *American Journal of Public Health, 72,* 55–57.

Rathbone-McCuan, E. (1976). Geriatric day care: A family perspective. *The Gerontologist, 16,* 517–521.

Rauckhorst, L. M. (1987). Health habits of elderly widows. *Journal of Gerontological Nursing, 13*(8), 19–22.

Raway, B. (1994). Pain behaviors and confusion in elderly patients with hip fracture. *Dissertation Abstracts International, 55,* 02B. (University Microfilms No. AAI94–18593)

Ray, C. (1991). Chronic fatigue syndrome and depression: Conceptual and methodological ambiguities. *Psychological Medicine, 21,* 1–9.

Rehm, L. P. (1977). A self-control model of depression. *Behavior Therapy, 8,* 787–804.

Reichenbach, V. R., & Kirchman, M. M. (1991). Effects of a multi-strategy program upon elderly with organic brain syndrome. In Anonymous, *The mentally impaired elderly* (pp. 131–151). Binghamton, NY: Haworth Press, Inc.

Reifler, B. V., Henry, R. S., Rushing, J., Yates, K., Cox, N. J., Bradham, D. D., & McFarlane, M. (1997). Financial Performance Among Adult Day Centers: Results of a National Demonstration Program, *Journal of the American Geriatrics Society, 45,* 146–153.

Reilly, A., Dracup, K., & Dattolo, J. (1994). Factors influencing prehospital delay in patients experiencing chest pain. *American Journal of Critical Care, 3,* 300–306.

Reilly, F. E. (1994). An ecological approach to health risk: A case study of urban elderly homeless people. *Public Health Nursing, 11,* 305–314.

Reisberg, B. (1984). Alzheimer's disease: Stages of decline. *American Journal of Nursing, 84,* 225–228.

Reisberg, B., Borenstein, J., Salob, S. P., Ferris, S. H., Franssen, E., & Georgotas, A. (1987). Behavioral symptoms in Alzheimer's disease: phenomenology and treatment. *Journal of Clinical Psychiatry, 48,* Suppl, 9–15.

Reisberg, B., Ferris, S. H., & deLeon, M. J. (1982). The global deterioration scale for assessment of primary degenerative dementia. *American Journal of Psychiatry, 139,* 1136–1139.

Resnick, B. (1989). Care for Life: A Faculty Practice With a Lifecare Community. *Nurse Practitioner Forum, 10,* 12–18.

Resnick, B. M. (1989). Care for life . . . even if a life care community is Utopia, the move can be a dramatic change. Here's how to smooth the transition. *Geriatric Nursing—American Journal of Care for the Aging, 10*(3), 130–132.

Resnick, B. (1998a). Functional performance of older adults in a long term care setting. *Clinical Nursing Research, 7,* 230–246.

Resnick, B. (1998b). Health care practices of the old-old. *American Academy Journal Nurse Practitioners, 10,* 147–155.

Resnick, B. (1999). Motivation in the older adult: Can a leopard change its spots? *Journal of Advanced Nursing, 29,* 792–799.

Resnick, B. (in press). Falls in a community of older adults: Putting research into practice. *Clinical Nursing Research.*

Resnick, B., Palmer, M. H., Jenkins, L., & Spellbring, A. M. (in press). Efficacy expectations and exercise behavior in older adults: A path analysis. *Journal of Advanced Nursing.*

Resnick, B., & Spellbring, A. M. (in press). Understanding what motivates older adults to exercise. *Journal of Gerontologic Nursing.*

Reuben, D. B., Silliman, R. A., & Traines, M. (1988). The aging driver: Medicine, policy and ethics. *Journal of the American Geriatrics Society, 36*(12), 1135–1142.

Rice, D., Fox, P. J., & Max, W. (1993). The economic burden of Alzheimer's disease care. *Health Affairs, 12*(2), 164–176.

Rice, K. M. (Ed.) (1989). *Taber's Cyclopedic Medical Dictionary.* Philadelphia: F. A. Davis Co.

Rice, V. H., Beck, C., & Stevenson, J. S. (1997). Ethical issues relative to autonomy and personal control in independent and cognitively impaired elders. *Nursing Outlook, 45,* 27–34.

Rich, M. W., Beckham, V., Wittenburg, C., Leven, C., Freddland, K., & Carney, R. (1995). A multidisciplinary intervention to prevent readmission of elderly patients with congestive heart failure. *The New England Journal of Medicine, 333,* 1190–1195.

Rich, M. W., Bosner, M. S., Chung, M. K., Shen, J., & McKenzie, J. P. (1992). Is age an independent predictor of early and late mortality in patients with acute myocardial infarction? *American Journal of Medicine, 92,* 7–13.

Richards, J. S., Nepomuceno, C., Riles, M., & Suer, Z. (1982). Assessing pain behavior: The UAB pain behavior scale. *Pain, 14,* 393–398.

Richards, K. C. (1993). *The effect of a muscle relaxation, imagery, and relaxing music intervention and a back massage on the sleep and psychophysiological arousal of elderly males hospitalized in the critical care environment.* Unpublished doctoral dissertation, The University of Texas, Austin.

Richardson, V. (1993). *Retirement counseling: A handbook for gerontology practitioners.* New York: Springer Publishing Co.

Richie, M. F. (1996). Meeting the challenge of disruptive behaviors in the nursing home. *Journal of Gerontological Nursing, 22*(11), 3.

Rigdon, I. S., Clayton, B. C., & Dimond, M. (1987). Toward a theory of helpfulness for the elderly bereaved: An invitation to a new life. *Advances in Nursing Science, 9*(2), 32–43.

Ring, C., Nayak, L., & Isaacs, B. (1988). Balance function in elderly people who have and who have not fallen. *Archives of Physical and Medical Rehabilitation, 69,* 261–264.

Robb, I. H. (1907). *Nursing: Its principles and practice for hospital and private use.* Toronto: J. A. Carveth.

Robbins, I., Lloyd, C., Carpenter, S., & Bender, M. P. (1992). Staff anxieties about death in residential settings for elderly people. *Journal of Advanced Nursing 17,* 548–553.

Roberts, B. L., Anthony, M. K., Matejczyk, M., & Moore, D. (1994). The relationship of social support to functional limitations, pain and well-being among men and women. *Journal of Women and Aging, 6,* 3–19.

Robichaud, L., Hebert, R., & Desrosiers, J. (1994). Efficacy of a sensory integration program on behaviors of inpatients with dementia. *The American Journal of Occupational Therapy, 48,* 355–360.

Robinson, A. D. (1994). Attitudes toward nursing home residents among aides of threed cultural groups. *Journal of Cultural Diversity, 1,* 16–18.

Robinson, I. (1988). Managing symptoms in chronic disease: Some dimensions of patients' experience. *International Disability Studies, 10,* 112–9.

Robinson, J. H. (1995). Grief responses, coping processes, and social support of widows: Research with Roy's model. *Nursing Science Quarterly, 8,* 158–164.

Rodrigues-Fisher, L., Bourguignon, C., & Good, B. V. (1993). Dietary fiber nursing intervention: Prevention of constipation in older adults. *Clinical Nursing Research, 2,* 464–477.

Roland, C. F., & Radnich, J. J. (1996). Screening a high-risk population for abdominal aortic aneurysm. *Journal of Vascular Nursing, 14*(2), 45–47.

Roper, N., Logan, W., & Tierney, A. (1996). *The elements of nursing: A model for nursing based on a model of living* (4th ed.). Edinburgh: Churchill Livingstone.

Rosen, W. G., Mohs, R. C., & Davis, K. L. (1984). A new rating scale for alzheimer's disease. *American Journal of Psychiatry, 141*, 1356–1364.

Rosenbaum, J. (1981). Widows and widowers and their medication use: Nursing implications. *Journal of Psychiatric Nursing and Mental Health Services, 19*, 17–19.

Rosenbaum, J. N. (1991). Widowhood grief: A cultural perspective: Greek-Canadian widows. *Canadian Journal of Nursing Research, 23*, 61–76.

Rosenfeld, P., Bottrell, M., Fulmer, T., & Mezey, M. (1999). Gerontological nursing content in baccalaureate nursing programs: Findings from a national survey. *Journal of Professional Nursing, 15*, 84–94.

Rosenkoetter, M., Garris, J., & Hendricksen, S. (1997). Perceptions of retirees: Depression in retirement. *Journal of Nursing Science, 2*, 142–152.

Rosenkoetter, M., & Garris, J. (1998). Psychosocial changes following retirement. *Journal of Advanced Nursing, 27*, 966–976.

Rosenstock, I. M. (1966). Why people use health services. *Milbank Memorial Fund Quarterly, 44*, 94–121.

Ross, D. G. (1993). Subjective data related to altered bowel elimination patterns among hospitalized elder and middle-aged persons. *Orthopaedic Nursing, 12*(5), 25–32.

Ross, D. G. (1995). Altered bowel elimination patterns among hospitalized elderly and middle-aged persons: Quantitative results. *Orthopaedic Nursing, 14*(1), 25–31.

Ross, L. A. (1997). Elderly patients' perceptions of their spiritual needs and care: A pilot study. *Journal of Advanced Nursing, 26*, 710–715.

Rossi, P. H. (1989). *Down and out in America: The origins of homelessness.* Chicago, IL: University of Chicago Press.

Rosswurm, M. A. (1989). Assessment of perceptual processing deficits in persons with Alzheimer's disease. *Western Journal of Nursing Research, 11*, 458–468.

Rosswurm, M. A. (1991). Attention-focusing program for persons with dementia. *Clinical Gerontologist, 10*(2), 3–16.

Rost, K., & Frankel, R. (1993). The introduction of the older patient's problems in the medical visit. *Journal of Aging and Health, 5*, 387–401.

Rovner, B. W., German, P. S., Broadhead, J., Morriss, R. K., Brant, L. J., Blaustein, J., & Folstein, M. F. (1990). The prevalence and management of dementia and other psychiatric disorders in nursing homes. *International Psychogeriatrics, 2*, 13–24.

Rovner, B. W., Lucas-Blaustein, J., Folstein, M., & Smith, S. W. (1990). Stability over one year in patients admitted to a nursing home dementia unit. *International Journal of Geriatric Psychiatry, 5*, 77–82.

Rovner, B., Steele, C. D., Shmuely, Y., & Folstein, M. F. (1996). A randomized trial of dementia care in nursing homes. *Journal American Geriatrics Society, 44*(1), 7–13.

Rowe, J., & Kahn, R. (1998). *Successful aging.* New York: Pantheon Books.

Rowles, G. D., & Dallas, M. (1996). Individualizing care: Family roles in nursing home decision making. *Journal of Gerontological Nursing, 22*(3), 20–25.

Roy, C., & Andrews, H. A. (1991). *The Roy Adaptation Model: The definitive statement.* Norwalk, CT: Appleton & Lange.

Roy, G., Gordon, S. G., & Cohen, S. T. (1997). An innovative school-based intergenerational model to serve grandparent caregivers. *Journal of Gerontological Social Work, 28*, 47–61.

Rozanski, A., Bailey, C. N., Krantz, D. S., Friedman, J., Resser, K. J., Morell, M., Hilton-Chaifen, S., Hestrin, L., Bietendorf, J., & Berman, D. (1986). Mental stress and the induction of silent myocardial ischemia in patients with coronary artery disease. *Circulation, 75*, 395–400.

Rubel, A. J., Reinsch, S., Tobis, J. & Hurrell, J. L. (1994). Adaptive Behavior Among Very Elderly Americans. *Physical & Occupational Therapy in Geriatrics, 12*(4), 67–80.

Ruchlin, H., Morris, S., & Morris, J. (1993). Resident medical care utilization patterns in continuing care retirement communities. *Health Care Financing Review, 14*, 151–161.

Ruffing-Rahal, M. A. (1991). Rationale and Design for Health Promotion with Older Adults. *Public Health Nursing, 8*, 258–263.

Ruiz, B. A., Tabloski, P. A., & Frazier, S. M. (1995). The role of gerontological advanced practice nurses in geriatric care. *Journal of the American Geriatrics Society, 44*(5), 6–11.

Rush, K. L., & Ouellet, L. L. (1993). Mobility: A concept analysis. *Journal of Advanced Nursing, 18*, 486–492.

Rush, K. L., & Ouellet, L. L. (1998). An analysis of elderly clients' views of mobility. *Western Journal of Nursing Research, 20*, 295–311.

Russell, C. (1994). Older adult care recipients' insight into their caregivers: "Beware the stone-faced elephant!" *Geriatric Nursing, 15*, 308–312.

Russell, C. (1996). Elder care recipients' care-seeking process. *Western Journal of Nursing Research, 18*, 43–62.

Ryan, C. (1997). Long term care employees; attitudes regarding feeding the older adult: a pilot study. *Journal of Nutrition for the Elderly, 16*(4), 17–25.

Ryan, E., Hamilton, J., & See, S. (1994). Patronizing the old: How do younger and older adults respond to baby talk in the nursing home? *International Journal of Aging and Human Development, 39*, 21–32.

Ryan, M. (1993). Caregiver stress and respite care. In L. M. Tepper & J. A. Toner (Eds.), *Respite Care: Programs, Problems and Solutions* (pp. 151–156). Philadelphia: Charles Press.

Rybash, J. M., Hoyer, W. J., & Roodin, P. A. (1986). *Adult cognition and aging: Developmental changes in processing, knowing, and thinking.* New York: Pergamon Press.

Ryden, M. B. (1988). Aggressive behavior in persons with dementia who live in the community. *Alzheimer Disease and Associated Disorders: An International Journal, 2*, 342–355.

Ryden, M., Bossenmaier, M., & McLachlan, C. (1991). Aggressive behavior in cognitively impaired nursing home residents. *Research in Nursing and Health, 14*(2), 87–95.

Ryden, M., & Feldt, K. (1992). Goal directed care: Caring for aggressive nursing home residents with dementia. *Journal of Gerontological Nursing, 18*(11), 35–42.

Ryden, M. B., Feldt, K. S., Oh, H. L, Brand, K. S., Warne, M., Nelson, J., & Gross, C (1999). Relationships between restraints, psychoactive medications, secured units, and aggressive cognitively impaired nursing home residents. *Archives of Psychiatric Nursing, 13*, 170–178.

Ryden, M., Snyder, M., Gross, C., Savik, K., Pearson, V., Krichbaum, K., & Mueller, C. (1999). Value-added outcomes: The use of advanced practice nurses in long-term care facilities. *Journal of the American Geriatrics Society* (in review).

Rudman, D., Alverno, L., & Mattson, D. E. (1993) A comparison of physically aggressive behavior in two VA nursing homes. *Hospital & Community Psychiatry, 44,* 571–575.

Sabat, S. R. (1998). Voices of Alzheimer's Disease sufferers: A call for treatment based on personhood. *Journal of Clinical Ethics, 9*(1), 35–48.

Safriet, B. (1992). Health care dollars and regulatory sense: The role of the advance practice nursing. *Yale Journal on Regulation, 9,* 417–487.

Sallout, H., Mayoral, W., & Benjamin, S. B. (1999). The aging esophagus. *Clinical Geriatric Medicine, 15,* 439–456.

Samarel, N., & Fawcett, J. (1992). Enhancing adaptation to breast cancer: The addition of coaching to support groups. *Oncology Nursing Forum, 19,* 591–596.

Sarna, L. (1989). *Impact of chemotherapy on the quality of life and functional states of older adults with non-small-cell lung cancer.* Unpublished doctoral dissertation, University of California, San Francisco.

Sarno, M. T. (1986). *Understanding Aphasia: A Guide for Family and Friends* (3rd ed.). New York: New York University Medical Education Center.

Sarno, M. T. (1998). *Acquired aphasia* (3rd ed.) (pp. 595–619). San Diego, CA: Academic Press.

Schell, E. S., & Kayser-Jones, J. (1999). The effect of role-taking ability on caregiver-resident mealtime interaction. *Applied Nursing Research, 12,* 38–44.

Scherb, C. A., Rapp, C. G., Johnson, M., & Maas, M. (1998). The nursing outcomes classification: Validation by rehabilitation nurses. *Rehabitation Nursing, 23,* 174 8, 191.

Schmidt, R. M. (1993). Health Watch: Health promotion and disease prevention in primary care. *Methods of Information in Medicine, 32,* 245–248.

Schoonmaker, L. (1998). Rehabilitation and prosthetic intervention/prosthetic pathwayis in managing the dysvascular patient. *Journal of Prosthetics & Orthotics, 10*(4), 82–84.

Schulz, R., O'Brien, A. T., Bookwala, J., & Fleissner, K. (1995). Psychiatric and physical effects of dementia caregiving: Prevalence, correlates, and causes. *The Gerontologist, 35,* 771–791.

Schumacher, H., Kippel, J., & Koopman, W. (Eds.). (1993). *Primer on the rheumatic diseases* (10th ed.). Atlanta: Arthritis Foundation.

Schwartz-Barcott, D., & Kim, H. (1986). A hybrid model for concept development. In P. Chinn (Ed.), *Nursing research: Methodology issues and implementation* (pp. 91–101). Rockville, MD: Aspen.

Scott, M., & Gelhot, A. R. (1999). Gastroesophageal reflux disease: Diagnosis and management. *Am Fam Physician, 59,* 1161.

Seeman, T. E., Kaplan, G. A., Knudsen, L., Cohen, R., & Guralnik, J. (1987). Social network ties and mortality among the elderly in the Alameda County Study. *American Journal of Epidemiology, 126,* 714–723.

Seeman, T., Mendes de Leon, C., & Ostfeld, A. (1993). Risk factors for coronary heart disease among older men and women: A prospective study of community-dwelling elderly. *American Journal of Epidemiology, 38,* 1037–1049.

Segall, M., & Wykle, M. (1988-89). The black families' experience with dementia. *Journal of Applied Social Sciences, 13,* 170–1191.

Select Committee on Aging, House of Representatives, U. S. Congress (1989). Healthcare Costs for America's Elderly 1977-1988. *U. S. Government Printing Office,* Washington, DC.

Seligman, M. (1975). Helplessness: On depression, development, and death. San Francisco: W. H. Freeman.

Sengstaken, E. A., & King, S. A. (1993). The problems of pain and its detection among geriatric nursing home residents. *Journal of the American Geriatrics Society, 41,* 541–544.

Shahin, W., & Murray, J. A. (1999). Esophageal cancer and Barrett's esophagus: How to approach surveillance, treatment, and palliation. *Postgraduate Medicine, 105,* 111–114, 119–122, 125–127.

Shanas, E. (1979). Social myth as hypothesis: The case of the family relations of old people. *Gerontologist, 19,* 3–9.

Shelkey, M., Sherman, K., Edwards, R., & Lantz, M. (1996). The dementia dog: Use of the in-residence service animal to empower and enable cognitively impaired nursing home residents [Abstract]. *The Gerontologist, 36* (Special issue 1), 274.

Sherman, B., Nisenboum, J. M., Jesberger, B. L., Morrow, C. A., & Jesberger, J. A. (1999). Assessment of dysphagia with the use of pulse oximetry. *Dysphagia, 14,* 152–156.

Sherman, S. R., & Newman, E. S. (1977). Foster-family care for the elderly in New York State. *The Gerontologist, 17,* 513–522.

Sherrell, K., Anderson, R., & Buckwalter, K. (1998). Invisible residents: The chronically mentally ill elderly in nursing homes. *Archives of Psychiatric Nursing, 12*(3), 131–139.

Sherrell, K., & Buckwalter, K. C. (1997). Geropsychiatry. Barriers to follow-up studies with the chronically mentally ill elderly in long-term care settings. *Journal of Gerontological Nursing, 23*(8), 37–40.

Sherwood, G. D. (1997). Meta-synthesis of qualitative analyses of caring: Defining a therapeutic model of nursing. *Advanced Practice Nursing Quarterly, 3*(1), 32–42.

Sherwood, S., & Morris, J. N. (1983). The Pennsylvania domiciliary care experiment: I. Impact on quality of life. *American Journal of Public Health, 73,* 646–653.

Siegel, P. A., Brackbill, R. M., & Heath, G. W. (1995). The epidemiology of walking for exercise: Implications for promoting activity among sedentary groups. *American Journal of Public Health, 85,* 706–710.

Siegel, S., & Rees, B. (1992). Preparing the public employee for retirement. *Public Personnel Management, 21,* 89–100.

Sifrim, D., Janssens, J., &, Vantrappen, G. (1996). Transient lower esophageal sphincter relaxations and esophageal body muscular contractile response in normal humans. *Gastroenterology, 110,* 659–68.

Silver, G. A. (1958). Beyond general practice: The health team. *Yale Journal of Biology and Medicine, 31,* 29–39.

Simmons, S. F., & Schnelle, J. F. (1999). Strategies to measure nursing home residents' satisfactions and preference related to incontinence and mobility care: Implications for evaluating intervention effects. *The Gerontologist, 39,* 345–355.

Simon, P. M., Schwartzstein, R. M., Weiss, J. W., Fencl, V., Teghtsoonian, M., & Weinberger, S. E. (1990). Distinguishable types of dyspnea in patients with shortness of breath. *American Review of Respiratory Disease, 142,* 1009–1014.

Simons, W., & Malabar R. (1995). Assessing pain in elderly patients who cannot respond verbally. *Journal of Advanced Nursing, 22,* 663–669.

Slaninka, S. C., & Galbraith, A. M. (1998). Health endings. A collaborative health promotion project for the elderly. *Journal of Gerontological Nursing, 24*(9), 35–42.

Slevin, K., & Wingrove, C. (1995). Women in retirement: A review and critique of empirical research since 1976. *Sociological Inquiry, 65,* 1–21.

Sloane, P. D., Davidson, S., Buckwalter, K., Lindsey, B. A., Ayers, S., Lenker, V., & Burgio, L. D. (1997). Management of the patient with disruptive vocalizations. *The Gerontologist, 37,* 675–82.

Sloane, P. D., Mathew, L. J., Scarborough, M., Desai, J. R., Koch, G. G., & Tangen, C. (1991). Physical and pharmacologic restraint of nursing home patients with dementia: Impact of specialized units. *JAMA, 265,* 1278–1282.

Smart, C. R., Hendrick, R. L., Rutledge, J. H., III, & Smith, R. A. (1995). Benefit of mammography screening in women ages 40–49 years. Current evidence from randomized controlled trials. *Cancer, 75,* 1619–1626.

Smets, E. M. A., Garssen, B., Schuster-Uitterhoeve, A. L. J., & de Haes, J. C. J. M. (1993). Fatigue in cancer patients. *British Journal of Cancer, 68,* 220–224.

Smiley, D. F., Gould, A. G., & Melby, E. (1931). *The principles and practice of hygiene.* New York: Macmillan.

Smith, C. E. (1993). Quality of life in long-term total parenteral nutrition patients and their family caregiver. *Journal of Parenteral and Enteral Nutrition, 17,* 501–506.

Smith, C. E. (1994a). A model of caregiving effectiveness for technologically dependent adults residing at home. *Advances in Nursing Science, 17,* 27–40.

Smith, C. E. (1994b). *Technological home care: Costs and quality of life.* Unpublished manuscript.

Smith, C. E. (1995). Technology and home care. In J. J. Fitzpatrick & J. S. Stevenson (Eds.), *Annual review of nursing research* (Vol. 13, pp. 137–167). New York: Springer Publishing.

Smith, C. E. (1996). Quality of life and caregiving in technological home care. In J. J. Fitzpatrick & J. Norbeck (Eds.), *Annual review of nursing research* (Vol. 14, pp. 95–118). New York: Springer Publishing.

Smith, D., Zhou, X., Weinberger, M., Smith, F., & McDonald, R. (1999). Mailed reminders for area-wide influenza immunization: A randomized controlled trial. *Journal of the American Geriatrics Society, 47,* 1–5.

Smith, M. C., Ellgring, H., & Oertel, W. H. (1997). Sleep disturbances in Parkinson's disease patients and spouses. *Journal of the American Geriatrics Society, 45,* 194–199.

Smith, S., Jepson, V., & Perloff, E. (1982). Attitudes of nursing care providers toward elderly patients. *Nursing & Health Care, 3,* 93–98.

Smith, S. C., Gilpin, E., Ahnve, S., Dittrich, H., Nicod, P., Henning, H., & Ross, J. (1990). Outlook after acute myocardial infarction in the very elderly compared with that in patients aged 65 to 75 years. *Journal of American College Cardiology, 16,* 784–792.

Smithard, D. G., O'Neill, P. A., England, R. E., Park, C. L., Wyatt, R., Martin, D. F., & Morris, J. (1997). The natural history of dysphagia following a stroke. *Dysphagia, 12,* 188–193.

Snowden, J. (1990). Validity of the Geriatric Depression Scale. *Journal of the American Geriatrics Society, 38,* 722.

Snowdon, D. A., Greiner, L. H., Mortimer, J. A., Riley, K. P., Greiner, P. A., & Markesbery, W. R. (1997). Brain infarction and the clinical expression of Alzheimer's disease. The Nun Study. *JAMA, 277,* 813–817.

Snyder, L. H., Rupprecht, P., Pyrek, J., Brekhus, S., & Moss, T. (1978). Wandering. *The Gerontologist, 18*(3), 272–280.

Snyder, M. (1993). The influence of interventions on the stress-health outcome linkage. In J. S. Barnfather & B. L. Lyon (Eds.), *Stress and coping: State of the science and implications for nursing theory, research and practice* (pp. 159–170). Indianapolis, IN: Sigma Theta Tau International.

Snyder, M., Egan, E. C., & Burns, K. R. (1995). Efficacy of hand massage in decreasing agitation behaviors associated with care activities in persons with dementia. *Geriatric Nursing, 16,* 60–63.

Social HMO Consortium (1998). National Bipartisan Commission on the Future of Medicare (Testimony of Walter Leutz).

Social Security Administration (1998). Table 1. C3.-OASDI benefits: Number and average amount of retired-worker benefits in current-payment status with and without reduction for early retirement, by sex, 1993–1997. *Social Security Bulletin, 61,* 80.

Society of Gastroenterology Nurses and Associates, Inc. (1998). *Gastroenterology nursing: A core curriculum* (2nd ed.). St. Louis: Mosby.

Soehren, P. M., & Schumann, L. L. (1994). Enhanced role opportunities available to the CNS/Nurse Practitioner. *Clinical Nurse Specialist, 8*(3), 123–127.

Solomon, C. G., Lee, T. H., Cook, E. F., Weisberg, M. C., Brand, D. A., Rouan, G. W., & Goldman, L. (1989). Comparison of clinical presentation of acute myocardial infarction in patients older than 65 years of age to younger patients: The Multicenter Chest Pain Study Experience. *The American Journal of Cardiology, 63,* 772–776.

Solon, J. A., Kilpatrick, N. S., & Hill, M. F. (1988). Aging-related education: A national survey. *Journal of Gerontological Nursing, 14*(9), 21–26, 38–39.

Sox, H. C. (1979). Quality of patient care by nurse practitioners and physician assistants: A 10 year perspective. *Annals of Internal Medicine, 91,* 459–468.

Spechler, S. J. (1992). Department of Veterans Affairs gastroesophageal reflux disease study group. Comparison of medical and surgical therapy for complicated esophageal reflux disease. *New England Journal of Medicine, 326,* 786.

Spechler, S. J. (1998). Does Helicobacter pylori infection contribute to gastroesophageal reflux disease? *Yale Journal of Biolgical Medicine, 71,* 143–148.

Spellbring, A. M., & Ryan, J. W. (1997). Measuring mobility and potential for falls. In M. Frank-Stromberg & S. J. Olsen (Eds.), *Instruments for clinical health-care research* (2nd ed.) (pp. 497–508). Boston, MA: Jones and Bartlett Publishers.

Spelman, C. C., Pate, R. R., Macera, C. A., & Ward, D. S. (1993). Self-selected exercise intensity of habitual walkers. *Official Journal of the American College of Sports Medicine, 25,* 1174–1179.

Spilker, B., Simpson, R. L. Jr., & Tilson, H. H. (1991). Quality of life bibliography and indexes: 1991 update. *Journal of Clinical Research in Pharmacoepidemiology, 6,* 205–266.

Spitzer, W. O., Sackett, D. L., Sibley, J. C., Roberts, R. S., Gent, M., Kergin D. J., Hackett, B. C., & Olynich, A. (1974). The Burlington randomized trial of the nurse practitioner. *The New England Journal of Medicine, 290,* 251–256.

Stachenfeld, N. S., DiPietro, L., Nadel, E. R., & Mack G. W. (1997). Mechanism of attenuated thirst in aging: Role of central volume receptors. *American Journal of Physiology, 272,* 148–57.

Stachenfeld, N. S., Mack, G. W. Takamata, A., DiPietro, L., & Nadel, E. R. (1996). Thirst and fluid regulatory responses to hypertonicity in older adults. *American Journal of Physiology, 271,* 757–65.

Stamatiadis, N. (1996). Gender effect on the accident patterns of elderly drivers. *Journal of Applied Gerontology, 15,* 8.

Stamford, B. (1994). Making a Splash. *Physician Sportsmedicine, 22,* 105.

Stanley, M., & Beare, P. (1999). *Gerontological nursing.* Philadelphia: F. A. Davis.

Stark, A. J., Kane, R. L., Kane, R. A., & Finch, M. (1995). Effect on physical functioning of care in adult foster homes and nursing homes. *The Gerontologist, 35,* 648–655.

Statistics. *Monthly Vital Statistics Report, 41*(7), Public Health Service, Hyattsville, MD.

Steele, C. M., Greenwood, C., Ens, I., Robertson, C., & Seidman-Carlson, R. (1997). Mealtime difficulties in a home for the aged: Not just dysphagia. *Dysphagia, 12,* 43–50.

Steele, R. G., & Fitch, M. I. (1996a). Coping strategies of family caregivers of home hospice patients with cancer. *Oncology Nursing Forum, 23,* 955–960.

Steele, R. G., & Fitch, M. I. (1996b). Needs of family caregivers of patients receiving home hospice care for cancer. *Oncology Nursing Forum, 23,* 823–828.

Steeman, E., Abraham, I. L., & Godderis, J. (1997). Risk profiles for insititutionalization in a cohort of elderly people with dementia or depression. *Archives of Psychiatric Nursing, 11,* 295–303.

Stephens, T., & Capersen, C. J. (1994). The demography of physical activity. In C. Bouchard, R. J. Shephard, & T. Stephens (Eds.), *Physical Activity, Fitness and Health.* Champion, IL: Human Kinetics Publishers.

Stevenson, T. (1997). Clinical. Drug therapy in the management of Parkinson's disease. *British Journal of Nursing, 6,* 144, 146–148.

Stewart, A. L., King, A. C., & Haskell, W. L. (1993). Endurance exercise and health-related quality of life in 50–65 year old adults. *The Gerontologist, 33,* 782–789.

Stolley, J. M., & Koenig, H. G. (1997). Religion/spirituality and health among elderly African Americans and Hispanics. *Journal of Psychosocial Nursing, 35*(11), 32–38, 45–46.

Strang, V., & Neufeld, A. (1990). Adult Day Care Programs, A Source for Respite. *Journal of Gerontological Nursing, 16*(11), 16–20.

Stratton, J. R., Levy, W. C., Cerqueira, M. D., Schwartz, R. S., & Abrass, I. B. (1994). Cardiovascular responses to exercise effects of aging and exercise training in health men. *Circulation, 89,* 1648–1655.

Steinhauer, M. B. (1982). Geriatric foster care: A prototype design and implementation issues. *The Gerontologist, 22*(3), 293–300.

Stromberg, L. (1998). *Hip Fracture in the Elderly: Social, Economic, and Psychological Aspects of Rehabilitation.* Stockholm, Sweden: Karolinska Institute.

Stone, R., Cafferata, G., & Sangl, J. (1987). Caregivers of the frail elderly: A national profile. *The Gerontologist, 27,* 616–626.

Strumpf, N. E., & Evans, L. K. (1988). Physical restraint of the hospitalized elderly: Perceptions of patients and nurses. *Nursing Research, 37,* 132–137.

Strumpf, N., & Tomes, N. (1993). Restraining the troublesome patient: An historical perspective on a contemporary debate. *Nursing History Review, 1*(1), 3–24.

Strumpf, N. E., & Whitney, F. W. (1994). Teaching collaborative skills to nurse practitioner students. In E. L. Sieglar & F. W. Whitney (Eds.), *Nurse-Physician Collaboration: Care of Adults and the Elderly* (pp. 159–167). New York: Springer Publishing Co.

Sullivan, E. J. (1995). *Nursing care of clients with substance abuse.* St. Louis: Mosby.

Sullivan, J. A. (1982). Research on nurse practitioners: process behind the outcome. *American Journal of Public Health, 72,* 8–9.

Sullivan-Marx, E., & Strumpf, N. (1996). Restraint-free care for acutely ill hospitalized patients. *AACN: Advanced Practice in Acute and Critical Care, 7,* 572–578.

Summer, C. H. (1998). Recognizing and responding. *American Journal of Nursing, 98*(1), 26–31.

Surgeon General's National Workshop on Hispanic/Latino Health. (1992). *Blueprint for improving Hispanic/Latino health: Implementation strategies* [Workshop proceedings]. Washington, DC: Office of the Surgeon General.

Sutton-Tyrrell, K., Alcorn, H. G., Herzog, H., Kelsey, S. F., & Kuller, J. H. (1995). Morbidity, mortality, and antihypertensive treatment effects by extent of atherosclerosis in older adults with isolated systolic hypertension. *Stroke, 26,* 1319–1324.

Sutton-Tyrrell, K., Alcorn, H. G., Wolfson, S. K., Kelsey, S. F., & Kuller, L. H. (1993). Predictors of carotid stenosis in older adults with and without isolated systolic hypertension. *Stroke, 24,* 335–361.

Swanson, E. A., Maas, M. L., & Buckwalter, K. C. (1993). Catastrophic reactions and other behaviors of Alzheimer's residents: Special unit compared with traditional units. *Archives of Psychiatric Nursing, 7*(5), 292–299.

Swanson, K. M. (in press). What's known about caring in nursing science: A literary meta-analysis. In A. S. Hinshaw, S. Feetham, & J. Shaver (Eds.), *Handbook of clinical nursing research.*

Svennson, O., Stromberg, L., Ohlen, G., & Lindgren, U. (1996). Prediction of the outcome after hip fracture in elderly patients. *Journal of Bone and Joint Surgery 78,* 115–118.

Swanson, E. A., Maas, M. L., & Buckwalter, K. C. (1994). Alzheimer's residents' cognitive and functional measures: Special and traditional care unit comparison. *Clinical Nursing Research, 3,* 27–41.

Szarka, L. A., & Locke, G. R. (1999). Practical pointers for grappling with GERD. Heartburn gnaws at quality of life for many patients. *Postgraduate Medicine, 105*(7), 88–90, 95–98, 103–106.

Szinovacz, M., & Harpster, P. (1994). Couples' employment/retirement status and the division of household tasks. *Journal of Gerontology: Social Sciences, 49,* S125–136.

Szinovacz, M., & Washo, C. (1992). Gender differences in exposure to life events and adaptation to retirement. *Journal of Gerontology: Social Sciences, 47,* S191–196.

Tabloski, P., Cooke, C., & Thoman, E. (1998). A procedure for withdrawal of sleep medication in elderly women who have been long-term users. *Journal of Gerontological Nursing, 24*(9), 20–28.

Tabloski, P. A., McKinnon-Howe, l., & Remington, R. (1995). Effects of calming music on the level of agitation in cognitively impaired nursing home residents. *Alternative Medicine Journal, March/April,* 27–32.

Taft, L. B., & Cronin-Stubbs, D. (1995). Behavioral symptoms in dementia: An update. *Research in Nursing and Health, 18,* 143–163.

Talley, N. J., Phillips, S. F., Melton, J., Wiltgen, C., & Zinsmeister, A. R. (1989). A patient questionnaire to identify bowel disease. *Annals of Internal Medicine, 111,* 671–674.

Talmadge, H., & Murphy, D. F. (1983). Innovative home care program offers appropriate alternative for elderly. *Hospital Progress, 64,* 50–51, 72.

Tappen, R. M. (1994). The effect of skill training on functional abilities of nursing home residents with dementia. *Research in Nursing & Health, 17,* 159–165.

Tappen, R., & Barry, C. (1995). Assessment of affect in advanced Alzheimer's disease: The Dementia Mood Picture Test. *Journal of Gerontological Nursing, 21*(3), 44–46.

Tariot, P. N., Mack, J. L., Patterson, M. B., Edland, S. D., Weiner, M. F., Fillenbaum, G., Blazina, L., Teri, L., Rubin, E., & Mortimer, J. A. et al. (1995). The Behavior Rating Scale for Dementia of the Consortium to Establish a Registry for Alzheimer's Disease. The Behavioral Pathology Committee of the Consortium to Establish a Registry for Alzheimer's Disease. *American Journal of Psychiatry, 152,* 1349–1357.

Tatara, T. (1993). Understanding the nature and scope of domestic elder abuse with the use of state aggregate data: Summaries of the key findings of a national survey of state APS and aging agencies. *Journal of Elder Abuse and Neglect, 5*(4), 35–57.

Taylor, C. B., Houston Miller, N., Killen, J. D., & DeBusk, R. F. (1990). Smoking cessation after acute myocardial infarction: Effects of a nurse-managed intervention. *Annals of Internal Medicine, 113,* 118–123.

Taylor, K., & Harned, T. L. (1978). Attitudes toward old people: A study of nurses who care for the elderly. *Journal of Gerontological Nursing, 4,* 43–47.

Taylor-Price, C. (1995). *The efficacy of structured reminiscence group psychotherapy as an intervention to decrease depression and increase psychological well-being in female nursing home residents.* Unpublished doctoral dissertation, Mississippi State University.

Tells, G. S., Polack, J. F., Ward, B. J., Kittner, S. J., Savage, P. J., & Robbins, J. (1994). Relation of smoking with carotid artery wall thickness and stenosis in older adults. The Cardiovascular Health Study (CHS) Collaborative Research Group. *Circulation, 90*(6), 29058.

Teresi, J., Holmes, D., Benenson, E., Monaco, C., Barrett, V., Ramirez. M., & Koren, M. J. (1993). A primary care nursing model in long-term care facilities: Evaluation of impact on affect, behavior and socialization. *Gerontologist, 33,* 667–674.

Teresi, J., Holmes, D., & Cohen, C. I. (1988). The physical well-being of old homeless men. *Journal of Gerontology, 43,* 121–128.

Teresi, J., Lawton, M. P., Holmes, D., & Ory, M. (1997). *Measurement in elderly chronic care populations.* New York: Springer Publishing Company.

Tesio, L., Alpini, D., Cesarani, A., & Perucca, L. (1999). Short form of the Dizziness Handicap Inventory: Construction and validation through Rasch analysis. *American Journal of Physical Medicine and Rehabilitation, 78,* 233–241.

Thomas, C. L. (Ed.). (1989). *Taber's Cyclopedic Medical Dictionary* (16th ed.). Philadelphia: F. A. Davis.

Thomas, C. L. (Ed.). (1997). *Taber's cyclopedic medical dictionary* (18th ed., p. 363). Philadelphia: F. A. Davis.

Thomas, D. W. (1995). Wandering: A proposed definition. *Journal of Gerontological Nursing, 21*(9), 35–41.

Thomas, D. W. (1997). Understanding the wandering patient: A continuity of personality perspective. *Journal of Gerontological Nursing, 23*(1), 16–24.

Thomas, D., Gao, D., Self, S., Allison, C., Toa, Y., Mahloch, J., Ray, R., Qin, Q., Presley, R., & Porter, P. (1997). Randomized trial of breast self examination in Shanghai: Methodology and preliminary results. *Journal of the National Cancer Institute, 89,* 355–365.

Thomas, D. W., Heitman, R. J., & Alexander, T. (1997). The effects of music on bathing cooperation for residents with dementia. *Journal of Music Therapy, 34,* 246–259.

Thomas, L. (1994). A comparison of the verbal interactions of qualified nurses and nursing auxiliaries in primary, team, and functional nursing wards. *International Journal of Nursing Studies, 31,* 231–244.

Thompson, C. L. (1990). Examination of walking distance by patients with chronic obstructive pulmonary disease. *American Review of Respiratory Disease, 141,* A326.

Thompson, C. L. (1997). Dyspnea, airway resistance, positive end expiratory pressure, heart rate, blood pressure, and mucus weight with tracheal suction in ICU patients. *Critical Care Medicine, 25*(Suppl.), A77.

Thompson, I. (1994). Woldenberg Village: An illustration of supportive design for older adults. *Experimental Aging Research, 20,* 239–244.

Thompson, L. (1996). Failure to wean: Exploring the influence of age-related pulmonary changes. *Critical Care Nursing Clinics of North America, 8,* 7–16.

Thomson, M., & Burke, K. (1998). A nursing assistant training program in a long term care setting. *Gerontology & Geriatrics Education, 19,* 23–35.

Thorne, S. E., & Robinson, C. A. (1988). Health care relationships: The chronic illness perspective. *Research in Nursing and Health, 11,* 293–300.

Thorpy, M. J. (1994). Classification of Sleep Disorders. In S. Chokroverty (Ed.), *Sleep Disorders Medicine: Basic Science, Technical Considerations & Clinical Aspects.* Boston: Butterworth-Heinemann.

Tinetti, M. E. (1986). Performance-oriented assessment of mobility problems in elderly patients. *Journal of American Geriatrics Society, 34,* 119–126.

Tinetti, M. E., Baker, D. I., McAvay, G., Claus, E. B., Garrett, P., Gottschalk, M., Koch, M. L., Trainor, K., & Horwitz, R. I. (1994). A multifactorial intervention to reduce the risk of falling among elderly people living in the community. *New England Journal of Medicine, 331*, 821–827.

Tinetti, M. E., & Ginter, S. F. (1988). Identifying mobility dysfunctions in elderly patients. *Journal of the American Medical Association, 259*, 1190–1193.

Tinker, G. M. (1981). Clinical presentation of myocardial infarction in the elderly. *Age and Ageing, 10*, 237–240.

Titler, M., & Mentes, J. (1999). Research utilization in gerontological nursing practice. *Journal of Gerontological Nursing, 25*, 6–9.

Toner, J. (1993). Concepts of respite care: A gerontologist's perspective. In L. Tepper & J. Toner (Eds.), *Respite care: Programs, problems and solutions* (pp. 123–131). Philadelphia: The Charles Press.

Torrance, G. W. (1987). Utility approach to measuring health-related quality of life. *Journal of Chronic Diseases, 40*, 593–603.

Travis, J. W., & Ryan, R. S. (1988). *The Wellness Workbook, 2nd ed.* Ten speed Press, Berkeley, CA.

Tresch, D. C. (1987). Atypical presentation of cardiovascular disorders in the elderly. *Geriatrics, 42*(10), 31.

Tripp-Reimer, T. (1994). *Gerontologic Nursing Interventions Research Center overview* (P30-NR03979). Iowa City: University of Iowa College of Nursing.

Tsukuda, R. A. (1990). Interdisciplinary collaboration: Teamwork in geriatrics. In C. K. Cassse, D. E. Riesenber, L. B. Sorenson, & J. R. Walsh (Eds.), *Geriatric Medicine* (pp. 668–675). New York: Springer.

Tsukuda, R. A. (1998). A perspective on health care teams and team training. In Siegler, E. L., Hyer, K., Fulmer, T., & Mezey, M. (Eds.), *Geriatric interdisciplinary team training* (pp 3–12). New York: Springer Publishing Co.

Tucker, J. S., Friedman, H. S., Tsai, C. M., & Martin, L. R. (1995). Playing with pets and longevity among older people. *Psychology and Aging, 10*, 3–7.

Tuckman, J., & Lorge, I. (1976). Attitudes toward old people. *Journal of Social Psychology, 37*, 249–260.

Turi, Z. G., Stone, P. H., Muller, J. E., Parker, C., Rude, R. E., Raabe, D. E., Jaffe, A. S., Hartwell, T. D., Robertson, T. L., & Braumwald, E. (1986). Implications for acute intervention related to time of hosptial arrival in acute myocardial infarction. *The American Journal of Cardiology, 58*, 203–208.

UCSF Symptom Management Faculty Group. (1992). *Symptom management proceedings: Symposium I and II.* San Francisco: UCSF School of Nursing.

Ugarriza, D. N., & Fallon, T. (1994). Nurses' attitudes toward homeless women: A barrier to change. *Nursing Outlook, 42*, 26–29.

United States Health Care Financing Administration. (1997a). [On-line]. Available: http://www.hcfa.gov/facts/F960100.htm

United States Health Care Financing Administration. (1997b). [On-line]. Available: http://www.hcfa.gov/medicaid/mover.htm

United States Health Care Financing Administration. (1997c). [On-line]. Available: http://www.hcfa.gov/medicaid/mservice.htm

United States Health Care Financing Administration. (1997d). [On-line]. Available: http://www.hcfa.gov/scripts/gotourl.exe#whatis

Uretsky, B. F., Farquhar, D. S., Berezin, A. F., & Hood, W. B. (1977). Symptomatic myocardial infarction without chest pain: Prevalence and clinical course. *The American Journal of Cardiology, 40,* 498–503.

U.S. Bureau of the Census. (1992). *1990 census of population: Vol. 1. Characteristics of the population.* Washington, DC: U.S. Government Printing Office.

U.S. Bureau of the Census. (1993a). Hispanic Americans today. *Current population reports* (P23-183). Washington, DC: U.S. Government Printing Office.

U.S. Bureau of the Census. (1993b). Poverty in the United States: 1992. *Current population reports* (P60-185). Washington, DC: U.S. Government Printing Office.

U.S. Bureau of the Census. (1999, May). *Current population reports: Coresident grandparents and grandchildren* [Series P–23, No 198]. Washington, DC: Author.

U.S. Bureau of the Census. (1997). *Marital status and living arrangements: March 1997 (update).* Current Population Reports, Series PPL–90 [On-line]. Available: http://www.aoa.gov/aoa/stats/profile

U.S. Department of Health and Human Services. (1990). *Healthy people 2000: Full report with commentary.* Boston: Jones & Bartlett.

U.S. Department of Health and Human Services, Public Health Service. (1990). *Healthy people 2000: National health promotion and disease prevention objectives.* Washington, DC: Author.

U.S. Department of Health and Human Services, National Center for Health Statistics. (1981). Characteristics of Nursing Home Residents, Health Status, and Care Received: National Nursing Home Survey, United States, May-December 1977. *Vital Health Statistics,* Series 13, No. 51, DHHS Pub. No. (PHS)81–1712.

U.S. Department of Health & Human Services. (1990). *Healthy people 2000: National health promotion and disease prevention objectives* (AHCPR Publication No. 90–50212).

U.S. Department of Health and Human Services. (1994). *Congestive heart failure: Evaluation and care of patients with left ventricular systolic dysfunction* (AHCPR Publication No. 94-0612). Rockville, MD: Author.

U.S. Department of Health and Human Services. (1995). *Cardiac Rehabilitation* (AHCPR Publication No. 96-0672). Rockville, MD: Author.

U.S. Preventive Services Task Force (1996). *Guide to clinical preventive services, 2nd ed.* Baltimore: Williams & Wilkins.

US TOO International, Inc. (1999). Louis Harris Survey: Perspectives on Prostate Cancer Treatments: Awareness, Attitudes and Relationships—A Study of Patients and Urologists. http://www.ustoo.com/louis.html.

Vacarro, F. J. (1988). Application of operant procedures in a group of institutionalized aggressive geriatric patients. *Psychology of Aging, 3,* 22–28.

Vachon, M. L. S. (1976). Grief and bereavement following the death of a spouse. *Canadian Psychiatric Association Journal, 21,* 35–43.

Vachon, M. L. S. (1987). *Occupational stress in the care of the critically ill, the dying and the bereaved.* Washington, DC: Hemisphere.

Vachon, M. L. S., Freedman, K., Forno, A., Rogers, J. Lyall, W. A. L., & Freeman, S. J. J. (1977). The final illness in cancer: The widow's perspective. *Canadian Medical Association Journal, 117,* 1151–1154.

Vachon, M. L. S., Lyall, W. A. L., & Freeman, S. J. J. (1978). Measurement and management of stress in health professionals working with advanced cancer patients. *Death Education, 1,* 365–375.

Vachon, M. L. S., Lyall, W. A. L., Rogers, J., Freedman-Letofsky, K., & Freeman, S. J. J. (1980). A controlled study of self-help intervention for widows. *The American Journal of Psychiatry, 137,* 1380–1384.

Vachon, M. L. S., Rogers, J., Lyall, W. A., Lancee, W. J., Sheldon, A. R., & Freeman, S. J. J. (1982). Predictors and correlates of adaption to conjugal bereavement. *The American Journal of Psychiatry, 139,* 998–1002.

Vachon, M. L. S., Sheldon, A. R., Lancee, W. J., Lyall, W. A., Rogers, J., & Freeman, S. J. J. (1982). Correlates of enduring distress patients following bereavement: Social network, life situation, and personality. *Psychological Medicine, 12,* 783–788.

Valanis, B., & Shortridge, L. (1987). Self-protective practices of nurses handling antineoplastic drugs. *Oncology Nursing Forum, 14*(3), 23–27.

Valanis, B. G., & Yeaworth, R. (1982). Ratings of physical and mental health in the older bereaved. *Research in Nursing and Health, 5,* 137–146.

Valanis, B., Yeaworth, R. C., & Mullis, M. R. (1987). Alcohol use among bereaves and nonbereaved older persons. *Journal of Gerontological Nursing, 13*(5), 26–32.

Valente, S. M. (1994). Messages of psychiatric patients who attempted or committed suicide. *Clinical Nursing Research, 3,* 316–333.

Vance, D. (1994). Barriers to use of services by older homeless people. *Psychological Reports, 75,* 1377–1378.

van Reekum, R., Simard, M., & Farcnik, K. (1999). Diagnosis of dementia and treatment of Alzheimer's disease: Pharmacologic management of disease progression and cognitive impairment. *Can Fam Physician, 45,* 945–952.

Van Rijswik, L. (1998). Assessing the risk of foot ulcers. *Home Healthcare Nurse, 16*(1), 25–33.

van Tilburg, T. (1992). Support networks before and after retirement. *Journal of Social and Personal Relationships, 9,* 433–445.

Venner, G., & Solitro-Seelbinder, J. (1996). Team management of congestive heart failure across the continuum. *Journal of Cardiovascular Nursing, 10*(2), 71–84.

Venters, H. D., Jr., Bonilla, L. E., Jensen, T., Garner, H. P., Bordayo, E. Z., Najarian, M. M., Ala, T. A., Mason, R. P., & Frey, W. H., 2nd. (1997). Heme from Alzheimer's brain inhibits muscarinic receptor binding via thiyl radical generation. *Brain Research, 764*(1–2), 93–100.

Verbrugge, L. M., & Jette, A. M. (1994). The disablement process. *Social Science Medicine, 38,* 1–14.

Verhaegen, P., Marcoen, A., & Goosens, L. (1992). Improving memory performance in the aged through mnemonic training: A meta-analytic study. *Psychology and Aging, 7,* 242–251.

Vinick, B., & Ekerdt, D. (1989). Retirement and the family. *Generations,* Spring, 1989.

Vinson, J., Rich, M., Sperry, J., Shah, A., & McNamara, T. (1990). Early readmission of elderly patients with congestive heart failure. *Journal of the American Geriatric Society, 38,* 1290–1295.

Vogelzang, J. L. (1999). Elusive Hunger. *Home Healthcare Nurse, 17,* 261–262.

Vogt, M. T., Cauley, J. A., Newman, Kuller, L. H., & Hulley, S. B. (1993). Prevalence and correlates of lower extremity arterial disease in elderly women. *American Journal of Epidemiology, 137*(5), S59–68.

Vogt, M. T., Wolfson, S. K., & Kuller, L. H. (1992). Lower extremity arterial disease and the aging process: A review. *Journal of Clinical Epidemiology, 45,* 529–542.

Volicer, L. (1997). Goals of care in advanced dementia: Comfort dignity, and psychological well-being. *American Journal of Alzheimer's Disease, 12,* 196–197.

Volicer, L., & Bloom-Charette, L. (1999). Assessment of quality of life in advanced dementia. In L. Volicer & L. Bloom-Charette (Eds.), *Enhancing the quality of life in advanced dementia* (pp. 3–20). Philadelphia, PA: Burnner/Mazel.

Volicer, L., Hurley, A. C., & Camberg, L. (1999). A model of psychological well-being in advanced dementia. *Journal of Mental Health and Aging, 5*(1), 83–94.

Volicer, L., Hurley, A. C., Lathi, D. C., & Kowall, N. W. (1994). Measurement of severity in advanced Alzheimer's disease. *Journal of Gerontology, 49,* M223–M226.

von Eschenbach, A., Ho, R., Murphy, G., Cunningham, M., & Lins, N. (1997). American Cancer Society Guideline for the Early Detection of Prostate Cancer: Update 1997. *CA: A Cancer Journal for Clinicians, 47*(5), 261–264.

Vullo-Navich, K., Smith, S., Andrews, M., Levine, A. M., Tischler, J. F., & Veglia, J. M. (1998). Comfort and incidence of abnormal serum sodium, BUN, creatinine, and osmolality in dehydration of terminal illness. *American Journal of Hospice Palliative Care, 15*(2), 77–84.

Wadd, L. (1983). Vietnamese postpartum practices: Implications for nursing in the hospital setting. *Journal of Gynecology Nursing, 12,* 252–258.

Wagner, J. S. (1996). Wandering and fall prevention: New solutions to a perennial problem. *Nursing 96, 26*(8), 24s–24t.

Walcott-McQuigg, J. A. (1995). The relationship between stress and weight-control behavior in African-American women. *Journal of the National Medical Association, 87,* 427–432.

Wald, A. (1997). Fecal incontinence: Three steps to successful management. *Geriatrics, 52*(7), 44–46, 49–52.

Wald, F. (1994). Finding a way to give hospice care. A nurse's diary. In I. B. Corless, B. B. Germino, & M. Pittman (Eds.), *Dying, death and bereavement: Theoretical perspectives and other ways of knowing* (pp. 31–47). Boston: Jones & Bartlett.

Walheim, G., Barrios, C., Stark, A., Bostrom, L., & Olsson, E. (1990). Post-operative improvement of walking capacity in patients with trochanteric hip fractures: A prospective analysis 3 and 6 months after surgery. *Journal of Orthopaedic Trauma, 4,* 137–143.

Walker, A. J., Pratt, C. C., & Eddy, L. (1995). Informal caregiving to aging family members: A critical review. *Family Relations, 44,* 402–411.

Walker, K. N., MacBride, A., & Vachon, M. L. S. (1977). Social support networks and the crisis of bereavement. *Social Science and Medicine, 11,* 35–41.

Walker, L., & Avant, K. (1983). *Strategies for theory construction in nursing.* Norwalk: Appleton-Century-Crofts.

Walker, S. N. (1989). Research agenda: Building s consensus on research questions. *American Journal of Health Promotion, 3,* 47–53.

Walker, S. N., Sechrist, K. R., & Pender, N. (1987). The Health Promoting Lifestyle Profile: Development and psychometric characteristics. *Nursing Research, 36,* 76–81.

Walker, T., Porter, M., Gruman, C., & Michalski, M. (1999). Developing individualized care in nursing homes: integrating the views of nurses and certified nurse aides. *Journal of Gerontological Nursing, 25*(3), 30–35.

Wallhagen, M. I., & Brod, M. (1997). Perceived control and well-being in Parkinson's disease. *Western Journal of Nursing Research, 19,* 11–31.

Wallsten, S. M. (1992). Geriatric mental health: A portrait of homelessness. *Journal of Psychosocial Nursing and Mental Health Services, 30*(9), 20–4, 38–9.

Wan, T. T. H., & Arling, G. (1983). Differential use of health services among disabled elderly. *Research on Aging, 5,* 411–431.

Ward, S. E., Berry, P. E., & Misiewicz, H. (1996). Concerns about analgesics among patients and family caregiver in a hospice setting. *Research in Nursing & Health, 19,* 205–211.

Ward, S. E., & Gordon, D. (1994). Application of the American Pain Society quality assurance standards. *Pain, 56,* 299–306.

Warner, S. L. (1987). A comparative study of widows' and widowers' perceived social support during the first year of bereavement. *Archives of Psychiatric Nursing, 1,* 241–250.

Warren, J. L., Bacon, W. E., Harris, T., McBean, A. M., Foley, D. J., & Phillips, C. (1994). The burden and outcomes associated with dehydration among US elderly, 1991. *American Journal of Public Health, 84,* 1265–1269.

Watson, J. (1988). *Nursing: Human science and human care: A theory of nursing.* New York: National League for Nursing.

Watson, J. (1995). Nursing's caring-healing paradigm as exemplar for alternative medicine? *Alternative Therapies in Health and Medicine, 1*(3), 64–69.

Watts, A. (1987). Stress in retirement and its management. *Stress Medicine, 3,* 205–210.

Watters, C. L. (1995). *An ethnographic study of reminiscence patterns in older adult females.* Unpublished doctoral dissertation. North Carolina State University.

Webb, W. B. (1987). Disorders of Aging Sleep. In W. Emser, D. Kurtz, & W. B. Webb (Eds.), *Interdisciplinary topics in gerontology: Sleep, aging, & related disorders* (pp. 1–12). New York: Karger.

Webb, D. J., Fayad, P. B., Wilbur, C., Thomas, A., & Brass, L. M. (1995). Effects of a specialized team on stroke care: The first two years of the Yale Stroke Program. *Stroke, 26,* 1353–1357.

Weber, N., & Schneider, P. (1993). Respite care for the visually impaired and their families. In L. Tepper & J. Tones (Eds.), *Respite care: Programs, problems and solutions* (pp. 62–77). Philadelphia: The Charles Press.

Wegman, J. A. (1987). Hospice home death, hospital death, and coping abilities of widows. *Cancer Nursing, 10,* 148–155.

Weinberg, N. (1995). Does apologizing help? The role of self-blame and making amends in recovery from bereavement. *Health and Social Work, 20,* 292–299.

Weinberger, M., Gold, D. T., Divine, G. W., Cowper, P. A., Hodgson, L. G., Schreiner, P. J., & George, L. K. (1993). Expenditures in caring for patients with dementia who live at home. *American Journal of Public Health, 83,* 338–341.

Weinberg, A. D., & Minaker, K. L. (1995) Dehydration: Evaluation and management in older adults. *JAMA, 274,* 1552–1556.

Weinberg, A. D., Pals, J. K., Levesque, P. G., Beal, L. F., Cunningham, T. J., & Minaker, K. L. (1994). Dehydration and death during febrile episodes in the nursing home. *Journal of the American Geriatric Society, 42,* 968–971.

Weinberg, A. D., Pals, J. K., McGlinchey-Berroth, R., & Minaker, K. L. (1994). Indices of dehydration among frail nursing home patients: Highly variable but stable over time. *Journal of the American Geriatric Society, 42,* 1070–1073.

Weiner, D. K., Ladd, K. E., Pieper, C. F., & Keefe, F. J. (1995). Pain in the nursing home: Resident versus staff perceptions. *Journal of the American Geriatrics Society, 43,* SA2.

Weiner, D. K., Peterson, B., & Keefe, E. J. (1999). Chronic pain-associated behaviors in the nursing home: Resident versus caregiver perceptions. *Pain, 80,* 577–588.

Weinrich, S. P., & Boyd, M. (1992). Education in the Elderly. *Journal of Geronotological Nursing, 18*(1), 15–20.

Weisensee, M. G., Kjervik, D. K., & Anderson, J. B. (1994). Impairment of short-term memory as a criterion for determination of incompetency. *Geriatric Nursing: American Journal of Care for the Aging, 15*(1), 35–40.

Weiss, S., & Davis, H. P. (1985). Validity and reliability of the collaborative practice scales. *Nursing Research, 34,* 299–305.

Wells, Y., & Jorm, A. (1987). Evaluation of a special nursing home unit for dementia sufferers: A randomized controlled comparison with community care. *Australian and New Zealand Journal of Psychiatry, 21,* 524–531.

Wetle, T., Walker, L., & Blechner, B. (1994). Developing model policies for implementing the Patient Self Determination Act in nursing homes [Special issue]. *Gerontologist, 14*(Suppl.), 251.

Whall, A. L., Black, M. E., Groh, C. J., Yandou, D. J., Kupferschmid, B. J., & Foster, N. L. (1997). The effect of natural environments upon agitation and aggression in late stage dementia patients. *American Journal of Alzheimer's Disease, 12,* 216–220.

Whetten-Goldstein, K., Sloan, F., Kulas, E., Cutson, T., & Schenkman, M. (1997). The burden of Parkinson's disease on society, family, and the individual. *Journal of the American Geriatrics Society, 45,* 844–849.

Whipple, B. (1982). *The G spot and other recent discoveries about human sexuality.* New York: Holt, Rinehart and Winston.

Wilhite, M. J., & Johnson, D. M. (1976). Changes in nursing student's stereotypic attitudes toward old people. *Nursing Research, 25,* 430–432.

Wilkinson, C. L. (1999). An evaluation of an educational program on the management of assaultive behaviors. *Journal of Gerontological Nursing, 25*(4), 6–11.

Williams, B. R., Nichol, M. B., Lowe, B., Yoon, P. S., McCombs, J. S., & Margolies, J. (1999). Medication use in residential care facilities for the elderly. *Annals of Pharmacotherapy, 33,* 149–155.

Williams, D. P., Wood, E. C., & Moorleghen, F. (1994). An in-service workshop for nursing personnel on the management of catastrophic reactions in dementia victims. *Clinical Gerontologist, 14,* 47–54.

Williams, J. S., & Engle, V. F. (1995). Staff evaluation of nursing home residents' competence. *Applied Nursing Research, 8,* 18–22.

Williams, R. B., Barefoot, J. C., Califf, R. M., Haney, T. L., Saunders, W. B., Pryor, D. B., Hlatky, M. A., Siegler, I. C., & Mark, D. B. (1992). Prognostic importance of social and economic resources among medically treated patients withe angiographically documented coronary artery disease. *Journal of the American Medical Association, 267,* 520–524.

Williams, T. F. (1988). Research and care: Essential partners in aging. *Gerontologist, 28,* 579–585.

Willis, D. A. (1997). Animal therapy. *Rehabilitation Nursing, 22*(2), 78–81.

Wilson, H., Hutchinson, S., & Holzemer, W. (1997). Salvaging quality of life in ethnically diverse patients with advanced HIV/AIDS. *Qualitative Health Research, 7,* 75–97.

Wilson, S. A. (1992). The family as caregivers: Hospice home care. *Family and Community Health, 15*(2), 71–80.

Wilson, S. A., & Daley, B. J. (1998). Attachment/Detachment: Forces influencing care of the dying in long term care. *Journal of Palliative Medicine, 1*(1), 21–34.

Wing, D. M., & Thompson, T. (1995). Causes of alcoholism: A qualitative study of traditional Muscogee (Creek) Indians. *Public Health Nursing, 12,* 417–423.

Wing, R., & Jeffery, R. (1995). Effect of modes of weight loss on changes in cardiovascular risk factors: Are there differences between men and women or between weight loss and maintenance? *International Journal of Obesity, 19,* 67–73.

Wing, R. R., Matthews, K. A., Kuller, L. H., Meilahn, E. N., & Plantinga, P. (1991). Waist to hip ratio in middle-aged women: Associations with behavioral and psychosocial factors and with changes in cardiovascular risk factors. *Arteriosclerosis and Thrombosis, 11,* 1250–1257.

Winningham, M., MacVicar, M., Bondoc, M., Anderson, J., & Minton, J. (1989). Effect of aerobic exercise on body weight and composition in patients with breast cancer on adjuvant chemotherapy. *Oncology Nursing Forum, 16,* 683–689.

Winningham, M. L., Nail, L. M., Burke, M. B., Brophy, L., Cimprich, B., Jones, L. S., Pickard-Holley, S., Rhodes, V., St. Pierre, B., Beck, S., Glass, E. C., Mock, V. L., Mooney, K. H., & Piper, B. (1994). Fatigue and the cancer experience: The state of the knowledge. *Oncology Nursing Forum, 21,* 23–36.

Wolfe, S. C., & Schirm, V. (1992). Medication counseling for the elderly: Effects on knowledge and compliance after hospital discharge. *Geriatric Nursing, 30,* 34–138.

Wolinsky, F. D., Stump, T. E., & Clark, D. O. (1995). Antecedents and consequences of physical activity and exercise among older adults. *Gerontologist, 35,* 451–462.

Wong, N. D., Cupples, L. A., Ostfeld, A. M., Levy, D., & Kannel, W. B. (1989). Risk factors for long-term coronary prognosis after initial myocardial infarction: The Framingham Study. *American Journal of Epidemiology, 130,* 469–480.

Woods, N. F. (1979). *Human sexuality in health and illness.* St. Louis: Mosby.

Woods, P., & Ashley, J. (1995). Simulated presence therapy: Using selected memories to manage problem behaviors in Alzheimer's Disease. *Geriatric Nursing, 16*(1), 9–14.

Woolf, S. (1994). Public health perspective: The health policy implications of screening for prostate cancer. *Journal of Urology, 152,* 1685–1688.

Wood, P., & Vogen, B. (1998). Feeding the anorectic client: Comfort foods and happy hour. *Geriatric Nursing, 19,* 192–194.

Woods, D. L., Craven, R., & Whitney, J. (1993). Effects of therapeutic touch on disruptive behaviors of individuals with dementia of the Alzheimer type [Abstract]. *The Gerontologist, 33* (Special Issue 1), 81.

Woods, P., & Ashley, J. (1995). Simulated presence therapy: Using selected memories to manage problem behaviors in Alzheimer's disease patients. *Geriatric Nursing, 16,* 9–14.

Work Group on Research and Evaluation of SCUs (WRESCU). (1996, November). *Alzheimer's disease special care units: Findings from the National Institute on Aging SCU WRESCU Investigators.* Paper presented at the 49th Annual Meeting of the Gerontological Society of America, Washington, DC.

World Health Organization (1959). *Concepts and cases in nursing ethics.* Broadview Press Ltd., Chicago, ILL.

World Health Organization. (1980). *International classification of impairment, disabilities and handicaps.* Geneva: Author.

World Health Organization, Health and Welfare Canada and Canadian Public Health Association, Ottawa Charter for Health Promotion. (1992). Presented at *International Conference on Health Promotion,* November.

Wright, L. K., Bennet, G., & Gramling, L. (1998). Telecommunication interventions for caregivers of elders with dementia. *Advances in Nursing Science, 20,* 76–88.

Wurzbach, M. E. (1996). Long-term care nurses' ethical convictions about tube feeding. *Western Journal of Nursing Research, 18,* 63–76.

Wykle, M. L., & Morris, D. L. (1994, May). Nursing care in Alzheimer's Disease. *Clinics in Geriatric Medicine,* Vol. 10, Number 2, pp. 351–365.

Yardley, L. (1998). Fear of imbalance and falling. *Reviews in Clinical Gerontology, 8,* 23–29.

Yardley, L., Beech, S., Zander, L., Evans, T., & Weinman, J. (1998). A randomized controlled trial of exercise therapy for dizziness and vertigo in primary care. *British Journal of General Practice, 48,* 1136–1140.

Yardley, L., & Beech, S. (1999). Nurse-delivered exercise therapy for dizziness. *Nursing Times, 95,* 51–51.

Yardley, L., Masson, E., Verschuur, C., Haacke, N., & Luxon, L. (1992). Symptoms, anxiety and handicap in dizzy patients: Development of the vertigo symptom scale. *Journal of Psychosomatic Research, 36,* 731–741.

Yarnold, B. (1999). Hip fracture: Caring for a fragile population. *American Journal of Nursing, 99,*(2), 36–41.

Yeaworth, R. C., & Valanis, B. (1985). Health status and resources of recently bereaved older persons. *Public Health Nursing, 2,* 232–244.

Yee, D. L., Capitman, J. A., Leutz, W. N., & Sceigaj, M. (1999). Resident-centered care in assisted living. *Journal of Aging and Social Policy, 10*(3), 7–26.

Yen, P. K. (1998). Don't forget the water! *Geriatric Nursing, 19,* 295–296.

Yesavage, J., Brink, T., Rose, T., Lum, O., Huang, V., Adey, M., & Leirer, V. (1983). Development and validation of a geriatric depression screening scale: A preliminary report. *Journal of Psychiatric Research, 17,* 37–49.

Young, C. (1993). Spirituality and the chronically ill Christian elderly. *Geriatric Nursing, 14,* 298–303.

Youssef, F. A. (1990). The impact of group reminiscence counseling on a depressed elderly population. *Nurse Practitioner, 15,* 32–38.

Yudofsky, S. C., Silver, J. M, & Hales, R. E. (1995). Treatment of agitation and aggression. In A. F. Shatzberg & C. B. Nemeroff (Eds.), *Textbook of psychopharmacology* (pp. 881–900). Washington, DC: American Psychiatric Press.

Yurchuck, R. E., & Brower, H. T. (1994). Faculty preparation for gerontological nursing. *Journal of Gerontological Nursing, 20*(1), 17–24.

Zalon, M. (1997). Pain in frail, elderly women after surgery. *Image: Journal of Nursing Scholarship, 29,* 21–26.

Zalon, M. L. (1993). Nurses' assessment of post-operative patients' pain. *Pain, 54,* 329–334.

Zanetti, O., Binetti, G., Magni, E., Rossini, L., Bianchetti, A., & Trabucchi, M. (1997). Procedural memory stimulation in Alzheimer's disease: Impact of a training programme. *Acta Neurologica Scandinavica, 95,* 152–157.

Zarit, S. H., Stephens, M. A. P., Townsend, A., & Greene, R. (1998). Stress reduction for family caregivers: Effects of adult day care use. *Journals of Gerontology Series B—Psychological Sciences & Social Sciences, 53B,* S267–277.

Zeltsman, D., & Kerstein, M. D. (1998). Sociology of care in patients with severe peripheral vascular disease. *American Surgeon, 2,* 175–177.

Zembrzuski, C. D. (1997). A three-dimensional approach to hydration of elders: Administration, clinical staff, and in-service education. *Geriatric Nursing, 18,* 20–26.

Zimmerman, D. R., Karon, S. L., Arling, G., Clark, B. R., Collins, T., Ross, R., & Sainfort, F. (1995). Development and testing of nursing home quality indicators. *Health Care Financing Review, 16,* 107–127.

Zorn, C. R. (1997). Factors contributing to hope among noninstitutionalized elderly. *Applied Nursing Research, 10,* 94–100.

Zorn, C. R., & Johnson, M. T. (1997). Religious well-being in noninstitionalized elderly women. *Health Care for Women International, 18,* 209–219.

Zuckerman, J., Fabian, D., Aharanoff, G., Kovel, K., & Frankel, V. (1993). Enhancing independence in the older hip fracture patient. *Geriatrics, 48,* 76–78.

Index